Brain Biochemistry and Brain Disorders

Philip G. Strange

Biological Laboratory, University of Kent

OXFORD NEW YORK TOKYO
OXFORD UNIVERSITY PRESS

Oxford University Press, Walton Street, Oxford OX2 6DP
Oxford New York
Athens Auckland Bangkok Bombay
Calcutta Cape Town Dar es Salaam Delhi
Florence Hong Kong Istanbul Karachi
Kuala Lumpur Madras Madrid Melbourne
Mexico City Nairobi Paris Singapore
Taipei Tokyo Toronto
and associated companies in
Berlin Ibadan

Oxford is a trade mark of Oxford University Press

Published in the United States by
Oxford University Press Inc., New York

A catalogue record for this book is available from the British Library

Library of Congress Cataloging in Publication Data
Strange, P. G. (Philip Gordon)
Brain biochemistry and brain disorders / Philip G. Strange.
Includes bibliographical references.
1. Brain—Pathophysiology.   2. Brain—Physiology.
3. Neuroanatomy.   4. Clinical biochemistry.   5. Brain—physiology.
I. Title.
[DNLM: 1. Affective Disorder—physiopathology.   2. Anxiety—
physiopathology.   3. Basal Ganglia Diseases—physiopathology.
4. Biochemistry.   5. Schizophrenia—physiopathology.   WL 307 S897b]
RC386.S73   1992   616.8' 047—dc20   91–46384
ISBN 0 19 854775 7

Printed in Great Britain by
Butler & Tanner, Frome and London

Preface

When I moved to Canterbury in 1986 I was asked to teach a specialist course for the final year B.Sc. Biochemistry students on a topic of my choice. I had no hesitation in choosing brain biochemistry and brain disorders as the topic. This had been a topic developing in my mind as a result of doing various pieces of unconnected teaching at the University of Nottingham Medical School. I have very much enjoyed teaching the course at Canterbury and as far as I can tell the course has been a great success with the students. It was therefore a natural progression for me to create a book out of the course to bring these ideas to a wider audience. Also there was no suitable textbook that covered similar ground but it was clear that the topic was of considerable current interest. So that is how this book began.

Writing the book has been great fun, very stimulating, and I have learned a lot. It has also been hard work. I need here to make a few comments about the structure of the book.

What really fascinates me and what I find really challenging is to understand the functions of the brain (both normal and disordered) in terms of the basic structures and processes contained in the brain. The book aims to show how normal and disordered brain function can be explained in this way with a particular emphasis on the biochemistry. In order to approach this I felt it was necessary to include chapters on the basic structure and function of the component parts of the brain and the first seven chapters provide this basic information. With this as a foundation the second half of the book describes six disorders of human brain and I have tried where possible to analyse each disorder and the related normal brain functions in terms of the basic processes described earlier. The chapters on disordered brain function are preceded by a general chapter on the methods used to study human brain function.

Some of the brain disorders I describe have prominent alterations of motor function and analysing changes in motor function in terms of changes in neuronal numbers provides no major philosophical conflicts. Most of the disorders I describe, however, also have prominent disturbances of what might broadly be called psychological or mental function and analysing these in terms of changes in number or function of neurones gets me in to much deeper philosophical water.

In order to be able to analyse psychological or mental disorders of brain function in terms of the basic processes contained therein I believe it is necessary to have some idea of how these basic processes relate to normal psychological or mental function. I therefore felt it was important to attempt to provide some relationship between the 'mind-type' functions of brain and these basic processes. To do this I have included a chapter on the mind–body problem which provides a central section relating the two parts of the book. Overall from the treatment given I hope I show how the brain may be described at a series of interrelated levels and that a full description can be achieved only by considering the different levels. These ideas about levels of description are stated more explicitly in the first chapter.

References in original literature appear in two ways. At the end of most chapters is a list of more general references (recommended reading). In the text, where information derives from these sources no reference is given. If, however, the information in the text derives from another more specific source, that source will be referenced in the text. These specific references are then brought together in the Bibliography at the end of the book. The material described in this book reflects in the most part information in references published up to the late summer of 1991. In the text I occasionally use the word 'he' or 'his' and it should be understood that this can equally refer to the female gender except where stated explicitly.

The book contains much information and I have attempted to make it as accurate as possible. I hope there are few errors but there are bound to be some and it would be a great help if anyone who spots errors could let me know so that corrections can be made.

Canterbury   P.G.S.
February 1992

Acknowledgements

I am indebted to a number of people who helped me in creating this book. Several people kindly gave me photographs for inclusion and the book is enhanced by these. I am most grateful to these individuals who are named in the appropriate figure legend.

A number of people kindly read parts or all of the manuscript and made helpful comments which enabled me to improve the final version: Anthony Baines, Paul Bolam, David Bowen, David Brown, Alan Crossman, Bill Deakin, Alec Dolby, Annette Dolphin, Mike Fairhurst, Barbara Grimwade, Kevin Hood, Peter Jenner, Andrew Lees, David Mann, Charles Marsden, John Parnevalas, Steven Rose, Margaret Strange, Peter Tyrer, and John Waddington. In addition there were several 'anonymous' readers approached by OUP who read part or all of the text. I am indebted to all of these.

Special thanks to Sue Davies who typed the manuscript with her usual superb efficiency, accuracy, and good humour.

Maggie Smith, Sue Morrish, and Margaret Strange helped me greatly in the development of some psychological concepts.

I should also like to thank the artist David Gardner who did the drawings from my originals, and the staff at Oxford University Press for all their help and support in the production of this book.

Credits

Several figures were taken from the published literature and the publishers and authors who gave permission are: **Fig. 2.11** (from Blakemore, C. (1977). *Mechanics of the mind*, Cambridge University Press); **Fig. 3.1** (from Sholl. D. A. (1956). *Organisation of the cerebral cortex*, Methuen); **Fig. 3.4** (from Lasek, R. and Black, M. M. (eds.) (1988). *Intrinsic determinants of neuronal form and function*. Copyright © Alan R. Liss, reprinted by permission of Wiley-Liss, a division of John Wiley and Sons Inc.); **Fig. 3.10** (from Alberts *et al.* (1989). *Molecular biology of the cell* (2nd edn.), Garland Publishing Inc.); **Fig. 5.3** (from Lapper, S. R. and Bolam, J. P. (1991). *Journal of Neuroscience Methods*, 39, 163–74, Elsevier Science Publishers BV); **Fig. 5.7** (Heuser, J. E. and Reese, T. S. (1981). *Journal of Cell Biology*, 88, 564–80, by copyright permission of the Rockefeller University Press); **Fig. 6.4** (from Olsen, R. W. and Tobin, A. J., *FASEB Journal*, 4, 1469–80, Federation of American Societies of Experimental Biology); **Fig. 7.2** (from Rakic, P. (1979). Genetic and epigenetic determinants of local neuronal circuits in the mammalian central nervous system. In *Neuroscience*, Fourth Study Program (ed. F. O. Schmitt and F. G. Worden), pp. 109–27, with copyright © permission from MIT press); **Fig. 7.3** (from Jean-Pierre Changeux (1983). *L'homme neuronal*, with copyright © permission from Librairie Artheme Fayard); **Fig. 7.20** (reprinted by permission from Zipser and Andersen (1988). *Nature* 331, 679–84, copyright © Macmillan Magazines Ltd.); **Fig. 9.1** (from Dodd, P. R., Hambley, J. W., Cowburn, R. F. and Hardy, J. A. (1988). A comparison of methodologies for the study of functional transmitter neurochemistry in human brain. *Journal of Neurochemistry*, 50, 1333–45); **Fig. 10.2** (from Ferry, G. (1987). *New Scientist*, 113, 56–50, with copyright © permission from New Scientist and Ivan Vaughan); **Fig. 12.2** (from Thomas, M. and Isaac, M. (1987). *Trends in Neurosciences*, 10, 306–7, Elsevier Trends Journals); **Fig. 12.5**, with copyright © permission from Dr. P. Luthert, Institute of Psychiatry, London; **Fig. 13.2** (from Seeman, P. (1981). Brain dopamine receptors. *Pharmacological Reviews*, 32, 230–87, copyright © permission from Williams and Wilkins).

Contents

1 *Introduction to brain function*

Suppose you have to run to catch a bus. Which bodily functions are called into play? You will have to run, so there will be a stimulation of muscle contraction. The stimulation of muscle contraction will consume ATP and the hormone adrenaline may be released into the blood to ensure that more ATP is made. During the run towards the bus there will be a careful coordination of sensory and positional information until you have successfully got on the bus. The whole exercise will require the formulation of an intention to catch the bus and the planning and execution of the intention. There may be a strong emotion attached to the event particularly if something else in your life depends on the bus journey. The events will be remembered for a shorter or longer period and may be recalled in vivid detail.

Essentially all of the actions described above are controlled and coordinated by our brains, so let me summarize what the brain does in our normal behaviour. The brain controls normal bodily function, that is, all the physical and physiological processes taking place in our bodies e.g. muscle contraction and hormone secretion. The brain is the site of our consciousness (our mind) and is therefore the source of our thoughts, plans, intentions, etc. The brain is also the seat of memory. Although this is only a brief summary of what the brain can do it emphasizes the central role of the brain in our behaviour.

The brain, however, can also malfunction. Suppose a person with Parkinson's disease wanted to catch the same bus. He or she would have great trouble initiating the running for the bus and once started would move rather slowly. Despite this, the thinking, planning, emotion, and memory will be largely unaffected for this individual. As we shall see later, in Parkinson's disease there is a fairly selective degeneration of a part of the brain concerned with the control of motor function. In the latter part of this book several other brain diseases where specific alterations of the brain activity lead to particular behavioural changes will be discussed.

Understanding the relation between the structure of the brain and the functions it generates and in particular how the brain can go wrong and lead to mental disease is one of the major challenges to present day scientists. This book sets out to describe the relationship between structure and function in the normal brain and how the relationship can be disturbed in disorders of the brain. Emphasis will be placed on the underlying biochemistry of normal and disturbed function but it will be a basic premise of the book that the brain may be described in a number of ways. Each means of description is valid in its own right and the different means are related to one another hierarchically. The different levels of description will be outlined here and covered in more detail in subsequent chapters.

1. *Overall neuroanatomy*: this reflects a purely visual description of the brain, its overall structure, and the key subdivisions.
2. *Cellular structure*: a description of the different cell types that make up the brain, their interrelationships, and their electrical and chemical properties.
3. *Subcellular structure*: a description of the internal workings of the brain cells.
4. *Functional level*: a description of the overall functions that the brain mediates as outlined earlier e.g. consciousness, thought, planning, and control of bodily functions.

It is the thesis of the book that the brain may be described in each of these four ways but that each descriptive level is related to the others. Understanding of a complex function will ultimately be achieved in terms of the four levels and in this way brain structure and function can be related. For example, consciousness (level 4) is likely to be a function of much of the physical brain (level 1) and will be due to the activity of groups of nerve cells (level 2) and their complex internal biochemical and electrical processes (level 3).

Neuroscientists tend to stay within levels 1–3 of description and formulate hypotheses about nerve cell function and interaction. Psychologists and philosophers concern themselves with level 4 of description and formulate their own particular theories about the function of the mind/brain. I hope that the treatment given here can begin to show how these different theories can be complementary and interlinked.

2 *Overall structure of the brain at the neuroanatomical level*

It is the intention in this chapter to convey an impression of the overall organization and three-dimensional structure of the brain. The treatment is not exhaustive, although the major substructures of the brain will be outlined particularly where these are important for later discussion. The reader is referred to the general references at the end of the chapter for a more detailed account of neuroanatomy.

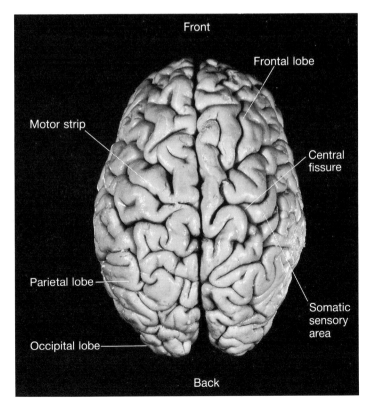

Figure 2.1 View of human brain from above.

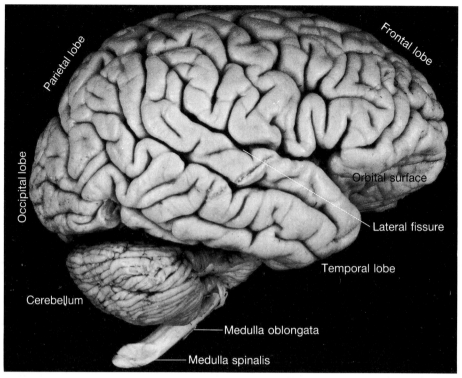

Figure 2.2   View of human brain from the side.

Structural and functional subdivision of the brain

Two external views of a human brain seen from the top and the side are shown in Figs 2.1 and 2.2 and certain features are immediately obvious. The top view illustrates the bilateral symmetry of the brain and its two cerebral hemispheres. In addition there are the characteristic infoldings and certain deeper clefts or fissures called sulci. There is often said to be a resemblance in this view to a large walnut. The brain material itself is pink-grey in colour and has the consistency of a thick porridge or pudding. The human brain is impressively large, weighing well over one kilogram. Comparisons of brain weight for other species are given in Table 2.1.

In the side view other structures are visible—the brain stem protruding from beneath and linking to the spinal cord, the cerebellum underneath and to the rear with a high degree of infolding, and the remainder which is often termed the cerebrum and consists of the two massive cerebral hemispheres.

The relative simplicity of the external views belies an enormous internal complexity exaggerated by the use of Latin names for naming the various internal structures. The internal structure is revealed in the two sections of the human brain shown in Figs 2.3

Table 2.1   Weight of brain for different species

	Weight of brain (g)
Human	1350
Monkey	105
Cat	30
Rabbit	14
Rat	2.5

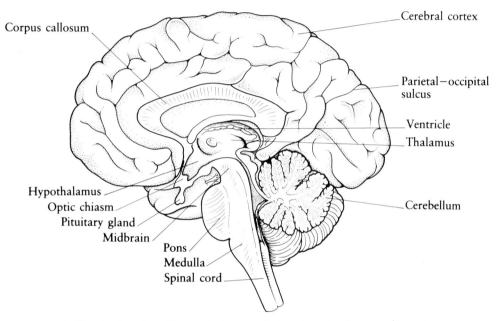

Figure 2.3   Mid-sagittal section of human brain (a vertical section taken between the eyes).

and 2.4. The mid-sagittal section (Fig. 2.3, a vertical section taken between the eyes) shows more detail of the infoldings of the cerebral cortex (the external layer of the cerebrum) and of the cerebellum. The entry of the brain stem into the brain and the components of the brain stem (medulla, pons, and midbrain) are visible as well as their linkage to the diencephalon (a collective name for the thalamus and hypothalamus). One can also see in section the corpus callosum, a set of nerve fibre tracts linking the two hemispheres, and a ventricle, a fluid-filled space within the brain which will be discussed further below.

In the coronal section (Fig. 2.4, a vertical section taken roughly through the ears) the symmetry of the two hemispheres is emphasized. Further internal structure is now visible and the interrelationships of the thalamus, hypothalamus, and the ventricles are clearer.

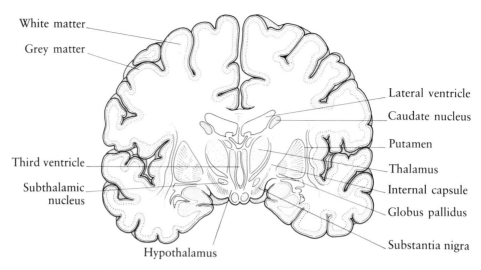

White matter
Grey matter
Lateral ventricle
Caudate nucleus
Putamen
Third ventricle
Thalamus
Subthalamic
nucleus
Internal capsule
Globus pallidus
Substantia nigra
Hypothalamus

Figure 2.4   Coronal section of human brain (a vertical section taken roughly through the ears).

New structures now visible are the caudate nucleus, globus pallidus, and putamen, collectively termed the corpus striatum, and part of a system called the basal ganglia and which is severely affected in Parkinson's disease (Chapter 10) and Huntington's disease (Chapter 11). A striking feature of the two sections is the division of the brain into regions of different colour and this is particularly apparent in the infoldings of the cerebral cortex. Within the cerebral cortex and elsewhere in the brain, there is the so-called grey matter, which contains neuronal cell bodies, and the white matter, which contains many myelinated axons of neurons (see Chapter 3).

It is, however, quite difficult to appreciate the three-dimensional interrelationships of the parts of the brain from these sections. Three further diagrams are shown, therefore, which attempt to illustrate this for some of the key structures. Fig. 2.5 shows the brain stem, cerebellum, diencephalon, and cerebrum, Fig. 2.6 shows the caudate nucleus and putamen in relation to the substantia nigra (these are important for control of movement and will be discussed in more detail in Chapter 10). Fig. 2.7 shows the hippocampus which plays a role in memory and the control of behaviour and will be discussed further in relation to Alzheimer's disease (Chapter 12) and schizophrenia (Chapter 13).

The sections shown in Figures 2.3 and 2.4 are taken from post-mortem material. Nowadays, however, using techniques such as magnetic resonance imaging we can obtain similar sections from a living human brain. A mid-sagittal section obtained in this way is shown in Fig. 2.8, revealing much the same information as the section taken post-mortem. Imaging techniques for studying the living human brain will be discussed in more detail in Chapter 9.

It should be becoming apparent that the brain is not a single organ but rather an

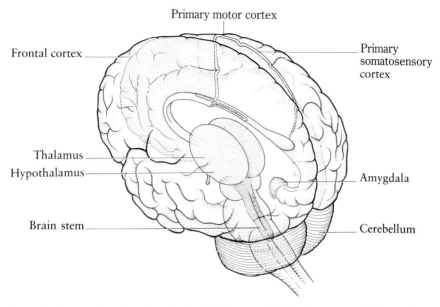

Figure 2.5 A diagram showing the relationship between the brain stem, cerebellum, diencephalon (thalamus and hypothalamus), and cerebrum.

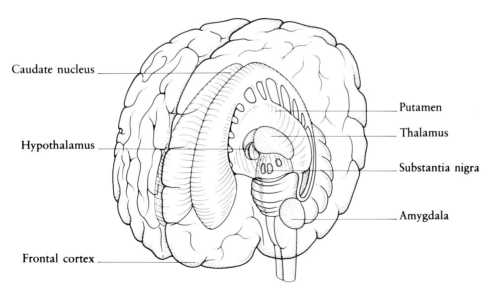

Figure 2.6 A diagram showing the relationship of the caudate nucleus, putamen, and substantia nigra.

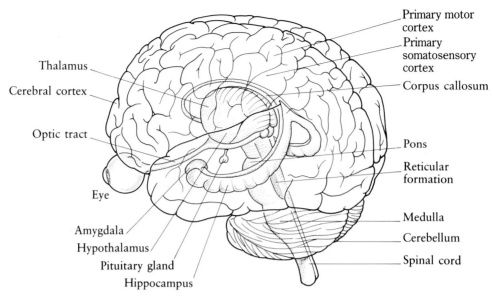

Figure 2.7   A diagram showing the hippocampus in relation to the rest of the brain.

assembly of smaller structures connected to one another as will be described later (Chapter 7). Indeed in some cases, subgroups of structures have been recognized, grouped according to their association with particular functions. An example is the so-called limbic system which is associated with emotion and is a group of structures consisting of the hippocampus, thalamus, hypothalamus, amygdala, septum, fornix, and the cingulate gyrus of the cerebral cortex.

In addition to grouping structures functionally, it has been recognized that certain structures may be further subdivided. This is particularly prominent and important for the cerebral cortex, the folded outer layer of each cerebral hemisphere. The cerebral cortex of each hemisphere may be divided into four lobes roughly delineated by sulci or clefts. The lobes are termed frontal, temporal, parietal, and occipital (after the adjacent bones of the skull) and are shown in Fig. 2.9. The sulci also separate the folds or gyri of the cerebral cortex e.g. parahippocampal gyrus which will be considered in more detail in Chapter 13. Each lobe may be further subdivided into regions although microscopy is required to establish the subdivisions. On the basis of cellular layering, Brodmann divided the cerebral cortex into about fifty discrete areas according to their cellular structure (Fig. 2.10). The boundaries of the lobes correspond well with boundaries between Brodmann's divisions. It is now clear that many of these divisions have functional relevance. Two examples of the functional relevance of the divisions of the cerebral cortex will be given here but for more detail refer to the general references and discussions in later chapters.

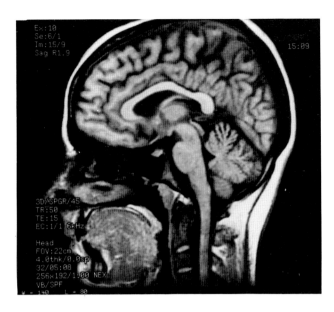

Figure 2.8 Mid-sagittal section of living human brain obtained by magnetic resonance imaging. This should be compared to Fig. 2.3. Courtesy of Dr. D. Shaw, General Electric.

The first example concerns the extensive studies that have been performed on the effect of electrical stimulation of the surface of the brain during neurosurgery. This has shown that a strip of cerebral cortex in front of the central sulcus (corresponding to Brodmann's area 4) is responsible for motor commands to the muscles. It is called the primary motor cortex (see Fig. 2.9) and can be further subdivided into areas controlling muscles in different parts of the body. The 'map' that results from this, or homunculus as it is called, is shown in Fig. 2.11. Areas of the body are not equally represented: regions of the body where great motor facility is required, e.g. hands, fingers, lips, and jaws, are represented in a disproportionately large way. Nevertheless this means that there exists in the brain a structural 'map' of the body in the motor cortex. Similar 'maps' exist in other parts of the brain, e.g. areas concerned with sensory input such as the primary somatosensory cortex (Figs. 2.9 and 2.11). This is an important principle for two reasons. First, information from the various organs converges on the brain in a highly organized manner. The final topographical representation of information in the cerebral cortex is reflected at all levels of information processing. Secondly, the brain can be seen to contain a representation of the world around us as depicted by our sensory apparatus. This latter point will become important when we consider theories of the mind (Chapter 8).

The second example of localization of function in cortical regions comes from studies on patients with the speech defect, Broca's aphasia. These patients can understand language and write it but cannot produce fluent language themselves. Such patients have damage to a specific region of the cerebral cortex of the left hemisphere corresponding to Brodmann's areas 44 and 45. This observation does not show that this region of the

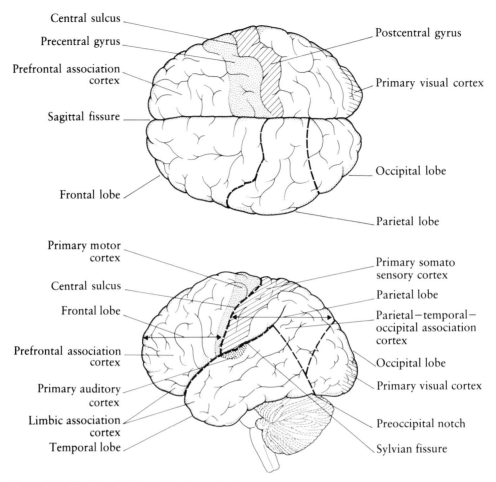

Central sulcus

Precentral gyrus

Prefrontal association
cortex

Sagittal fissure

Frontal lobe

Postcentral gyrus

Primary visual cortex

Occipital lobe

Parietal lobe

Primary motor
cortex

Central sulcus

Frontal lobe

Prefrontal association
cortex

Primary auditory
cortex

Limbic association
cortex

Temporal lobe

Primary somato
sensory cortex

Parietal lobe

Parietal–temporal–
occipital association
cortex

Occipital lobe

Primary visual cortex

Preoccipital notch

Sylvian fissure

Figure 2.9   The lobe divisions of the human brain.

brain is solely responsible for language. It does show, however, that this region of the brain participates in the expression of language and it further emphasizes the functional subdivisions of the cerebral cortex. In fact it is now known that several discrete regions of the cerebral cortex are responsible for the various aspects of language.

Thus it seems likely that within the brain, information is passed from region to region and overall behavioural function may depend on several regions cooperating. With a complex function such as language, different aspects of the function are processed in parallel and finally converge on a single output area. The concept of parallel processing in distributed areas is very important for a modern view of brain function.

In summary, areas of the cerebral cortex can be identified with certain aspects of the body, e.g. motor cortex for muscle control, somatosensory cortex for sensory input,

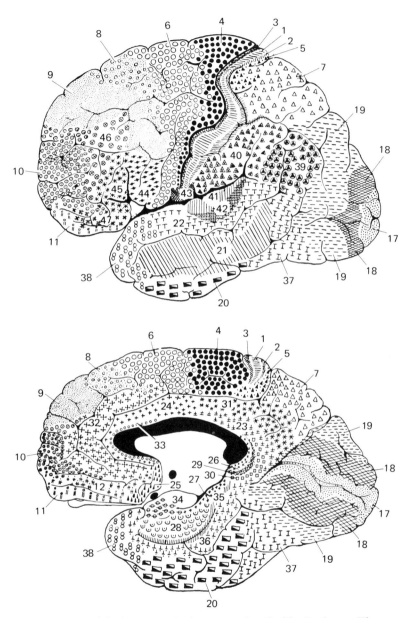

Figure 2.10 The divisions of the human cerebral cortex as described by Brodmann. The upper view is a view from the side externally, the lower view is a view from the side in a mid-sagittal section, the front is to the left in both sections.

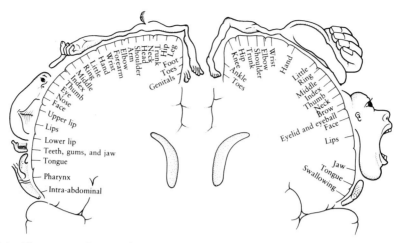

Figure 2.11 The motor and sensory homunculi. On the right is a view of the primary motor cortex on the right side of the brain sliced coronally. The representation of the parts of the body or motor homunculus is shown. On the left a similar diagram is shown but for the primary somatosensory cortex (see Fig. 2.9 for the boundaries of these regions). Redrawn from Blakemore (1977) with permission.

visual cortex for visual input, etc. There are also large areas of the cerebral cortex which cannot be identified with specific functions and which presumably perform more complex syntheses of information; these are referred to as association areas (see Fig. 2.9) and are highly developed in man compared with other species. This presumably reflects the greater cognitive capacity of man relative to other species.

Thus we may develop a picture of the brain as composed of a number of discrete regions cooperating to provide the overall functional activity. Within regions further subdivisions are apparent and these again cooperate. Brain function can, therefore, be seen to be due to cooperative performance of the whole organ rather than to the isolated actions of individual parts.

The blood supply to the brain and the cerebrospinal fluid

The brain is richly supplied with blood vessels derived ultimately from the internal carotid arteries. Each cerebral hemisphere can be divided into discrete regions with respect to blood supply and each of these regions is supplied by a particular cerebral artery. These branch on the surface of the brain, supplying the cerebral cortex, and also send smaller penetrating branches into the deeper structures of the brain. The capillaries branch widely and with this branching it has been proposed that each nerve cell is no more than 40–50 μm from a capillary. This is important as the brain is a great consumer of energy and so needs to be well nourished with glucose and oxygen. Indeed, although the brain constitutes only 2 per cent of the body by weight, it receives about 15 per cent of the blood pumped by the heart and consumes about 20 per cent of the total body oxygen and glucose usage. In order to supply this there is a rapid throughput of blood in the brain. The high consumption of oxygen and glucose by the brain reflects the high levels of oxidative metabolism by nerve cells and emphasizes the need for an extensive, efficient blood supply.

There is a problem, however, in the supply of nutrients to the brain directly from the blood. Although the composition of the blood is controlled, it does fluctuate, for example in response to dietary changes. Because nerve cell function is critically dependent on the ionic concentrations in extracellular fluid, the brain cannot tolerate even small changes in the composition of extracellular fluid. Therefore the brain and nerve cells are surrounded by a fluid compartment that is separate from the blood although linked to it and dependent on it. This compartment consists of extracellular fluid which forms the actual external medium of the nerve cells. The extracellular fluid is in equilibrium with cerebrospinal fluid. The cerebrospinal fluid fills the ventricles of the brain, surrounds the spinal cord and acts as a lining of the skull so that the brain effectively floats in it. The ventricles form an interconnecting set of cavities within the hemispheres.

Cerebrospinal fluid is formed from blood largely by secretion from a network of capillaries in the ventricles called the choroid plexus but also from cerebral capillaries elsewhere. It is a low protein fluid resembling an ultrafiltrate of plasma. The extracellular fluid/cerebrospinal fluid compartment is separated from the blood by an operational barrier called the blood–brain barrier. This barrier is partly a mechanical one, due to tight junctions between endothelial cells lining cerebral capillaries and epithelial cells at the choroid plexus. The tight junctions prevent movement of material between cells but there are also selective transport mechanisms in the cells that maintain the composition of the fluid, permitting entry of certain substances, for example glucose and certain amino acids, and removing others.

As well as being essential for the proper function of brain cells, the existence of a blood–brain barrier has practical consequences. For example in certain diseases such as meningitis and systemic lupus erythematosus, the blood–brain barrier may be less effective so that substances such as drugs (e.g. penicillin) or antibodies that are normally excluded can enter the cerebrospinal fluid. A second example concerns the treatment of Parkinson's disease, in which there is a deficiency of dopamine in parts of the brain (Chapter 10). Whereas it would be desirable to treat parkinsonian patients with dopamine, this substance does not cross the blood–brain barrier. L-DOPA, a precursor of dopamine, does, however, cross the barrier and is successfully used to treat the disease as will be discussed later.

Recommended reading

Goldstein, G. W. and Betz, A. L. (1986). The blood–brain barrier. *Scientific American*, **255**(3), 70–8.

Kandel, E. R. and Schwartz, J. H. (1985). *Principles of neural science*. (2nd edn). Elsevier, New York.

Kuffler, S. W., Nicholls, J. G., and Martin, A. R. (1984). *From neuron to brain*. Sinauer Associates Inc., Sunderland, MA.

Niewenhuys, R., Voogd, J., and van Huijzen, C. (1981). *The human central nervous system a synopsis and atlas*. Springer-Verlag, New York.

Spector, R. and Johanson, C. E. (1989). The mammalian choroid plexus. *Scientific American*, **261**(5), 48–53.

3   *Cellular structure of the brain*

In Chapter 2 the overall structure of the brain and its division into functionally discrete but interdependent regions were described. All of these regions are composed of cells; there are two principal kinds of cell in the brain—neurones, which are the 'business cells' of the brain in which major information transfer occurs, and neuroglial cells whose role is more passive but nevertheless essential to overall brain function.

There is some further diversity within the neuronal and neuroglial cell populations but the functional diversity of different brain regions is more a result of differing interconnections of similar cells. Therefore we may consider the individual cells of the brain as building blocks responsible for brain function which is generated via their very complex interconnections.

Neurones

The neurone, as I have said, is the 'business cell' of the brain and the human cerebral cortex contains about 10^{10} neurones, the whole brain probably containing about 10^{12}. The number of neurones already suggests considerable complexity but the neuronal interconnections multiply this complexity many times over. The neurones of the brain can be visualized with a number of histological methods, but the Golgi stain (Fig. 3.1), which stains only a small percentage (1–5 per cent) of the cells, reveals a striking picture of the morphology of individual neurones. Figure 3.2 highlights the main features of a generalized neurone i.e. the cell body (also called soma or perikaryon) whose diameter varies in the region of 10–50 μm, the finger-like projections of the cell body called dendrites which often have spines, and the long cable-like structure called the axon.

We may appreciate some of the properties of neurones by taking some specific examples. Within the cerebral cortex there is a class of neurone called a pyramidal cell (so called because of the shape of its densely staining cell body, see also Chapter 7). Pyramidal cell axons can connect regions of the cerebral cortex to another region of the cerebral cortex, to another part of the brain, or to the spinal cord and so may be centimetres or hundreds of centimetres in length. A second heterogeneous class of neurone is found in the cerebral cortex and is collectively termed stellate (the cells have a star-like appearance) or non-pyramidal cells. These non-pyramidal cells do not send axons out of the cerebral cortex: they are involved in the intrinsic function of the tissue and are termed

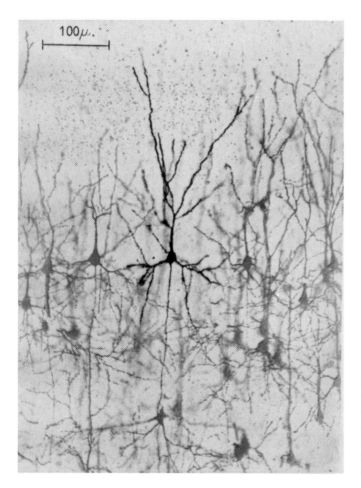

Figure 3.1 The pattern of neurones in the cerebral cortex of cat as visualized by Golgi stain. (From Sholl (1956) with permission. The image of the pyramidal cell has been enhanced photographically).

interneurones. Further examples of interneurones will be described in other chapters. Where the axon of a neurone branches, the branches are termed axon collaterals and enable one neurone to influence several target cells. Another example of a neurone that will be considered in detail later in relation to disease is the mesostriatal dopamine cell which has cell bodies in the substantia nigra and axons stretching a few centimetres to reach the striatum (see Chapters 5 and 10).

The axon is often surrounded by a specialized, discontinuous lipid–protein coat called myelin, interrupted by regular breaks called nodes of Ranvier. The structure and formation of myelin will be considered later in this chapter and the importance of the nodes of Ranvier in signal transmission in Chapter 4. The myelin coat gives the axon a white appearance and the colour of the white matter of the cerebral cortex (see Chapter 2) is due to the many myelinated axons leaving the tissue. The colour of the grey matter is due to neuronal cell bodies.

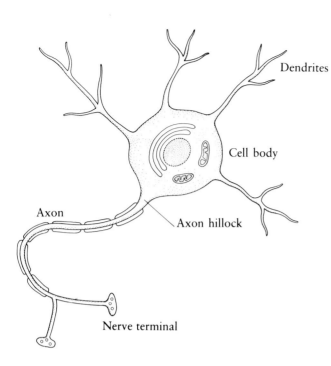

Figure 3.2 Key features of a neurone. Neurones in different brain regions differ in their relative structures, but certain key features can be discerned as shown above. The diagram is not to scale—the cell body may be *c*.20 μm in diameter whereas the nerve terminal may be *c*.0.5 μm across. Dendrites and the axon may branch and stretch distances many times the diameter of the cell body.

The axon terminates when it reaches either another cell body or a dendrite of another cell. Here it widens to form a nerve terminal. The nerve terminal does not touch the adjacent cell, rather there is a gap of about 20–30 nm. This specialized cell–cell junction is called a synapse and its function will be considered in more detail later in this chapter and in subsequent chapters.

Subcellular structure of the neurone

Looking at neurones under higher magnification reveals further features. These are summarized in Fig. 3.3. The neuronal cell body contains the organelles that typify all cells:

1. *The nucleus* contains the DNA, and is packaged together with certain proteins to form chromatin. The chromatin in neurones is less tightly packed than in non-neuronal cells; this is consistent with a high level of transcription.
2. *The nucleolus* is a prominent feature within the nucleus and is involved actively in ribosome synthesis and in the transfer of RNA to the cytosol. There is evidence that mRNA for specific proteins can be targeted to particular parts of the neurone, for example mRNA for microtubule associated protein-2 (MAP-2) is targeted at dendritic processes. This targeting presumably helps maintain the structural differentiation of the neurone.

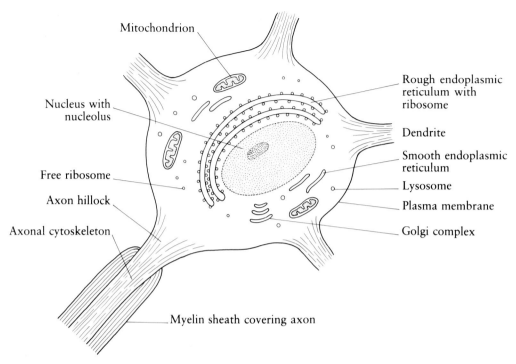

Figure 3.3   The cell body of a neurone and its constituent parts. Typical subcellular features of a neuronal cell body are shown, but omitted from this diagram for clarity are the nerve terminals that would form many synapses on to both the cell body and dendrites. See Fig. 3.10 for this detail. Also omitted is the cytoskeleton of the cell body.

3. *Mitochondria* supply energy for the cell in the form of ATP. As outlined in Chapter 2 and described in detail in Chapter 4, the brain consumes large amounts of ATP. Interference with mitochondrial ATP generation can lead to neuronal death (Chapter 10).

4. *Smooth endoplasmic reticulum* is involved in lipid synthesis and in protein glycosylation.

5. *Rough endoplasmic reticulum* is formed from the attachment of ribosomes to the smooth endoplasmic reticulum; these ribosomes are the site of protein synthesis (mainly membrane proteins) and the reticulum allows transport of these proteins around the cell and participates in their glycosylation.

6. *The Golgi complex* is near the nucleus and is responsible for protein glycosylation, membrane assembly, and protein sorting.

7. *Lysosomes* are associated with the degradation of all kinds of cellular debris.

8. *The plasma membrane* bounding the neurone itself is a membrane of typical structure, about 7 nm thick, composed of a bilayer of phospholipid with some cholesterol and glycolipids and integral (intrinsic) and peripheral (extrinsic) mem-

brane proteins. The phospholipid composition of neuronal membranes is similar to that of other cells and the lipid bilayer provides an impermeable barrier for many substances so that movement across the membrane depends on specialized proteins. One very minor membrane phospholipid, phosphatidylinositol bisphosphate, plays a critical role in transmembrane signalling by some receptors (Chapter 6). Peripheral membrane proteins are those attached to the inner or outer face of the lipid bilayer or to integral membrane proteins in the bilayer by ionic interactions. Fodrin (see below) is a good example of this class of protein; it is attached to the inner face of the membrane. Integral membrane proteins are those that penetrate deeply into the bilayer or completely through it. Many of the proteins responsible for the unique function of the neurone are of this class, e.g. neurotransmitter receptors and voltage sensitive ion channels. This class of protein is also dependent on the membrane for its stability and orientation and the precise phospholipid composition around the proteins may be important.

9. *The cytosol* is the fluid remaining which contains enzymes responsible for the metabolism of the cell and some free ribosomes which make proteins for the cytosol.

These are the typical components found in almost every cell in the body. The reader is referred to the recommended reading at the end of the chapter for a more detailed description of their properties.

Neurones do, however, have specific organelles not found in other cells and these are associated with specific functions. They are dealt with in a little more detail in subsequent sections.

Neuronal cytoskeleton

In terms of its shape and function, the neurone is a highly differentiated cell with its cell body, axon, and nerve terminal each of characteristic shape and function. The shape and function of the neurone are dependent on the neuronal cytoskeleton (Fig. 3.4). Although all cells have some kind of cytoskeleton, the neuronal cytoskeleton is of a particular form. It is a structure composed of a series of fibrous proteins that give strength to the axon and provide a scaffold for its assembly as well as providing mechanisms for the specific location of membrane proteins.

The scaffold for assembly of the axon is provided by microtubules, neurofilaments (the neuronal members of the intermediate filament family), and microfilaments (actin). Two broad divisions of the axonal cytoskeleton have been recognized (Lasek 1988) (Fig. 3.4). The internal cytoskeleton consists of microtubules and neurofilaments along the length of the axon with the shorter actin filaments intermingled with these longer fibrous proteins. There are also cross-bridges linking the microtubules and neurofilaments so that a supporting structure for the axon is provided. The microtubules are thought to provide a track for the movement of vesicular material via fast axonal

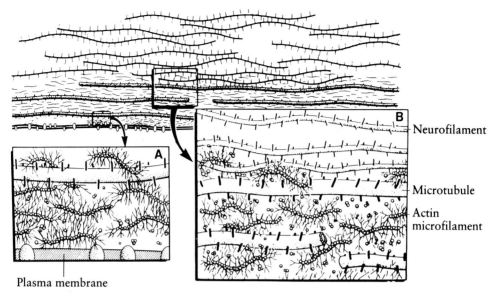

Figure 3.4 The neuronal cytoskeleton. The diagram (taken from Lasek 1988 with permission) shows the two divisions of the cytoskeleton in an axon. The internal cytoskeleton (see insert on the right) consists of microtubules, neurofilaments, and actin microfilaments along the length of the axon linked by cross bridges. The cytoskeleton near the axonal membrane (cortical cytoskeleton) (see insert on the left) is largely due to actin microfilaments linked to microtubules internally and to the plasma membrane via fine filaments including fodrin. These fine filaments in turn provide for sites of localization of proteins in the axonal membrane e.g. Na^+ channels at nodes of Ranvier (Srinivasan *et al.* 1988).

transport (see below). The microtubule/neurofilament array also undergoes a slow translocation down the axon (slow axonal transport, see later).

The part of the cytoskeleton near the axonal membrane (cortical cytoskeleton) (Fig. 3.4) consists of actin microfilaments linked internally to microtubules and to the plasma membrane via a network of fine filamentous proteins including the protein fodrin (a brain form of spectrin (Bennett 1985)). This protein provides sites for the attachment and location of integral membrane proteins either via direct interactions, e.g. the neuronal cell adhesion molecule (N-CAM), or indirectly via another protein, called ankyrin in the case of sodium channels. This latter interaction may provide a means for concentrating Na^+ channels at nodes of Ranvier (Srinivasan *et al.* 1988; Baines 1990). It seems likely that other proteins such as receptors will also be shown to be associated with the cytoskeleton. The synaptic postsynaptic density, a densely staining region on the postsynaptic side of synapses (see below), is also likely to be composed of cytoskeletal and other proteins to which receptors may attach. Interaction of synaptic vesicles with components of the cytoskeleton at nerve terminals is also likely and would provide a means for concentrating vesicles in the terminal prior to release of neurotransmitter. It seems that there may be linkage of vesicles to actin and fodrin filaments in the nerve terminal via the protein synapsin I (Landis *et al*. 1988; Hirokawa *et al*. 1989); the mechanisms involved are considered in more detail in Chapter 5.

We may therefore view the cytoskeleton as a protein network providing strength to the neurone and specificity in localizing specific components at particular points. The cytoskeleton has a slightly different composition in different parts of the neurone, for example axons and dendrites, and this may be a way of providing different structural and functional units for the neurone.

It has been widely speculated that the filamentous structures seen in certain degenerative diseases e.g. tangles (paired helical filaments) in Alzheimer's disease (Chapter 12) are related to cytoskeletal proteins. There is no simple relationship although one of the microtubule-associated proteins (tau) has been shown to be a component of Alzheimer's disease tangles.

Vesicular components of the neurone

Two principal vesicular structures are seen within neurones:

1. *Synaptic vesicles*: within the nerve terminal there are a number of small smooth vesicles (30–100 nm) containing the neurotransmitter substance. In Chapter 5 the role of these vesicles in neurotransmitter release will be outlined.
2. *Coated vesicles*: these are vesicles found within the nerve terminal as well as in other regions of the neurone. They have a fuzzy coat composed principally of the protein clathrin and are thought to be involved in retrieval and recycling of membrane components including synaptic vesicles. In Chapter 6 the role of coated vesicles in the turnover of receptor proteins will be discussed.

Axonal transport

The distinctive shape of the neurone provides problems with its function in that the main machinery for the synthesis and degradation of macromolecules and organelles is in the cell body and yet there is a substantial metabolic activity along the axon and particularly at the nerve terminal which is separated from the cell body by the long axon and where neurotransmitter release occurs by exocytosis. This metabolic activity is important under all circumstances but is given additional importance during a growth phase. Therefore there must be a continuous provision of new materials from the cell body of the neurone to the nerve terminal and a continuous retrieval of material. The process is called axonal transport and represents a continuous flow of material down the axon towards the nerve terminal (anterograde) and back to the cell body (retrograde) (Fig. 3.5).

Axonal transport may be divided into two broad classes according to speed, although there is much heterogeneity within the two classes (Grafstein and Forman 1980; Lasek *et*

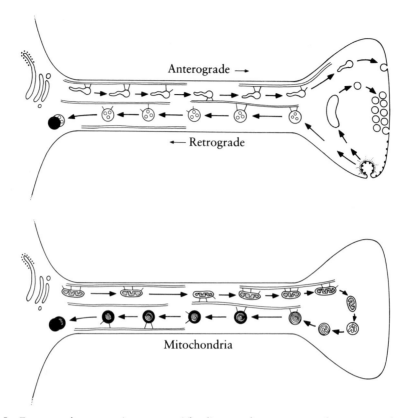

Figure 3.5 Fast axonal transport in neurones. The diagram shows anterograde transport of vesicles and vesiculotubular structures (upper) and mitochondria (lower) from their site of biosynthesis in the cell body to the nerve terminal. The microtubules in the axon act as guides for transport and axonal smooth endoplasmic reticulum (not shown) is important here also. The vesicles and vesiculotubular structures have diameters of 50–80 nm (Tsukita and Ishikawa 1980). Retrograde transport in the reverse direction occurs as larger membranous organelles (diameter 100–500 nm) termed multivesicular bodies. These transport membranous material retrieved by endocytosis from the nerve terminal membrane as well as organelles and degradation by lysosomes then occurs in the cell body. Anterograde transport provides for synthesis of synaptic vesicles which release neurotransmitter. The generation of large and small synaptic vesicles is not shown in this diagram but is considered in more detail in Chapter 5 (Fig. 5.8).

al. 1984). Fast axonal transport (both anterograde and retrograde) occurs at a rate of 200–400 mm day^{-1} and consists of the movement of vesicles, tubular structures, organelles, enzymes for neurotransmitter synthesis, and neurotransmitter-containing vesicles as well as retrieved recycled organelles and vesicles in the form of larger multivesicular bodies. Movement occurs along tracks that may be formed from microtubules in association with axonal smooth endoplasmic reticulum. The molecular basis of fast axonal transport is rapidly being established and two different motor molecules, dynein and kinesin, are known to be responsible for movement in the retrograde and anterograde directions respectively. The neurone is basically a specialized secretory cell with neurotransmitter release being its principal secretory activity. Fast axonal transport is important in maintaining this secretory activity.

Fast axonal transport (retrograde) is also important in enabling nerve terminal organelle degradation to occur in cell body lysosomes. In addition it provides a continuous source of information to the cell body on the state of the nerve terminal, provides for the uptake of growth factors, and may provide a route for the uptake of toxins and viruses.

Slow axonal transport or axoplasmic flow (largely anterograde) seems to involve some kind of physical translocation of the entire cytoskeleton and transport rates of 1 mm day^{-1} for microtubules, neurofilaments, and fodrin and 2–4 mm day^{-1} for structural and metabolic proteins (microfilaments, clathrin, fodrin, and soluble enzymes) have been measured. The function of slow axoplasmic flow is not clear but it may provide new cytoskeletal material for the nerve terminal.

Neuronal death and remodelling

The mature human cerebral cortex contains about 10^{10} neurones and once maturity has been reached there is no scope for growth of new neurones although there can be remodelling of dendritic connections. There seems to be a continuous loss of cells from the brain once maturity has been reached. The cell loss is different in different brain regions and quite difficult to estimate; age-related losses of between 10 and 60 per cent in terms of neuronal cell density have been reported for human cerebral cortex from early adulthood to late old age. Cell loss is, however, very variable from individual to individual. Any changes in cerebral volume, which also decreases, will magnify the total cell loss (Coleman and Flood 1987).

As well as cell death there is evidence for a reduction in the extent of the dendritic branching which would also reduce neuronal function. In contrast, some neurones show an increased dendritic branching with ageing, perhaps as a compensatory mechanism for loss of adjacent cells. Thus the overall picture is a much more dynamic one than that implied by a simple loss of neurones with ageing. Superimposed on these normal age dependent changes are the specific cell losses which occur in disease processes like Alzheimer's disease (Chapter 12), Huntington's disease (Chapter 11), and Parkinson's disease (Chapter 10).

The function of the neurone—electrical signalling and synaptic (chemical) transmission

The purpose of the neurone is to generate and transmit electrical impulses (signals) and, together with its highly differentiated structure, it is this electrical excitability that sets the neurone apart from other cells. A specialized part of the neuronal cell body, the axon hillock or initial segment (see Fig. 3.2), is capable of generating an electrical signal (called the action potential, which will be discussed in more detail in Chapter 4). The action potential can travel down the axon (more efficiently if the axon is myelinated) until it reaches the nerve terminal.

At the nerve terminal the electrical signal cannot jump across the synaptic cleft (the gap at the synapse between the nerve terminal and adjacent cell). Rather, its arrival triggers the release of a chemical substance called a neurotransmitter (Chapter 5). This is contained in the synaptic vesicles in the nerve terminal and by a process resembling secretion the neurotransmitter is released into the synaptic cleft. The chemical neurotransmitter interacts with the cell or part of the cell on the far side of the synapse via specific receptors (Chapter 6) and alters the electrical excitability of this postsynaptic cell; in this way information is passed from cell to cell. This may be in the form of a new electrical impulse in the postsynaptic cell or a change (positive or negative) in the ability of the postsynaptic cell to generate another electrical impulse. Much of the detail of these processes will be covered in the next few chapters.

This kind of chemical transmission between neurones at synapses is the major form of transmission in the mammalian nervous system. At a very small minority of sites in the mammalian nervous system and also more frequently in lower vertebrates and invertebrates, a second form of cell–cell communication is seen based on electrical synapses. The two cells are bridged by a gap junction which allows an electrical change in one cell to spread with little attenuation into the neighbouring cell. In this way assemblies of neurones may become activated together. This form of transmission is, however, so minor in the mammalian nervous system that I shall restrict discussion to chemical synaptic transmission.

The synapse and its morphology

The typical synapse consists of the junction (20–30 nm) between a nerve terminal and another cell (Fig. 3.6). In the brain this can be on to the cell body (axo-somatic), a dendrite or one of its spines (axo-dendritic), or another axon near the nerve terminal (axo-axonic) (Fig. 3.7). Occasionally an axon can form a synaptic contact before the nerve terminal; such contacts are termed en passant synapses. The functional consequences of the various interactions are quite different. For example, axo-dendritic synapses may affect impulse passage in the dendrite whereas axo-somatic interactions, which will be closer to the site of generation of new electrical impulses, may have a larger effect upon this new impulse. Inhibitory interactions are often of this class. Axo-axonic synapses seem to be associated with controlling neurotransmitter release.

At the microscopic level certain key features of the synapse can be discerned (Fig. 3.8). On the presynaptic side there are mitochondria, which are important for energy generation, synaptic vesicles containing the neurotransmitter, vesicles coated with

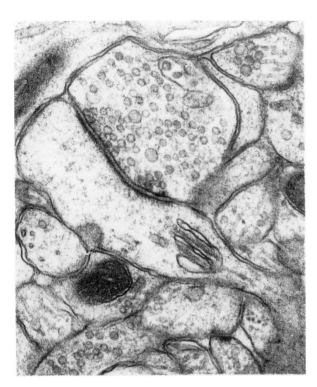

Figure 3.6 A synapse as seen in the electron microscope. The picture shows an axon terminal forming a synapse with a dendritic spine in the visual cortex of the rat. The magnification is 53 000× and the axon terminal containing vesicles can be seen in the upper half of the picture. (Courtesy of Dr. J. Parnevalas.)

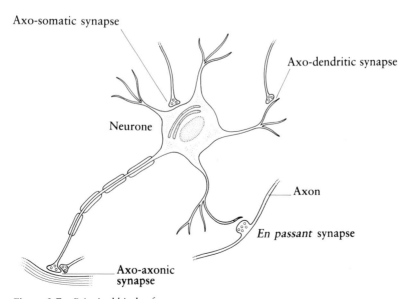

Axo-somatic synapse

Axo-dendritic synapse

Neurone

Axon

En passant synapse

Axo-axonic synapse

Figure 3.7 Principal kinds of synapse.

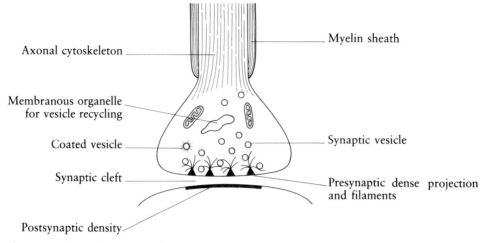

Axonal cytoskeleton

Myelin sheath

Membranous organelle
for vesicle recycling

Coated vesicle

Synaptic vesicle

Synaptic cleft

Presynaptic dense projection
and filaments

Postsynaptic density

Figure 3.8   Detailed structure of a synapse.

clathrin, membranous structures involved in retrieval of membrane, and the presynaptic grid with accompanying dense projections which may guide the vesicles as they approach the presynaptic membrane to release their contents. The presynaptic dense projections may be formed from collapsed cytoskeletal elements, the collapse being artefactual in the preparation of the sample for microscopy (Landis *et al.* 1988). On the postsynaptic side there is the postsynaptic thickening or density which seems likely to be important in the holding of receptor proteins in their correct positions. The importance of these structures will be discussed in Chapter 5 where neurotransmitter release is considered in more detail.

Morphologically different synapses have been distinguished at the electron microscopic level and termed Gray's Type I and Gray's Type II (Fig. 3.9). Type I synapses are often excitatory; they have a cleft of about 30 nm with presynaptic dense projections, round synaptic vesicles, and an extensive postsynaptic density so that the synapse has an asymmetric appearance. Type II synapses are often inhibitory with a cleft of 20 nm, fewer dense projections, oval, flattened vesicles, and modest postsynaptic and presynaptic densities so that the synapses appear symmetrical.

Although the diagrams of synapses shown here indicate a single presynaptic cell making contact with the postsynaptic cell, this is misleading as a postsynaptic cell can receive many inputs, both excitatory and inhibitory, both on to the dendrites and on to the cell body (Fig. 3.10). For example, the Purkinje cell of the cerebellum may receive more than 10^5 synaptic contacts on to its extensively branched dendrites. This enormous complexity at the synaptic level adds greatly to the complexity generated by the number of cells.

In the peripheral nervous system at autonomic postganglionic synapses a different

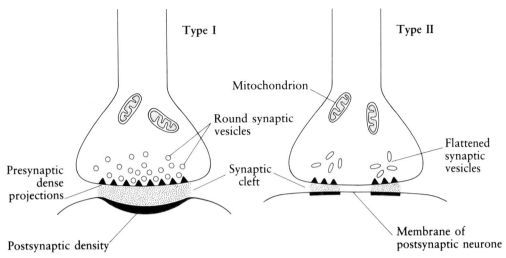

Figure 3.9 Gray's Type I and Type II synapses. Type I synapses are characterized by a more extensive post-synaptic density and round synaptic vesicles. They appear asymmetric because there is an asymmetric distribution of pre- and postsynaptic densities. Type II synapses show modest postsynaptic and presynaptic densities and oval flattened vesicles; they appear symmetrical because the pre- and postsynaptic densities are comparable in size. Type I synapses are often excitatory whereas Type II synapses are often inhibitory.

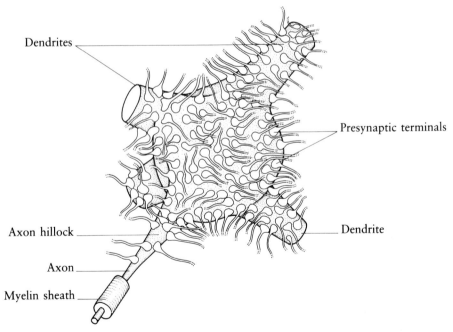

Figure 3.10 Synaptic interactions of a typical neurone. The diagram (taken from Alberts *et al.* 1989 with permission) illustrates the number and complexity of the synaptic interactions that a typical neurone receives on to its cell body and dendrites.

kind of synaptic organization has been recognized with much less synaptic specialization. The axons of the neurones here branch widely and have many small swellings or varicosities. Neurotransmitter release occurs from vesicles contained within the varicosities and there is little presynaptic specialization. There is also no postsynaptic density and the synaptic cleft is up to 400 nm wide. The extensive branching and numerous varicosities seem designed to provide widespread release of the neurotransmitter which can then affect a large target field via diffusion given the larger synaptic separation. Specificity of action will be guaranteed by the presence of specific receptor molecules. These kind of synapses have often been described for monoamine or peptide neurotransmitters.

For some time, particularly in neurones dependent on the monoamine neurotransmitters dopamine, noradrenaline, and 5-hydroxytryptamine, it had been assumed that similar neuronal systems occurred in the central nervous system where the purpose of the neurone is to influence a wide target area. It is true that for such systems the neurone produces a very widely branching axon and has many varicosities, but more recent work has shown that typical synapses do occur in a highly organized manner in most cases, so these systems in the brain may be more conventional than had been suspected (Parnevalas and Papadopoulos 1989). Nevertheless, such widely branching neurones may have a functional significance which will be discussed in Chapter 7 and they are important in certain diseases e.g. Parkinson's disease (Chapter 10).

Whereas there is no firm evidence for peripheral-type diffuse synaptic actions within the brain, there are some specific examples of neurones with no postsynaptic cell close by—these are typified by the neurosecretory cells of the hypothalamus. For example, a class of cell in the hypothalamus contains the monoamine dopamine as a neurotransmitter but upon activation the dopamine is released into the portal circulation. After passage in the blood to the anterior pituitary gland, the dopamine reaches its specific receptors. This is an extreme example of 'action at a distance'.

Neuroglial cells

Although the neurones are the 'business cells' of the brain, they are surrounded and outnumbered by a second class of cell collectively termed neuroglial cells or glia. Estimates of the relative number of glial cells and neurones vary but in monkey striate cortex the ratio is 2:1. Neuroglial cells do not have the electrically excitable membrane of the neurone but they nevertheless perform important maintenance functions. Neuroglial cells generally provide the bulk of the brain, comprising up to half its volume and separating and supporting the neurones, but not in a rigid way. Neuroglial cells each possess the complement of typical subcellular organelles already outlined for neurones. They can be divided into two different groups: microglial cells and macroglial cells, the latter being further subdivided into astrocytes, oligodendrocytes, and ependymal cells.

These groups of cells are quite similar in size (astrocytes and oligodendrocytes have cell bodies 5–8 μm in diameter whereas microglia can be slightly smaller, 4–8 μm), they differ in their morphology and function.

Astrocytes

Astrocytes possess long narrow cellular processes which give the cells their star-like appearance. The cellular processes often contact both capillaries and neurones via so-called end feet (Fig. 3.11). Two classes of astrocyte have been described. *Fibrous astrocytes* are packed with gliofilaments made largely of glial fibrillary acidic protein, and are found mainly in white matter where they are positioned between bundles of myelinated axons. *Protoplasmic astrocytes* have fewer filamentous structures and are found mainly in grey matter between neuronal cell bodies where they constitute a large part of the bulk of the tissue.

Owing to the contacts that astrocytes make with capillaries and neurones, it has been suggested that astrocytes may play a role in conducting nutrients from the blood to neurones. Although this is an attractive hypothesis, the evidence in support of it is not extensive. Other roles for astrocytes may be the removal by active transport of released neurotransmitters, the provision of substances for neurotransmitter synthesis, e.g. glutamine for GABA and glutamate synthesis, and the buffering of extracellular

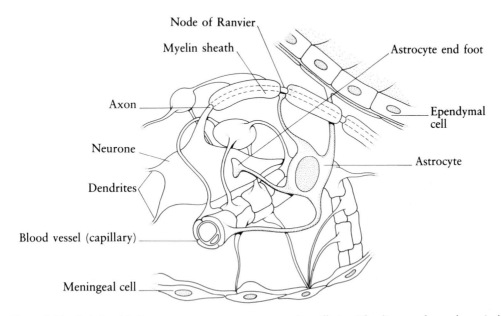

Figure 3.11 Relationship between astrocytes, neurones, and capillaries. The diagram shows the typical interactions between astrocytes, capillaries, and neurones.

potassium ions following depolarization of neurones. It seems likely that astrocytes perform a kind of monitoring role on substances gaining access to the neuronal extra-cellular fluid.

The astrocytes form a fairly dense surrounding for the capillaries so that substances emerging from the capillaries must pass through the small spaces between the astrocytes before gaining access to the neurones. Thus these substances are subject to the astrocyte uptake systems and the glial cells can be seen as providing a protection system for the neurones preventing the influence of a number of substances on neuronal activity. Nevertheless, these structures do not form the basis of the blood–brain barrier (Chapter 2), which is formed by tight junctions between endothelial and epithelial cells at the blood vessel wall. There is therefore a double control mechanism for the composition of neuronal extracellular fluid. Substances which are allowed via facilitated diffusion to pass the blood–brain barrier are then subjected to additional monitoring by this glial filter system.

Oligodendrocytes

Oligodendrocytes are found in both grey and white matter. In white matter they are responsible for forming the insulating myelin sheath around the axon (Fig. 3.12). In grey matter they may contribute to neuronal maintenance and may also provide myelin for axons coursing through the grey matter. In the periphery these functions are fulfilled by an analogous cell type called a Schwann cell. The myelin is formed by the outgrowth of the plasma membrane of the oligodendrocyte which wraps around the axon many times, excluding extracellular fluid from between the layers of plasma membrane and thus

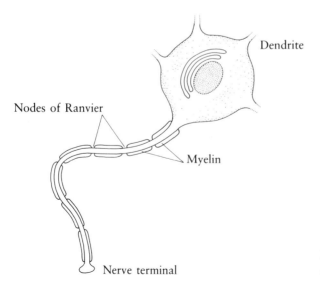

Figure 3.12 Myelin sheath and nodes of Ranvier.

generating a highly insulating coating for the axon (Fig. 3.13). This highly insulating coating, which is interrupted at the nodes of Ranvier, is important for efficient transmission of the electrical impulse as will be discussed in Chapters 4 and 7. The precise composition of the myelin membrane is different from that of glial cell membranes in that it has a greater proportion of lipid. The lipids in the myelin are also different from typical glial lipids and myelin contains two major specific protein components, myelin basic protein and myelin proteolipid protein.

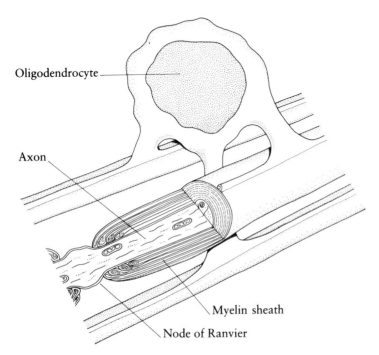

Figure 3.13 Formation of myelin sheath around axons by oligodendrocytes. The diagram shows the oligodendrocyte membrane wrapping round an axon to form the myelin sheath. Each oligodendrocyte can contribute to myelination of more than one axon.

Ependymal and microglial cells

Ependymal cells are a class of cell that line the inner surfaces of the brain in the ventricles. They are usually considered along with other neuroglial cells and appear to be involved in the exchange of material with the surrounding cerebrospinal fluid. Microglia show some resemblance to the macrophages of other parts of the body and seem to play a role in removing cell debris via phagocytosis following damage to the brain.

Other roles that have been proposed for neuroglial cells are as follows: (1) neuroglial cells may contribute to the guidance of growing neurones; (2) damage to brain tissue leads to proliferation of neuroglial cells which, unlike neurones, retain the ability to divide. Such proliferation is called gliosis and is due to an increased number of astrocytes, oligodendrocytes, and microglia. These are involved in removal of debris and eventually the formation of scar tissue. Glial cell proliferation may occur in some of the degenerative diseases of the brain where neurones are lost, e.g. Huntington's disease (Chapter 11) and Alzheimer's disease (Chapter 12).

Extracellular space

The extracellular space in the grey matter of the central nervous system is between 12 and 25 per cent of the tissue volume; this is much lower than is generally found elsewhere, for example in liver it is 30–40 per cent of tissue volume. This must reflect the tight packing of cells in the central nervous system provided by the neuroglial cells being closely apposed to neurones. The extracellular space contains the extracellular fluid of neurones and functionally the lower extracellular space means that substances released from neurones reach higher concentrations more quickly. The neuronal and neuroglial transport systems can, however, quickly deal with this, maintaining a constant neuronal extracellular environment. This is important in maintaining consistent neuronal function.

Recommended reading

Alberts, B., Bray, D., Lewis, J., Raff, M., Roberts, K., and Watson, J. D. (1989). *Molecular Biology of the Cell* (2nd edn). Garland, New York.

Allen, R. D. (1987). The microtubule as an intracellular engine. *Scientific American*, **256**(2), 26–33.

Bradford, H. F. (1986). *Chemical neurobiology*. Freeman, New York.

Kimelberg, H. K. and Norenberg, M. D. (1989). Astrocytes. *Scientific American*, **260**(4), 44–52.

McGeer, P. L., Eccles, J. C., and McGeer, E. G. (1987). *Molecular neurobiology of the mammalian brain* (2nd edn). Plenum Press, New York.

Shepherd, G. M. (1988). *Neurobiology* (2nd edn). Oxford University Press.

Siegel, G., Agranoff, B., Albers, R. W., and Molinoff, P. (1989). *Basic neurochemistry* (4th edn). Raven Press, New York.

Smith, C. U. M. (1989). *Elements of molecular neurobiology*. Wiley, Chichester.

4 *Electrical signalling in neurones*

The plasma membranes of all cells in the body are polarized, that is they are said to have a membrane potential. This is true for both neurones and neuroglial cells. What is important for the function of the neurone and for the brain as a whole is that in addition to possessing a membrane potential, the membrane of the neurone is electrically excitable. This electrical excitability forms the basis for all message transmission in the mammalian brain from the cell body along the axon and to the nerve terminal of neurones. In this chapter, the basis of the membrane potential will be dealt with first, and then the basis of the electrical excitability of the neuronal membrane and its consequences will be considered.

The resting membrane potential of cell membranes

The plasma membranes of both neuroglial cells and neurones are polarized, there being an excess of negative charge inside and a corresponding positive charge outside. This membrane potential is the result of an unequal distribution of ions across the plasma membrane coupled with the selective permeability of the plasma membranes to certain of these ions.

In most cells, and this is certainly true of neurones and neuroglial cells, the intracellular and extracellular fluids differ in their contents of certain ions. Typically the concentration of sodium ions is higher extracellularly than intracellularly and the concentrations of potassium ions differ in the opposite direction (some typical concentrations are given in Fig. 4.1). Although these ions are present at different concentrations inside and outside of the cell, at any time the total concentration of positive and negative ions on either side of the membrane balance so that there is strict charge neutrality either side of the membrane. Also the concentrations of ions on either side of the membrane are such that osmotic balance is maintained.

Now a cell membrane normally has a very low permeability to any charged species, but in the membrane of the cell there are protein channels selective for certain ions. These allow a low level of passive diffusion of ions down their concentration gradients. The membrane of the neuroglial cell possesses channels that are selective for potassium ions

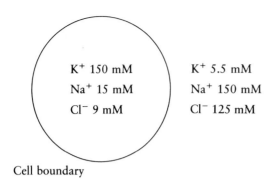

K⁺ 150 mM

Na⁺ 15 mM

Cl⁻ 9 mM

K⁺ 5.5 mM

Na⁺ 150 mM

Cl⁻ 125 mM

Cell boundary

Figure 4.1 Typical intracellular and extra-cellular concentrations of certain ions for neurones and neuroglial cells. The figures are for cat motor neurones taken from Smith (1989) and are representative for many cells in the nervous system. The concentrations of other ions will be such as to maintain charge neutrality on each side of the membrane and osmotic balance across the membrane.

and so the membrane has a low selective permeability for potassium ions. To a first approximation the same is true for neurones although this statement will be qualified slightly later.

The selective permeability to potassium ions means that these ions will tend to leak out of the cell down their concentration gradient (Fig. 4.1). This will alter the charge balance leading to a separation of charges so that the inside of the membrane will become slightly negatively charged and the outside positively charged. The membrane therefore becomes polarized. This diffusion of potassium ions will continue and the polarization will increase until the electrical effect of the membrane potential created in this way balances the tendency of the potassium ions to leak out of the cell. At this point a steady state is reached and the membrane potential across the cell membrane is termed the resting membrane potential. Whereas this derivation of the resting membrane potential is accurate for neuroglial cells, the actual situation in the neurone is more complex. The neuronal membrane also has a low but significant permeability to sodium ions again due to the presence of passive protein channels which in this case are selective for sodium ions. This sodium ion permeability is generally much lower than the potassium ion permeability. In consequence the resting membrane potential of the neurone, while dominated by the potassium ion permeability and distribution, will be slightly less negative than that of a neuroglial cell owing to the diffusion of sodium ions into the cell. Neuronal membranes are also permeable to chloride ions but in most cells these are distributed passively in response to the overall resting membrane potential.

If the membrane were selectively permeable only to potassium ions, then the resting membrane potential could be maintained indefinitely. If, however, there is also a signifi-cant sodium ion permeability, then at rest there must be flux of potassium ions out of the cell and sodium ions in to the cell. This would eventually lead to the dissipation of the transmembrane ionic concentration gradients that lead to the resting potential. There-fore there is a need for a restorative system; this is provided by a membrane pump. This is an integral membrane protein that pumps sodium ions out of the cell and potassium ions in, thus maintaining the ionic gradients. The pumping is carried out at the expense of

ATP hydrolysis so the Na^+/K^+ pump is often referred to as the Na^+/K^+ ATPase. The action of this pump is the basis of the large requirement of the brain for energy in the form of ATP in turn derived from oxidative metabolism of glucose (Chapter 2).

As a result of the processes described above, the membrane of neuroglial cells is polarized, negative inside, at a membrane potential of about -75 mV whereas for a typical neurone the membrane potential is slightly less at about -60 mV. As we shall see below the neuronal membrane potential can under certain circumstances become less negative, in which case it is said to be depolarized. Alternatively it can become more negative or hyperpolarized.

In summary, the resting membrane potential in the neurone is a result of the unequal distribution of ions across the plasma membrane together with the selective permeability of the membrane to certain ions, principally potassium. The unequal distribution of ions across the membranes is maintained by the pumping action of the Na^+/K^+ ATPase.

Excitability of the neuronal membrane

The principal physical property that sets the neurone apart from other cells is the electrical excitability of its plasma membrane. This electrical excitability can be seen by considering a typical neuronal membrane and its associated membrane potential. If the resting cell (membrane potential -60 mV) is depolarized by a brief stimulus of current to a membrane potential of -45 mV or more, then a, now classical, series of events is observed.

A rapid and large depolarization of the membrane follows that produced by the stimulating current. The membrane in fact reverses potential to about $+30$ mV; this occurs over about 0.75 ms. Almost as rapidly, the membrane repolarizes, reaching its previous resting potential. It may undershoot slightly (to -80 mV) before steadying at the normal resting level. These events are depicted in Figure 4.2 and are collectively referred to as the action potential. In some neurones the action potential is dominated by the depolarizing phase followed by a slower repolarization. The basis of these differences will be explored below. The action potential or nerve impulse is responsible, as will be described below, for most of the electrical signalling and information transfer in the brain.

Molecular basis of the action potential

Careful study of the electrical events involved in the action potential has shown that the depolarizing phase of the action potential is due to increased permeability of the membrane to sodium ions, whereas in the rapid repolarizing phase the membrane loses its permeability to sodium ions but becomes permeable to potassium ions (Fig. 4.3). The molecular basis of these changes is the presence in neuronal membranes of selective

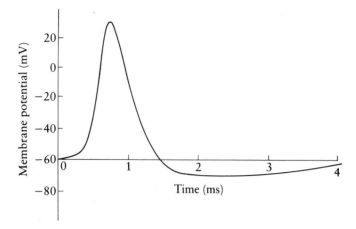

Figure 4.2 The action potential. The trace shows the action potential that might typically be recorded using an intracellular electrode from a squid giant axon, a popular tissue for such studies owing to the ease of manipulation (Hodgkin and Huxley 1952). The trace shows a rapid re-polarization phase.

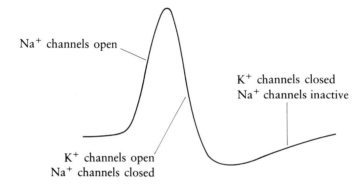

Figure 4.3 Ionic basis of the action potential (see Fig. 4.2).

protein channels for sodium ions and potassium ions; these channels are normally closed but can open in response to changes in the neuronal membrane potential. These ion channels are therefore termed voltage-sensitive ion channels.

The effect of the stimulating current and the small depolarization from -60 mV to -45 mV is sensed by the voltage-sensitive Na^+ channels some of which open. This increases the permeability of the membrane to sodium ions, some sodium ions enter the cell and a further depolarization occurs. This leads to the opening of more Na^+ channels and further depolarization until the membrane potential is dominated by the sodium ion gradient and becomes positive ($+30$ mV). The process is autocatalytic in that once enough Na^+ channels are opened by a small depolarization, all the available voltage-sensitive Na^+ channels will open and a full depolarization will occur. There is said to be a threshold depolarization which if exceeded will always lead to a full depolarization. The threshold potential represents the point at which the rate of entry of sodium ions through voltage-sensitive Na^+ channels exceeds the rate of exit of potassium ions through resting

K^+ channels. At this point there is a net entry of positive ions, further depolarizing the cell membrane so that the autocatalytic process can occur. Typically a threshold of −45 mV is seen for mammalian neurones. When the membrane is depolarized a second property of the voltage-sensitive sodium channel emerges—the channels inactivate (close again) in response to the depolarization and stay inactive until the membrane repolarizes.

In many neurones a rapid repolarizing phase ensues; an exception to this is mammalian myelinated axons. Here the rapid depolarization is followed by a slower repolarization (Fig. 4.4). This reflects the inactivation of the Na^+ channels and the slow (2 ms) repolarization reflects leakage of potassium ions out across the membrane through the same K^+ channels involved in generating the resting membrane potential.

Where a rapid repolarization occurs (Figs 4.2 and 4.3), this is due to the presence of additional voltage-sensitive K^+ channels in the neuronal membrane. These open in response to membrane depolarization but more slowly than the Na^+ channels. The opening of the K^+ channels allows the membrane to become more permeable to potassium ions and the membrane repolarizes. When the membrane potential has reached its normal resting value these K^+ channels close but there may be a small under-shoot in the membrane potential as they react somewhat slowly to the change in potential. These voltage-sensitive K^+ channels are critical in enabling a rapid resetting of the membrane potential to occur after an action potential has been triggered. These channels are not present in mammalian myelinated axons (Fig. 4.4), accounting for the slower repolarization. The repolarization mechanism based on voltage-sensitive K^+ channels is found extensively in invertebrates but is also found in the neuronal cell body in vertebrates and in vertebrate unmyelinated axons. In the excitable membranes (axon hillock)

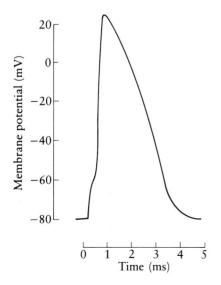

Figure 4.4 The action potential in a mammalian myelinated axon. The trace is typical of that seen in a rabbit myelinated axon (Chiu *et al.* 1979) and shows the slower repolarization phase typical of a tissue that lacks voltage-sensitive K^+ channels. Compare the time course with that of Figs 4.2 and 4.3 for invertebrate axons.

of some mammalian central neurones (e.g. pyramidal cells of the hippocampus), a slightly different mechanism again is used for repolarization. The majority of the repolarization in these cells can be accounted for by the initial depolarization of the membrane leading to opening of voltage sensitive Ca^{2+} channels. The influx of Ca^{2+} ions then triggers the opening of fast Ca^{2+}-dependent K^+ channels which leads to membrane repolarization. There is also some contribution from voltage-sensitive K^+ channels (Storm 1987).

Although the amounts of sodium ions and potassium ions moving across the membrane during a single action potential are not great, repetitive firing of action potentials in a small diameter axon will change the transmembrane ionic gradients. The Na^+/K^+ pump therefore is very important here in restoring the sodium and potassium ion gradient after action potential firing. This is performed at the expense of hydrolysis of ATP.

Experimentally it is observed that after a neurone has triggered an action potential there is a short (1–2 ms) refractory period during which further action potentials cannot be generated. In the mammalian myelinated axon this corresponds to the period required for the reversal of Na^+ channel inactivation while the membrane repolarizes. If voltage-sensitive K^+ channels are present, the refractory period (corresponding to Na^+ channel inactivation and increased neuronal membrane potassium ion permeability) is rather shorter (≈ 1 ms). Thus the presence of the voltage-sensitive K^+ channels makes the neurone ready more quickly to fire another action potential.

An action potential is an 'all or none' phenomenon. Once the membrane has been depolarized past its threshold point, a full action potential will always result. Fractions of an action potential are not possible so that in terms of information content the action potential contains only a single piece of information. As will be described in Chapter 7, this means that information is encoded in the frequency of action potential triggering.

In summary, voltage-sensitive, ion-selective channels in the neuronal plasma membrane give rise to the action potential, the main information signal in the nervous system. The structures of these channels are beginning to be understood and they are complex integral membrane proteins (Catterall 1988; Maelicke 1988; Miller 1991).

Propagation of the action potential

The action potential as described so far is a static phenomenon, but we know from Chapter 3 that electrical messages in neurones are conveyed down axons. In fact the neuronal membrane is so constructed that the action potential can move along the membrane and down the axon. This is due to the voltage-sensitive nature of the Na^+ channels in the neuronal membrane and the electrical properties of the neuronal membrane.

If we reconsider the initial depolarizing phase of the action potential, then when the voltage-sensitive Na^+ channels are open, a current moves across the membrane carried by sodium ions. Although the Na$^+$ channels that are open will be present at a discrete point in the membrane where depolarization has occurred, the electrical effects are more widespread. There is some passive spreading of the depolarization along the internal face of the membrane on either side of the initial depolarized segment (Fig. 4.5). This spread of the depolarization will be due to outward flow of current across the membrane dissipating the inward flow due to the depolarizing current. This will be due to potassium ions gradually leaking out across the membrane and the currents result in so-called 'local circuits'. These properties are often referred to as the cable-like properties of the neuronal membrane. The size of the current flowing and the resulting depolarization diminishes as the distance from the initial depolarizing point increases. Although this passive spread of the depolarization provides a means for some propagation of the action potential, it does not allow for rapid unidirectional transmission of the action potential. This is provided by the presence in the neuronal membrane of the voltage-sensitive Na$^+$ channels.

To understand action potential transmission, let us consider a point on the neuronal membrane where a local depolarization has occurred due to the opening of sodium channels (Fig. 4.6). The depolarization will spread passively along the membrane due to the local circuit currents. As the depolarization at the start has exceeded the threshold for action potential generation, then the spreading depolarization must also have exceeded the threshold for some distance away from the initial depolarizing point. If voltage-sensitive Na$^+$ channels are present at sufficient density, then where neighbouring pieces of neuronal membrane are depolarized below threshold, action potential generation will

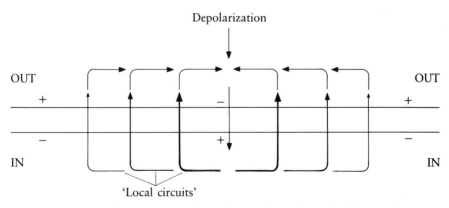

Figure 4.5 Passive spread of depolarization along the axonal membrane. The diagram shows a section of one side of the axonal membrane with a depolarization at one point, for example by injection of a small amount of current from an electrode. The amount of current is not enough to trigger an action potential but it causes a small depolarization of the membrane that spreads along the membrane. The magnitude of the depolarization decays exponentially as shown by the decreasing thickness of the arrows. The resulting currents are termed 'local circuits'. Similar 'local circuits' are present when the membrane is depolarized past the threshold for action potential generation (Fig. 4.6).

Direction of progagation of action potential ⟶

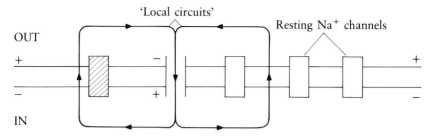

A few milliseconds later

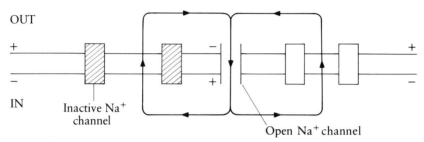

Figure 4.6 Propagation of the action potential. The upper diagram shows a section through one side of the axonal membrane with a depolarization at one point such that sodium channels are open and 'local circuit' currents (see Fig. 4.5) are set up. As the depolarization is above the threshold, then at points adjacent, the depolarization will spread and will remain above the threshold for some distance. Na$^+$ channels within this distance will open owing to their voltage-sensitive nature and the action potential will spread. In principle this mechanism provides for spread of the action potential in both directions away from the initial depolarization point. As explained in the text, however, owing to the geometry of neurones and the excitability of the axonal membrane compared with the neuronal cell body (see Fig. 4.7) and the inactivation of the voltage-sensitive Na$^+$ channels after their brief opening, action potential propagation occurs unidirectionally. The diagram shows the action potential moving from left to right with inactivated sodium channels behind the action potential and channels ready for depolarization ahead of it. In the lower diagram the same membrane is shown a few milliseconds later with the action potential having moved to the right. Behind the wave of action potential, mechanisms described in the text will restore the membrane potential to its resting state and also allow Na$^+$ channels to return to their resting state.

occur in those pieces of membrane. A full depolarization will then occur in the neighbouring membrane, leading to further passive spread of the depolarization and further propagation of the action potential. The 'all or none' character of the action potential ensures that a complete signal is propagated at all times.

For information transfer in the nervous system, the action potential must be propagated unidirectionally down the axon of a neurone from a cell body to the nerve terminal. In an individual neurone the action potential arises in a specialized part of the

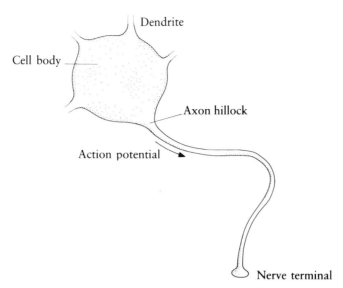

Figure 4.7 Axon hillock as the site of action potential generation. The diagram shows the axon hillock or initial segment, which is the excitable area of the neuronal cell body where action potential generation occurs. The various inputs to the dendrites and cell body alter the membrane potential felt by the axon hillock and action potentials are generated accordingly. The neuronal cell body is usually unable to generate action potentials; this fact, together with the excitable nature of the axonal membrane, ensures that action potentials generated in the axon hillock travel away from the axon hillock down the axon. The inactivation of Na$^+$ channels behind the wave of action potential also contributes to this unidirectionality.

cell body near the origin of the axon called the axon hillock or initial segment (Fig. 4.7). The action potential then propagates down the axon and this is unidirectional in part owing to the geometry of the cell body and axon and in part because of the refractory period that follows action potential generation. Once the action potential has started moving in one direction, that is down the axon, it will continue in that direction as the Na$^+$ channels will be inactive for a short time after firing an action potential and so only those in advance of the signal will be available for propagation. Also, the neuronal cell body does not have the ability to generate action potentials as it has very few voltage-sensitive Na$^+$ channels, so backwards spread from the axon hillock is prevented. Action potential propagation proceeds at speeds of between 0.2 and 120 ms^{-1} depending on the axon. Action potential propagation is faster in larger diameter axons but a very considerable increase in propagation is achieved by coating the axon with the myelin sheath (see below). Behind the wave of propagating action potential there will be either a delayed opening of voltage-sensitive K$^+$ channels or a leakage out of the potassium ions through resting K$^+$ channels if voltage-sensitive K$^+$ channels are absent as in mammalian myelinated axons. Either mechanism will lead to repolarization of the membrane. The sodium channels then return to their resting state and the membrane is ready for further action potential propagation. Propagation of action potentials will lead to further flux of sodium and potassium ions and will require a Na^+/K^+ pump activity and ATP hydrolysis to restore the transmembrane ion gradients.

Action potential propagation in myelinated axons

Although the above mechanism of action potential propagation is efficient, it can be made more efficient in two ways. The size of the axon is one factor that determines the efficiency of propagation so that a large diameter (0.6 mm) axon such as the squid giant axon conducts rapidly. In mammals, however, axons are smaller but the passive spread of the action potential depolarization is improved by providing the axon with an insulating coat, the myelin sheath (Fig. 3.12). Myelin is such a good insulator that it reduces the leakage of the potassium ions in advance of the inward Na^+ current which would otherwise occur during the depolarizing phase of the action potential so that the depolarization can spread further away along the axon. As the myelin sheath is not continuous but is interrupted by nodes of Ranvier about 1 mm apart, the spread of the depolarization need only be from one node to the next. This does, however, restrict the need for Na^+ channels to the nodes and this is indeed where they are concentrated, there being none between the nodes. Therefore a depolarization leading to an action potential at one node can spread passively to the next node where action potential generation can occur, thus reinforcing the signal which spreads to the next node (Fig. 4.8). The action potential therefore jumps from node to node and propagation is said to be saltatory (after the Latin for to leap: *saltare*). This arrangement speeds up action potential propagation (a non-myelinated axon of diameter 0.5–1.0 mm conducts at about 20 m s^{-1} whereas a myelinated axon of diameter 20 μm conducts at 120 m s^{-1}), there is less movement of sodium ions and thus less requirement for ATP to pump the ions back, and it requires fewer sodium channels along the membrane. In mammalian myelinated axons as described above there are no voltage-sensitive K^+ channels at the nodes, so repolarization of the membrane occurs after the action potential has passed, by inactivation of the sodium channels and leakage of the potassium ions back out of the membrane (Chiu *et al*. 1979).

Mammalian nerve fibres vary in size considerably. Myelinated fibres are generally 2–20 μm in diameter and conduct at velocities between 12 and 120 m s^{-1}. Unmyelinated fibres are also seen, with diameters of 0.2–1μm and conduction velocities of 0.2–2 m s^{-1}. The faster conducting nerve fibres are generally seen where the information must be transferred quickly, as in motor neurones and some sensory fibres, whereas slower conducting unmyelinated nerve fibres are seen in some sensory pathways and in the central nervous system where the effects of the neurone are more modulatory. These points will be discussed again in Chapter 7.

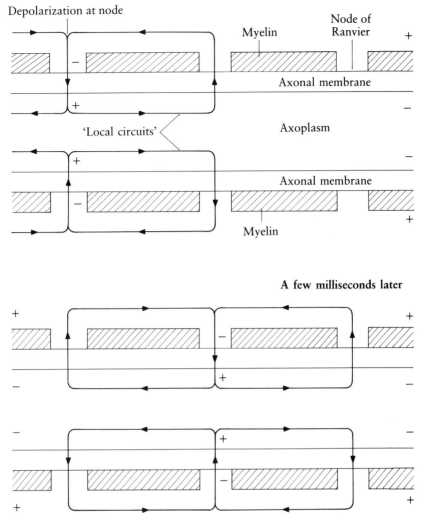

Figure 4.8 Myelin sheath and fast action potential propagation. A section through a myelinated axon is shown with, in the upper diagram, a depolarization at a node of Ranvier due to opening of voltage-sensitive Na^+ channels. The depolarization spreads via local circuit currents along the axon to the next node when a further depolarization occurs (lower diagram) reinforcing the signal. The spread of the depolarization is much greater than in Figs 4.5 and 4.6 owing to the insulating properties of the myelin sheath.

Events at the nerve terminal

The mechanisms described above provide for rapid propagation of the action potential down the axon until it reaches the nerve terminal. The arrival of the wave of depolarization at the nerve terminal leads to activation of a further set of voltage-sensitive ion channels. These are selective for calcium ions and open in response to the arrival of the wave of depolarization. As a result, calcium ions enter the nerve terminal down their concentration gradient and the nerve terminal cytosolic calcium ion concentration, which is normally very low, may increase up to one hundred fold. The increased calcium ion concentration causes the synaptic vesicles in the nerve terminal to fuse with the nerve terminal membrane, releasing the chemical neurotransmitter contained in the vesicles into the synaptic cleft (Fig. 4.9). There it diffuses to the postsynaptic membrane which contains receptor proteins specific for the neurotransmitter. Because the neurotransmitter is released from vesicles each containing a certain amount of the substance, the release appears to be in packets or quanta. These processes will be considered in more detail in Chapter 5.

The combination of the neurotransmitter with its specific receptor in the postsynaptic membrane leads to a change in the postsynaptic neurone. The changes that occur will be considered in more detail in Chapter 6 but the possibilities will be summarized here. Some receptors are coupled directly to ion channels in the postsynaptic membrane forming ligand-gated ion channels. These produce a rapid electrical change in the postsynaptic membrane, within a few milliseconds.

There are two classes of rapid electrical change that are possible here (Fig. 4.10). In one case the receptor opens an ion channel selective for both sodium and potassium ions. This depolarizes the membrane and the effect is said to be excitatory (excitatory postsynaptic potential or EPSP) as it depolarizes the membrane to the threshold for action potential triggering. In the brain, glutamate is the principal excitatory neurotransmitter.

In the other case, the ion channel is selective for chloride ions and opening of such a channel hyperpolarizes the membrane slightly. This is said to be inhibitory (inhibitory

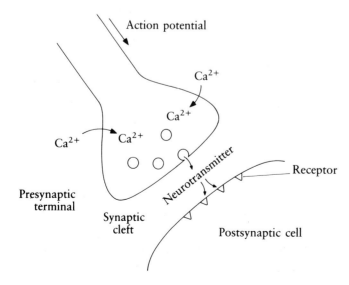

Figure 4.9 Neurotransmitter release at the synapse. The action potential arrives at the nerve terminal and the depolarization opens voltage-sensitive Ca^{2+} channels. The resultant increase in intraterminal Ca^{2+} triggers release by exocytosis of the neurotransmitter stored in synaptic vesicles. The neurotransmitter diffuses to specific neurotransmitter receptors on the postsynaptic cell and the combination of neurotransmitter and receptor leads to changes in the electrical excitability of the postsynaptic cell.

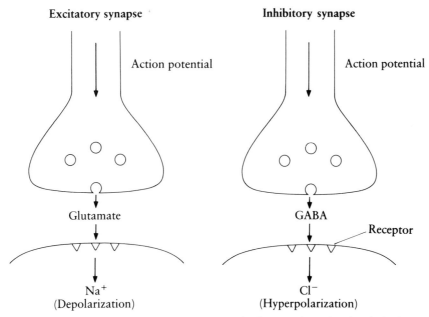

Figure 4.10 Fast neurotransmitter actions at synapses. The diagram shows fast depolarization and hyperpolarization in postsynaptic cells due to release of different neurotransmitters and their interaction with specific receptors. Acetylcholine (excitatory) and glycine (inhibitory) also play minor roles as fast neurotransmitters in the nervous system.

postsynaptic potential or IPSP) as it renders the membrane less excitable. γ-amino butyric acid (GABA) is the principal inhibitory neurotransmitter in the brain.

Another group of receptors at synapses act much more slowly and here the time-scale is from seconds to minutes. These receptors frequently alter the concentrations of chemicals in the postsynaptic cell called second messengers, e.g. cyclic AMP, inositol trisphosphate, and diacylglycerol (Fig. 4.11). These may in turn alter membrane ionic permeabilities via a series of stages and their speed of action means that they must be involved in slower modulatory events in neurones. Some slow acting receptors are also linked more directly to ion channels. The properties of the ligand-gated ion channels and receptors linked to second messengers will be considered in more detail in Chapter 6.

Integration by neurones—encoding of action potentials

Much of our discussion above has over-simplified what actually occurs at neurones in the brain. A typical neurone receives hundreds or perhaps thousands of inputs from other neurones terminating as synapses on its cell body and dendrites (Fig. 3.10). Each input will have some effect on the neuronal membrane potential and the different effects are integrated to produce a net membrane potential. This is then translated into a new

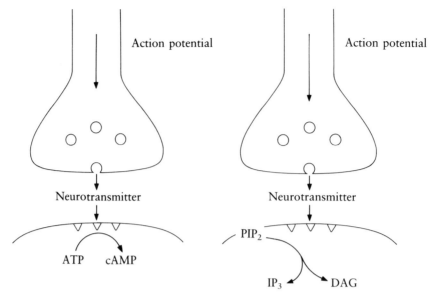

Figure 4.11 Slow neurotransmitter actions at synapses. The diagram shows the interactions of slow neurotransmitters with postsynaptic receptors to alter levels of the second messenger molecules cyclic AMP (cAMP) or inositol trisphosphate (IP$_3$) and diacyl glycerol (DAG) (generated from the membrane phospholipid phosphatidyl inositol bisphosphate (PIP$_2$)). Several neurotransmitters can have effects on both systems dependent on the postsynaptic receptor subtype present. For example noradrenaline via α_1 adrenergic receptors activates PIP$_2$ breakdown, via α_2-adrenergic receptors inhibits cAMP generation and via β-adrenergic receptors activates cAMP generation. As described in Chapter 6 there are also some slow effects of neurotransmitters on the postsynaptic membrane potential. These can be due to the effects of second messengers altering the activities of membrane ion channels or more direct effects on ion channels. The mechanistic details of this will be discussed later.

form by the specialized region of the cell body close to the axon called the axon hillock (or initial segment) (Fig. 4.7). This has specialized electrical properties which enable it to convert the net postsynaptic potential into a particular frequency of action potential firing. In most neurones there is a basal level of action potential firing and the net neuronal membrane potential modulates this. Thus the picture as described above of a neurone being driven past its threshold and firing an action potential is rather misleading. This is occurring all the time as the membrane potential oscillates and action potentials fire when the membrane potential is driven below the threshold. The net membrane potential due to all the neuronal inputs makes it easier or more difficult for the membrane potential to be driven past the threshold and the action potential frequency alters accordingly. This emphasizes the role of the action potential as the informational currency of the brain; the frequency of firing represents the information patterns.

 The qualities of the inputs that influence the net membrane potential will be considered in more detail in Chapter 7 but are noted here. Four qualities can be discerned:

(1) *frequency* of action potential firing in an input axon;
(2) the *sign* of the input to a neurone i.e. excitatory or inhibitory;
(3) the *spatial pattern* of the inputs to a neurone—axo-dendritic and axo-somatic inputs have rather different effects (see also Chapter 3);
(4) the *time course* of the effect of an input on the neuronal cell body can be either fast or slow.

The neurone therefore carries out a complex integration of the inputs impinging on it and fires action potentials accordingly.

Recommended reading

Aidley, D. J. (1989). *The physiology of excitable cells* (3rd edn). Cambridge University Press.
Alberts, B., Bray, D., Lewis, J., Raff, M., Roberts, K., and Watson, J. D. (1989). Molecular biology of the cell (2nd edn). Garland, New York.
Kandel, E. R. and Schwartz, J. H. (1985). *Principles of neural science*. Elsevier, New York.
Kuffler, S. W., Nicholls, J. G., and Martin, A. R. (1984). *From neuron to brain*. (2nd edn.) Sinauer Associates Inc., Sunderland, MA.

5   *Chemical signalling at the synapse—synaptic transmission*

The previous chapter described in detail how electrical signals could be transmitted along axons of neurones in the form of a propagating action potential. This electrical signal eventually reaches the nerve terminal and synapse where the neurotransmitter is released to cross the synaptic cleft and reach the postsynaptic membrane, which continues the electrical signalling in the adjacent postsynaptic cell. Therefore signalling in the brain consists of electrical signals linked together by chemical signals. The chemical signalling at the synapse is often referred to as synaptic transmission.

In this chapter the processes involved in chemical signalling at the synapse and the criteria which must be fulfilled for a substance to be considered as a neurotransmitter will be discussed in detail. This discussion is important for the later chapters on brain disorders as some of these disorders may be due to disturbances of synaptic transmission and the drugs that are used to treat the disorders mostly act at specific sites at or near synapses.

An overview of chemical signalling at the synapse

In Fig. 5.1 a diagram shows the key stages in chemical signalling at the synapse by neurotransmitters (synaptic transmission). The arrival of the electrical signal (action potential) at the nerve terminal triggers fusion of the synaptic vesicles, containing neurotransmitter, with the presynaptic membrane; the neurotransmitter is then released into the synaptic cleft. Here it diffuses until it reaches specific receptors on the postsynaptic membrane of the adjacent neuronal cell body, dendrite, or nerve terminal. The three types of synapse involved are known as axo-somatic, axo-dendritic, and axo-axonic respectively (Chapter 3). The neurotransmitter combines with its receptor, activating a transduction mechanism which causes a change in the excitability of the postsynaptic membrane (Chapters 4 and 6). The action of the neurotransmitter must be terminated in some way in order to limit the actions of the neurotransmitter and to allow for rapid repetitive signalling; typically this is achieved either by removing the neurotransmitter from the

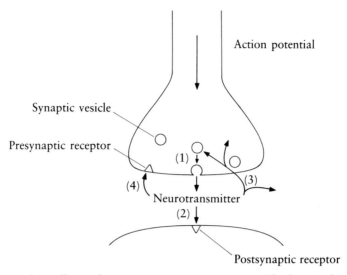

Figure 5.1 Chemical signalling at the synapse (synaptic transmission). The diagram shows the key stages in synaptic transmission: (1) release of neurotransmitter in response to depolarization of nerve terminal by the action potential; (2) interaction of neurotransmitter with postsynaptic receptor to cause a change in the postsynaptic cell; (3) the action of the neurotransmitter is terminated by either taking it back into the nerve terminal or by destroying it in the synaptic cleft; (4) presynaptic receptors may exist to control release of the neurotransmitter.

synapse or by degrading it *in situ*. Neurotransmitter release is often modulated by receptors (presynaptic receptors) on the presynaptic cell (nerve terminal) that inhibit (or in some cases stimulate) neurotransmitter release. This general scheme will be considered in more detail below.

A number of substances have been discovered that conform to the above scheme to a greater or lesser degree and so can be considered as neurotransmitters; they are listed in Table 5.1. A set of criteria can be laid down (Table 5.2) which ideally should be satisfied if a substance is to be considered a neurotransmitter. Some of these criteria are quite difficult to satisfy in the brain, mainly owing to access problems so that it may not be easy to establish definitively that a substance is a neurotransmitter in the brain. Nevertheless for a number of the substances in Table 5.1 many of the criteria are satisfied. For the more recently discovered substances (most of the neuropeptides fall into this category), fewer of the criteria are satisfied although many of these substances are thought to be neurotransmitters; this is an area of active current research.

Neurotransmitters and neuromodulators

It seems clear that in most cases neurotransmitters are released at clear synapses with closely apposed pre- and postsynaptic membranes. As pointed out in Chapter 3,

Table 5.1   Established and putative neurotransmitters in the brain

---

A. *Small molecule neurotransmitters*
    Fast   acetylcholine, γ-aminobutyric acid (GABA), glutamate (aspartate), glycine,
           5-hydroxytryptamine
    Slow acetylcholine, adenosine, adrenaline, ATP, dopamine, GABA, glutamate, histamine,
           5-hydroxytryptamine, noradrenaline

B. *Neuropeptides*
    angiotensin II, bombesin, bradykinin, carnosine, CGRP, cholecystokinin, corticotropin (ACTH),
    corticotropin releasing factor, dynorphin, β-endorphin, gastrin, leucine enkephalin, LHRH,
    melanotropin (α-MSH), methionine enkephalin, neurokinin A, neurokinin B, neuropeptide Y,
    neurotensin, somatostatin, substance P, TRH, vasopressin, vasoactive intestinal peptide (VIP)

The more established small molecule neurotransmitters are given, divided into the fast and slow categories (Chapters 6 and 7). Neuropeptides are generally slow acting and only for a few of the substances shown is it certain that they act as neurotransmitters. The list of neuropeptides contains several substances for which the evidence for neurotransmitter function is very slight. For more details of these see the general references at the end of the chapter.

however, this was not always thought to be so and some substances were thought to act more diffusely. Although this does not now seem to be generally so in the brain, there are examples of some substances released from neurosecretory cells into the blood stream with no close postsynaptic target. In addition, as I shall speculate in Chapter 10, when the system is perturbed, as in Parkinson's Disease, there may be some diffusion of the released neurotransmitter dopamine away from the synaptic sites of release even in the brain. Also, some neurotransmitters act quickly and others more slowly; this subdivision has been included in Table 5.1. Neuropeptides may be a further class acting even more slowly.

Table 5.2   Criteria for classifying a substance as a neurotransmitter

---

1. The substance is present in neurones, together with biosynthetic enzymes and is stored in vesicles found in nerve terminals.
2. The substance is released from neurones upon depolarization of the nerve terminal. Release is Ca^{2+} dependent.
3. Receptors for the substance are present at the synapse on the postsynaptic cell and combination of the substance with the receptor alters the excitability of the postsynaptic cell.
4. Application of the substance exogenously elicits similar effects upon cell excitability as does electrical stimulation of the presynaptic cell leading to synaptic release of the substance.
5. The action of the synaptically released and exogenously supplied substance can be blocked by specific antagonists.
6. A mechanism exists at the synapse for termination of the action of the substance.
7. Receptors specific for the substance exist upon the nerve terminal (presynaptic receptors) and these limit the release of the substance.

These considerations of space and time have led people to question the use of the term neurotransmitter and to apply the term neuromodulator to certain substances. In some cases the term neuromodulator is used to hide frank ignorance about the status of the candidate neurotransmitter. It may, however, be used more genuinely to denote a substance that indeed modulates neurones or other cells in the nervous system but not necessarily by synaptic release close to that neurone. For example, the neuromodulatory action could be to facilitate or reduce (pre- or postsynaptically) the actions of an identified neurotransmitter. The neuromodulator could be released with the neurotransmitter (see section on neurotransmitter coexistence below).

It is therefore perhaps best to reserve the term neurotransmitter for any substance released at a synapse which acts on a neighbouring postsynaptic cell and satisfies many of the criteria outlined above (Table 5.2). The speed of the response and the synaptic specialization and distance would then be secondary qualifications applied to this broad descriptive term.

Details of the individual stages of synaptic transmission

In this section the behaviour of one neurotransmitter, dopamine, will be analysed in more detail in order to exemplify the principles outlined in Table 5.2. It is beyond the scope of this book to give full details of neurotransmission by other substances and the reader is referred to the reading list at the end of this chapter. However, where other neurotransmitters differ in principle from dopamine, the differences will be outlined and Table 5.3 gives the key components of other neurotransmitter systems. Dopamine has been chosen as the example because of its importance along with other monoamine neurotransmitters, e.g. noradrenaline and 5-hydroxytryptamine, in the later discussion of brain disorders (Chapters 10–15).

Extensive neuroanatomical tracing of pathways containing dopamine has shown that there exist in the brain several neuronal systems in which dopamine is presumed to act as a neurotransmitter. These comprise a number of short pathways including the tuberohypophysial dopamine cells which project from the arcuate and periventricular nuclei into the intermediate lobe of the pituitary gland and the median eminence. The latter nerve terminals secrete dopamine into the portal circulation to influence anterior pituitary gland prolactin secretion. This is the neurosecretory pathway referred to previously. For more detail of these short dopamine-containing pathways consult the reviews by Moore and Bloom (1978), Lindvall and Bjorklund (1982) and Cooper *et al.* (1986).

There are also longer dopamine-containing neuronal pathways (Fig. 5.2). These form a major set of neurones with cell bodies in the substantia nigra and ventral tegmental area of the brain innervating a variety of midbrain and cortical regions and

Table 5.3 Properties of well defined neurotransmitter systems

Neurotransmitter	Precursors	Synthetic enzymes	Means of termination of action	Receptors	Agonists	Antagonists
Acetylcholine	choline, acetate	choline acetyl-transferase	acetylcholinesterase	nicotinic; muscarinic M₁, M₂, M₃	Carbamoylcholine; nicotine (nicotinic); muscarine (muscarinic) oxotremorine (muscarinic)	α-bungarotoxin (nicotinic); tubocurarine (nicotinic); atropine (muscarinic); pirenzepine (M₁); scopolamine (muscarinic)
Dopamine	tyrosine	tyrosine hydroxylase; aromatic L-amino acid decarboxylase	uptake; monoamine oxidase; catechol O-methyltransferase; aldehyde dehydro-genase	D₁; D₂	apomorphine, 6,7-dihydroxy amino tetralin (ADTN)	SCH23390 (D₁); domperidone (D₂); sulpiride (D₂) (see also Table 5.4)
Excitatory amino acids (glutamate, aspartate)	glutamine; 2-oxoglutarate	glutaminase; aspartic acid and ornithine amino transferases	uptake; glutamine synthetase (glial); oxidation (neuronal)	NMDA;AMPA; KA; L-AP4; ACPD	NMDA (NMDA); AMPA, quisqualate (AMPA); KA (KA); L-AP4 (L-AP4); quisqualate, ACPD (ACPD)	MK801 (NMDA); CPP (NMDA); CNQX (AMPA and KA)
GABA	glutamate	glutamic acid decarboxylase	uptake; GABA aminotransferase; succinic acid semialdehyde dehydrogenase	GABA_A; GABA_B	muscimol (GABA_A); baclofen (GABA_B); benzo-diazepines (modulate GABA_A)	bicuculline (GABA_A)
Glycine	serine	serine hydroxy methyltransferase	uptake	glycine	glycine	strychnine

	Precursor	Synthesis enzymes	Degradation/uptake enzymes	Receptor subtypes	Agonists	Antagonists
Histamine	histidine	histidine decarboxylase	histamine methyl transferase, monoamine oxidase, aldehyde dehydrogenase	H_1; H_2; H_3	2-methyl histamine (H_1); 4-methyl histamine (H_2); dimaprit (H_2); N-methylhistamine (H_3)	mepyramine (H_1); cimetidine (H_2); ranitidine (H_2); thioperamide (H_3)
5-Hydroxytryptamine	tryptophan	tryptophan-5-hydroxylase; aromatic L-amino acid decarboxylase	uptake; monoamine oxidase; aldehyde dehydrogenase	5-HT_1 sub-types A–D; 5-HT_2; 5-HT_3	8OH-DPAT and spiroxatrine (5-HT_{1A}); RU24969 (5-HT_{1B}); LSD (5-HT_{1C} and 5-HT_2)	spiperone (5-HT_{1A} and 5-HT_2); cyanopindolol (5-HT_{1B}); ketanserin, mianserin, and mesulergine (5-HT_{1C} and 5-HT_2); ondansetron(5-HT_3)
Noradrenaline/ Adrenaline	tyrosine	tyrosine hydroxylase; aromatic L-amino acid decarboxylase; dopamine β-hydroxylase (noradrenaline-N-methyl transferase)	uptake; monoamine oxidase; catechol O-methyl transferase; aldehyde dehydrogenase	α_1; α_2; β_1; β_2	isoprenaline (β); methoxamine (α_1); clonidine (α_2)	prazosin (α_1); idazoxan (α_2); propranolol (β)
Enkephalins/ endorphin, dynorphin	—	enzymes of protein synthesis	neuropeptidases	κ; μ; δ; σ	enkephalins (δ); β-endorphin (μ, δ); dynorphin (κ); morphine (μ)	naloxone (μ)

Details are given of the key components of certain well defined neurotransmitter systems. The information is by no means exhaustive, particularly with respect to the number of agonists and antagonists cited and subtypes of receptors. The agonists shown are where possible selective for the receptor subtype indicated, otherwise it can be assumed that they are not selective. For each receptor subclass the natural agonist can be assumed to be active. Mechanistic details of the different receptors are found in Table 6.1.

Abbreviations: ACPD, 1-aminocyclopentyl-1,3-dicarboxylate; AMPA, α-amino-3-hydroxy-5-methyl-isoxazole-4-propionate; CNQX, 6-cyano-7-nitro-quinoxaline-2,3-dione; CPP, 3,3(2-carboxypiperazin-4-yl)propyl-l-phosphate; KA, kainic acid (kainate); LAP4, L-2-amino-4-phosphonobutyrate; LSD, lysergic acid diethylamide; MK801, dibenzocycloheptenimine; NMDA, N-methyl-D-aspartic acid; 8OH-DPAT, 8-hydroxy-2-(dipropyl)aminotetralin; RU24969, 5-methoxy-3-(1236-tetrahydro-4-pyridinyl)-1H-indole; SCH23390, 7-chloro-2,3,4,5-tetrahydro-3-methyl-5-phenyl-1H-3-benzazepine-7-ol.

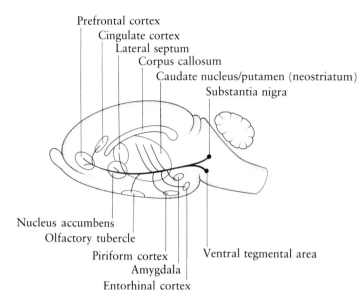

Prefrontal cortex
Cingulate cortex
Lateral septum
Corpus callosum
Caudate nucleus/putamen (neostriatum)
Substantia nigra

Nucleus accumbens
Olfactory tubercle
Piriform cortex   Ventral tegmental area
Amygdala
Entorhinal cortex

Figure 5.2 Dopamine neuronal pathways in rat brain. The principal long dopamine neuronal pathways in rat brain are shown. Several of the shorter neuronal pathways are omitted for clarity but for further details consult the reviews by Moore and Bloom (1978), Lindvall and Bjorklund (1982) and Cooper *et al.* (1986).

collectively constituting a major meso-telencephalic dopamine system. The principal pathways are:

(1) neurones with cell bodies in the substantia nigra (pars compacta) and to a limited extent the ventral tegmental area and nerve terminals in the caudate nucleus, putamen, and globus pallidus;

(2) neurones with cell bodies in the ventral tegmental area and nerve terminals in the nucleus accumbens;

(3) neurones with cell bodies in the substantia nigra and ventral tegmental area with nerve terminals in the olfactory tubercle, septum, interstitial nucleus of the stria terminalis, amygdala, piriform cortex, entorhinal cortex, and several regions of the frontal lobe.

A variety of names have been used for the different divisions of this dopamine system so a newcomer to the literature may be confused. In early studies two groupings were defined and termed the nigrostriatal system (those neurones linking the substantia nigra and caudate nucleus/putamen (neostriatum)) and mesolimbic system (those neurones linking the ventral tegmental area to limbic regions, e.g. nucleus accumbens, olfactory tubercle, and amygdala). More recently, with the discovery of additional areas of nerve terminals, two different groupings were defined termed the mesostriatal system (comprising groups (1) and (2) above, the nucleus accumbens can be considered as a ventral extension of the striatum (Chapter 2)) and the mesocortical system (group (3) above). This latter terminology will be used in subsequent discussions.

The precise description used is not important as it seems that within each cell group there is a fairly precise topographical organization. Thus cell bodies in, for example, a discrete part of the substantia nigra project to a discrete terminal field and the whole system can be viewed as being a large group of related but topographically distinct neurones.

This topography is further emphasized by the recent description of compartments within the neostriatum (caudate nucleus/putamen) termed the striosomes and the extra-striosomal matrix (Fig. 5.3). These are histochemically distinct regions of the striatum that are known to be neurochemically distinct and to receive distinct projections from subgroups of mesostriatal dopamine neurones (Gerfen 1984; Jimenez Castellanos and Graybiel 1987; Graybiel 1990). Therefore the innervation of the striatum is highly organized and this must reflect its function. This will be considered again later (Chapter 7).

The synaptic interactions of the mesostriatal cells in the striatum have been examined extensively. Earlier work showed that the pathway branched widely in the striatum with numerous varicosities (swellings) containing vesicles as well as some conventional nerve terminals. Little synaptic specialization was observed, suggesting a diffuse innervation and release of neurotransmitter, but more recent studies (Freund *et al.* 1984) have shown clear synapses of mesostriatal nerve terminals on to striatal neurones characterized by

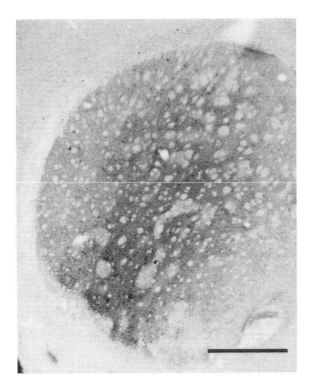

Figure 5.3 Compartmentalization of the striatum into striosomes and extra-striosomal matrix. The figure shows a section through rat striatum and the scale bar is 1 mm. The striosomes are the lighter areas embedded in the darker extrastriosomal matrix. Taken from Lapper and Bolam (1991) with permission.

their medium size and spiny dendrites. These synapses are of the symmetrical (Type II, inhibitory) type and about half are on to dendritic spines and half on to dendritic shafts and cell bodies of the striatal medium size spiny neurones. Thus the dopamine innervation may be influencing the ability of these cells to be excited by other inputs both generally (shafts and cell bodies) and more specifically (spines). This will be examined in more detail in Chapter 7.

Much of the above information has been obtained on rat brain or the brains of other common laboratory animals but is presumed to be directly applicable to human brain. There may, however, be differences in detail between these different species related to the evolution of higher functions in man (see for example Berger *et al.* 1991; Foote and Morrison 1987). Although dopamine neuronal systems exemplify many of the general principles of neuronal organization, there are some additional ones and it is useful to outline the different kinds of neurone that are seen more generally in the brain. These fall into four categories:

(1) long ascending/descending pathways with cell bodies in discrete well identified brain nuclei, e.g. acetylcholine-, dopamine-, 5-hydroxytryptamine-, and noradrenaline-containing neurones;
(2) pathways as in (1) but with cell bodies widely distributed, e.g. amino acid (GABA, glutamate)-containing neurones;
(3) intra-regional pathways (interneurones), e.g. intracortical somatostatin neurones;
(4) neurosecretory pathways, e.g. tuberohypophysial dopamine neurones (see above).

In the next section the different aspects of chemical transmission will be considered, based on the list given in Table 5.2.

Synthesis and storage of the neurotransmitter

The catecholamine, dopamine, is synthesized within dopamine neurones in a series of steps (Fig. 5.4) starting from the amino acid tyrosine which is taken up from the blood stream across the blood–brain barrier by a carrier mediated process. The first step in the pathway, the conversion of tyrosine to 3,4-dihydroxyphenylalanine (L-DOPA) is carried out by the enzyme tyrosine hydroxylase, which is the rate-limiting enzyme for catecholamine synthesis. The enzyme is specific and stereospecific, oxidizing efficiently only L-tyrosine and requires molecular oxygen, Fe^{2+}, and as a cofactor, tetrahydropteridine. The enzyme is found in the cytosol of dopamine neurones in the cell body and nerve terminals although some of the enzyme may also be bound to membranes. It is also the rate-determining step in noradrenaline and adrenaline biosynthesis in neurones containing those substances.

As it is a rate-determining enzyme, its regulation is important and alteration of the rate

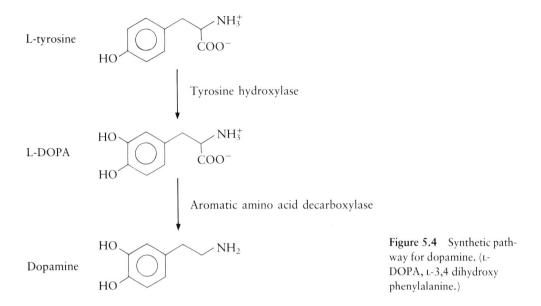

L-tyrosine

Tyrosine hydroxylase

L-DOPA

Aromatic amino acid decarboxylase

Dopamine

Figure 5.4 Synthetic pathway for dopamine. (L-DOPA, L-3,4 dihydroxy phenylalanine.)

of tyrosine hydroxylation changes levels of the catecholamine products of the pathways. Acute regulation of the enzyme is achieved by feedback inhibition of the enzyme by the catecholamine products, e.g. dopamine. Hence depletion of dopamine by release will lead to increased tyrosine hydroxylation whereas a build up of dopamine (due to a reduction in release or suppression of metabolism, for example by administration of a monamine oxidase inhibitor) will suppress hydroxylation. It is also possible to inhibit tyrosine hydroxylase activity by pharmacological intervention and hence alter catecholamine levels. For example amino acid analogues such as α-methyl-p-tyrosine are competitive inhibitors of tyrosine hydroxylation suppressing catecholamine synthesis.

Acute regulation of tyrosine hydroxylase *in vivo* also seems to be achieved by phosphorylation of the enzyme leading to enzyme activation. This phosphorylation may be important for the observed activation of the enzyme following electrical stimulation (depolarization) of catecholamine neurones which could be a means of increasing catecholamine synthesis in neurones actively releasing dopamine in addition to reduced feedback inhibition by dopamine. Phosphorylation could be triggered by increased levels of Ca^{2+} following depolarization, the Ca^{2+} acting via a calmodulin-dependent protein kinase (Zigmond *et al*. 1989). Chronic regulation of the enzyme with long term changes in synthesis of enzyme molecules also occurs following prolonged increases in the activity of catecholamine neurones. As will be shown later in the final section of this chapter, tyrosine hydroxylase activity can also be affected by released dopamine via presynaptic dopamine receptors. Thus regulation of tyrosine hydroxylase is exceedingly complex but seems to be designed to maintain a constant functional level of dopamine.

The concentrations of tyrosine available are such that tyrosine hydroxylase is generally saturated with its substrate (tyrosine). This means that changes in plasma tyrosine levels do not usually affect catecholamine synthesis. In other neurotransmitter systems this pattern may not obtain. For example, the rate-limiting enzyme for 5-hydroxytryptamine synthesis, tryptophan hydroxylase, is not generally saturated with its substrate (tryptophan). Therefore changes in plasma tryptophan levels will affect the rate of 5-hydroxytryptamine synthesis. This property of the 5-hydroxytryptamine neuronal systems has been exploited in the treatment of depression (Chapter 14).

The second step in the pathway to dopamine is the decarboxylation of L-DOPA to dopamine by the enzyme DOPA decarboxylase. The enzyme is found in the cytosol in cell bodies and nerve terminals and requires pyridoxal phosphate (derived from vitamin B_6) as a cofactor. This enzyme not only acts on L-DOPA, but will also decarboxyate other naturally occurring aromatic L-amino acids, including histidine, phenylalanine, tyrosine, tryptophan, and 5-hydroxytryptophan. Therefore this enzyme should rather be termed 'aromatic L-amino acid decarboxylase'. A decarboxylation also occurs in the biosynthetic pathway for 5-hydroxytryptamine (decarboxylating 5-hydroxytryptophan) but this is due to a slightly different enzyme from the one found in catecholamine neuronal systems. Nevertheless, the broad specificity of the enzymes means that after administration of 5-hydroxytryptophan, 5-hydroxytryptamine can arise in dopamine nerve terminals as well as 5-hydroxytryptamine terminals; this can complicate the interpretation of experiments.

Dopamine is synthesized in dopamine neurones by these two enzymic steps, i.e. tyrosine hydroxylase and aromatic L-amino acid decarboxylase, whereas in neurones using noradrenaline or adrenaline as neurotransmitter, additional enzymes are present to convert dopamine into the other catecholamines.

The dopamine synthesized by this route is then stored in membrane bounded vesicles (see Fig. 3.6 and 5.6) which are thought to be assembled in the cell body and transported down the axon to the nerve terminal where they are found in large numbers. Dopamine synthesis can also occur at the terminal to replenish vesicle contents and in fact the major proportion of dopamine synthesis in a dopamine neurone occurs at the terminal. Where there are also varicosities these have large numbers of vesicles containing dopamine.

The properties of these vesicles in central neurones have not been extensively studied but considerable knowledge on vesicle structure has come from related peripheral sympathetic systems. For example in the vas deferens, noradrenaline-containing nerves contain large (100 nm) and small (50 nm) vesicles, frequently with a densely staining core which is thought to be the catecholamine. Both the small and large vesicles seem to be active in neurotransmitter release and the small population contains ATP in addition to the catecholamine. The larger vesicles also contain proteins, some of which are called chromogranins. Dense cored vesicles of different sizes have been described in dopamine neurones and it is assumed that their properties are similar. The origin and function of these two classes of vesicle is considered below.

The vesicles possess a specific, ATP-dependent uptake mechanism in their membrane which enables them to take up and concentrate catecholamine from the cytosol. Thus dopamine synthesized in the cytosol either in the cell body or nerve terminal can be taken up but, because the storage vesicles are concentrated at the nerve terminal, dopamine is found predominantly in the nerve terminal region. The alkaloid reserpine is a useful pharmacological agent that prevents storage of catecholamines in vesicles. Therefore newly synthesized catecholamines are metabolized and not released so that there is an irreversible depletion of the neurotransmitter stores. The stimulant amphetamine causes release of catecholamine by a Ca^{2+} independent effect on the vesicle membrane which may involve effects on pH gradients (Sulzer and Rayport 1990).

In cholinergic neurones small vesicles are seen containing the neurotransmitter acetylcholine and lacking the dense core. At the neuromuscular junction and in the brain these are about 50 nm in diameter whereas in *Torpedo* electric organ, vesicles of 90 nm diameter have been described which contain acetylcholine, ATP, and protein. Vesicles containing neuropeptides are mostly of the large (100 nm) variety and show dense cores; they may also contain a second coexisting neurotransmitter (see below).

The general pattern outlined for dopamine holds for most of the small molecule neurotransmitters, i.e. a precursor often taken up from the bloodstream is converted by biosynthetic enzymes into the neurotransmitter. It is presumed although not always proven that vesicular storage then takes place and the vesicles containing the neurotransmitter arrive at the nerve terminal by axonal transport. Table 5.3 lists the precursors and biosynthetic enzymes for some key neurotransmitters.

A slightly different synthetic route is used for the neuropeptides; this can be exemplified by considering the pentapeptide neurotransmitters Leu-enkephalin and Met-enkephalin. In this case a large (263–267 amino acid) precursor (pro-enkephalin A) is synthesized on ribosomes. It contains six Met-enkephalin sequences and one Leu-enkephalin sequence. These are then released by proteolytic cleavage to process the precursor to the mature neuropeptides (Fig. 5.5). Similar principles hold for other neuropeptides, that is their synthesis takes place as part of a much larger polypeptide precursor and proteolytic cleavage follows to release the active species.

As the protein synthetic machinery of the cell is used for synthesis of neuropeptides, this must occur on ribosomes in the neuronal cell body. The precursor neuropeptide is then packaged into vesicles via the Golgi complex and transported to the nerve terminal by axonal transport. Cleavage to release the mature neuropeptide can occur during axonal transport. This is a clear distinction from the more classical neurotransmitters which can be synthesized in the nerve terminal. Therefore whereas for a neurotransmitter such as a catecholamine, depletion via release can be countered by local synthesis in the nerve terminal, for a neuropeptide, replenishment depends on synthesis in the cell body in the form of a large polypeptide precursor and the relatively slow process of axonal transport.

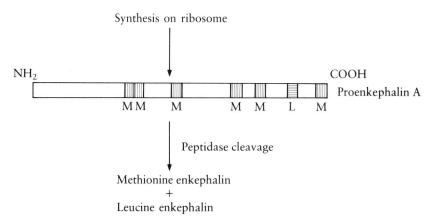

Figure 5.5 Synthetic pathway for a neuropeptide. The synthetic pathway for the enkephalins is shown from the precursor pro-enkephalin A which contains six Met-enkephalin (M) sequences and one Leu-enkephalin (L) sequence. Pairs of basic amino acids which form consensus cleavage sites for proteolytic processing are found on each side of the enkephalin sequences and are indicated by heavy lines.

Coexistence of more than one neurotransmitter

For many years it had been assumed that a particular neurone contained only one neuro-transmitter which defined that class of neurone and that neurotransmitter was present at all synapses formed by that neurone. This idea is often referred to as Dale's principle after the British pharmacologist Henry Dale who first suggested the idea in 1935. With the discovery of neuropeptides it has become increasingly clear that the principle needs to be modified. There are now many examples of neurones which contain a small molecule neurotransmitter and a neuropeptide or an adenine nucleotide both of which have synaptic effects. This phenomenon has been called coexistence and may be widespread. For example, a population of the mesostriatal and mesocortical dopamine cells has been shown to contain, in addition to the neurotransmitter dopamine, the neuropeptide cholecystokinin. It is, however, only a proportion of the total population of dopamine cells that contains cholecystokinin, suggesting some subdivision of function. There are many examples of this coexistence of neurotransmitters and neuropeptides and the significance of the phenomenon in the brain is far from clear. It does seem, however, that Dale's principle must be modified so that a particular neurone can still be chemically homogeneous at each of its nerve terminals but may contain more than one releasable active substance.

There are currently many unanswered questions relating to the phenomenon of co-existence. For example, it is known that in some cases the coexisting substances are stored in the same large (100 nm) vesicles and released together whereas in other cases the coexisting substances are stored in separate vesicles and so could be released differentially. What would be the functional consequences of coexistence and release of more than one substance? This must provide for a considerable increase in the complexity of the signalling patterns at a synapse, particularly if one substance acts more slowly than the others. Thus the slower acting substance could modify the release by acting pre-synaptically or amplify or reduce the effect of the faster acting substance by acting post-synaptically. This takes us back to the discussion earlier about distinctions between neurotransmitters and neuromodulators which becomes considerably more blurred if this kind of arrangement exists. The plethora of possibilities offered by coexistence is considered in more detail in the reviews by Lundberg and Hokfelt (1983) and Jones and Hendry (1986) and although the phenomenon increases the complexity of synaptic transmission it also may provide for many new sites of drug action for drug companies to investigate.

Neurotransmitter release

The conventional view of neurotransmitter release is that Ca^{2+} influx triggered by the arrival of the action potential at the nerve terminal and opening of voltage-sensitive Ca^{2+} channels leads to release of neurotransmitter by exocytosis of the synaptic vesicles (Fig. 5.6). Such a scheme is difficult to verify in detail for neurones in the brain, although some information is now becoming available. Most of our knowledge on this, however, comes from more accessible model systems such as acetylcholine release from cholinergic neurones at the frog neuromuscular junction and *Torpedo* electric organ, or noradrenaline release from chromaffin granules in the adrenal medulla, or from vesicles in the vas deferens (for reviews see the recommended reading at the end of the chapter).

In many cases specialized sites of neurotransmitter release have been recognized in the central nervous system that have been termed active zones (Smith and Augustine 1988). These are regions of the presynaptic membrane about 500 nm across which have dense projections forming a synaptic grid with associated cytoskeletal filaments (see the discussion of synapses in Chapter 3). Synaptic vesicles are located close to the active zone which is often in register with a specialized postsynaptic region with a concentration of postsynaptic receptors (postsynaptic density). Extracellular material is also found between the two specialized regions. Active zones of this form are now well defined in the central nervous system. They seem to be found particularly where rapid synaptic function is required and so are seen at synapses dependent on fast neurotransmitters and receptors, e.g. acetylcholine, GABA, glutamate/aspartate, and glycine, although they have also been described for slow neurotransmitters, e.g. 5-hydroxytryptamine, dopamine, and neuropeptides. Active zones of a slightly different structure have also been described at the neuromuscular junction (Heuser *et al.* 1979). It is thought that the trigger for neurotransmitter release is influx of Ca^{2+} through voltage-sensitive Ca^{2+} channels also located in the active zone at the presynaptic membrane. This leads to exocytosis via

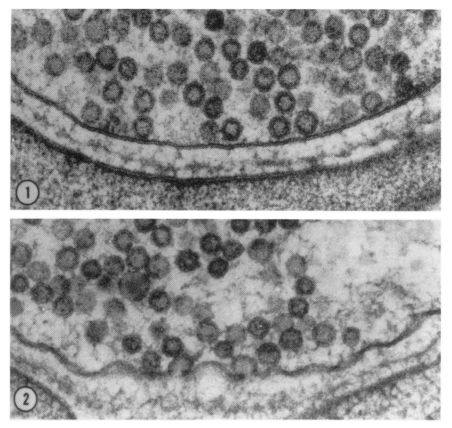

Figure 5.6 Exocytosis for release of neurotransmitter at the synapse. The figure shows: (1) a section through an active zone at the frog neuromuscular junction at rest showing synaptic vesicles and (2) a section through the same tissue that has received a 5.2 millisecond stimulation to release neurotransmitter. In the stimulated tissue many pockets are visible in the presynaptic membrane. These are likely to be due to vesicles that have released their contents after fusing with the presynaptic membrane. Taken from Heuser and Reese (1981) with permission.

fusion of the synaptic vesicle with the presynaptic membrane. The contents of the synaptic vesicle are then emptied into the synaptic cleft.

The concept of vesicular release was originally developed to account for the observed pattern of acetylcholine release at the neuromuscular junction. This seemed to occur in packets or quanta and it was suggested that one quantum of acetylcholine corresponded to the contents of one vesicle (estimated as several thousand molecules for acetylcholine or glutamic acid (Riveros *et al*. 1986) and about a thousand for noradrenaline). Vesicular release is also consistent with the release of other messenger molecules such as hormones, e.g. insulin, which occurs by exocytosis. Thus neurones can be considered as specialized secretory cells. The speed of the exocytosis process is, however, rather low and this has prompted the suggestion of other hypotheses including vesicular release without actual exocytosis and non-vesicular release from a cytoplasmic pool (see for example Almers and Tse 1990). Nevertheless, electron microscopy has shown vesicles fusing with the presynaptic membrane in peripheral nervous tissues, and very rapid exocytosis of vesicles (5 ms after stimulation) has been demonstrated at the frog neuromuscular junction (Fig. 5.6). The speed of the process may in part reflect vesicles being ready in the correct position to fuse close to the active zone, perhaps attached in some way to the presynaptic specialized structures. It may also reflect the presence of calcium channels at the active zones so that the Ca^{2+} signal is delivered directly to the waiting vesicles. The precise mode of action of the Ca^{2+} ions in triggering release is at present unknown and a variety of Ca^{2+} sensors have been considered (Augustine *et al.* 1987) but no firm conclusion has been reached. One protein whose phosphorylation state is increased by the increased level of Ca^{2+} ions is synapsin I (via a calmodulin-sensitive protein kinase). It is thought that synapsin I normally holds vesicles in a depot pre-release state by attaching them to the cytoskeleton in the presynaptic terminal, thus preventing their participation in the release process (Fig. 5.7). Phosphorylation disrupts the interaction with the cytoskeleton allowing vesicles to move to a second releasable pool nearer the active zone where they are thought to be either free or held by cross-linkage to the

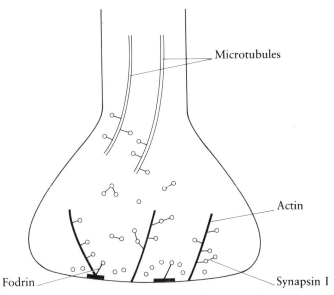

Figure 5.7   Role of the cytoskeleton in neurotransmitter release. Synaptic vesicles are shown attached to microtubules and actin filaments and to one another via synapsin I cross-bridges. Thinner strands (fodrin?) link synaptic vesicles to the presynaptic membrane. Ca^{2+} influx upon nerve terminal depolarization leads to phosphorylation of synapsin by Ca^{2+}/calmodulin dependent protein kinase and this detaches synaptic vesicles from actin ready for release at the next discharge of the terminal. The vesicles ready for release are either free or linked to fodrin but close to the presynaptic membrane.

protein fodrin but ready for release (Hirokawa *et al.* 1989). Thus synapsin I phosphorylation is not the trigger for release; rather, as stated earlier, the trigger is some as yet unknown Ca^{2+} dependent process which must act on the releasable vesicle pool held in position close to the active zone.

A further problem with exocytosis concerns the potential expansion of the postsynaptic membrane following vesicle-membrane fusion. This seems to be counteracted by endocytosis of vesicles to retrieve membrane (Boarder 1989; de Camilli and Jahn 1990) (Fig. 5.8). Those vesicles undergoing endocytosis are first seen as vesicles surrounded by a fuzzy coat of a protein called clathrin (coated vesicles) which later become smooth vesicles. These smooth vesicles can either be reused as synaptic vesicles after refilling or recycled to the cell body via axonal transport in multivesicular bodies for degradation. Refilling is only possible for classical neurotransmitters whose biosynthetic enzymes are available in the nerve terminal. For peptide neurotransmitters, refilling requires recycling to the cell body which is the only site of synthesis of the neuropeptides via their precursors.

These ideas can now be brought together to explain the functions and origins of the different kinds of vesicles observed in nerve terminals (Boarder 1989; de Camilli and Jahn 1990). Vesicles arrive at the nerve terminal via axonal transport; these are of the large (100 nm) dense core variety. They will contain some amine neurotransmitters but can take up more from synthesis at the terminal. They may also contain a neuropeptide precursor synthesized in the cell body and are active in the release of peptide and amine when they arrive at the terminal. At the nerve terminal there is endocytosis of vesicular

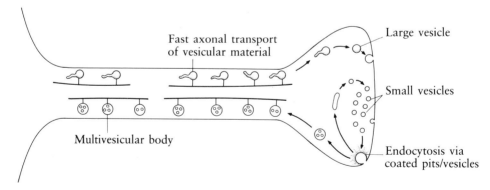

Figure 5.8 Events involved in exocytosis and endocytosis of vesicles at the nerve terminal. The diagram shows vesicles arriving by fast axonal transport at the nerve terminal. These will be large (100 nm) and may contain neuropeptide and amine neurotransmitter. They can take up more amine from the cytosol and are active in release by exocytosis. Recycling of vesicular material occurs by endocytosis of coated vesicles. These lose their fuzzy coat and are either recycled to the cell body via fast axonal transport of multivesicular bodies or provide small vesicles (50 nm) which take up amine neurotransmitter for further release (see also Fig. 3.5).

material and after loss of the clathrin coat some of these vesicles are seen as small clear vesicles (50 nm); these are able to take up amine neurotransmitter synthesized in the cytosol giving them a dense core. These smaller vesicles are also active in amine neurotransmitter release. The small vesicles do not contain neuropeptide as this is made in the cell body. This is shown in the form of a diagram in Fig. 5.8.

Although there is some information emerging on the details of neurotransmitter release from brain neurones, much is still argued by analogy with the more accessible model systems. It will continue to be difficult to obtain detailed information on release from brain neurones and indirect methods will continue to be useful. For example, much indirect evidence for neurotransmitter release comes from the use of brain slice preparations or synaptosomes (pinched off nerve terminals). These can be shown to release neurotransmitters, e.g. dopamine, upon depolarization; the process is Ca^{2+} dependent.

Somewhat more direct information can be obtained by sampling dopamine and its metabolites near the site of release using a push–pull cannula where fluid is pulsed into the brain down a cannula and out again to remove released substances. Other techniques used are *in vivo* voltammetry with electrodes for electrochemical detection of released dopamine inserted into the appropriate brain region or intracerebral microdialysis using a cannula containing a microdialysis probe. These methods may be used to detect release of dopamine and metabolites *in vivo* (O'Neill and Fillenz 1985; Beneviste 1989; Stamford 1989).

None of these approaches provides any detailed knowledge about the release processes, for example, they do not show actual synaptic release, rather they measure neurotransmitter overflow, but at present they are the best available approaches. Despite these reservations no observations have been made that conflict with the general scheme outlined above of a Ca^{2+} dependent vesicular release process for most neurotransmitters.

Interaction of neurotransmitter with postsynaptic receptor

The neurotransmitter dopamine diffuses, after it is released, to its specific receptors which are integral membrane proteins located in the postsynaptic membrane. The structures and mechanisms of such receptors will be dealt with in much more detail in Chapter 6. The postsynaptic receptors upon binding dopamine cause a change in the postsynaptic cell which leads to alterations in the membrane excitability. In the case of dopamine these changes are slow and involve the interaction of several protein species, leading to alterations of second messenger systems or slow ion channels. For other receptors, as outlined in Chapter 4, rapid alterations of ion channel activity follow receptor activation. Again these distinctions will be developed in more detail in Chapter 6.

For most neurotransmitters it is now clear that there is more than one species of receptor specific for the particular neurotransmitter. These are usually distinct bio-chemically, have different pharmacological specificities, and are associated with different functions. This is exemplified by the receptors for dopamine where D_1 and D_2 receptors have been described whose properties are outlined in Table 5.4. Although the immediate biochemical effects of receptor activation by dopamine are reasonably well understood for each receptor, how these lead to changes in cell excitability is less well understood. This will be considered in more detail in Chapter 6.

Table 5.4 Dopamine receptor subtypes

Subtype	Agonists		Antagonists	
	Selective	Non-selective	Selective	Non-selective
D_1	SKF38393		SCH23390	
		apomorphine		(+)-butaclamol;
		dopamine		flupenthixol
D_2	quinpirole		domperidone;	
	N-0437		haloperidol;	
			sulpiride	

The application of gene cloning techniques has identified multiple D_1-like and D_2-like receptors (reviewed in Strange 1990, 1991*a*). Although these multiple forms do differ pharmacologically, the selectivity of existing compounds does not at present justify a subclassification beyond that given in this table for functional purposes.

Abbreviations: N-0437, 2-[N-*n*-propyl-*N*-2-(2-thenyl)ethylamino]5-hydroxytetralin; SCH23390, 7-chloro-2,3,4,5-tetrahydro-3-methyl-5-phenyl-1*H*-3-benzazepine-7-o1; SKF38393, 2,3,4,5-tetrahydro-7,8-dihydroxy-l-phenyl-1*H*-3-benzazepine.

The efficiency of synaptic transmission must depend in part on the localization of the postsynaptic receptors. This has been well described for the neuromuscular junction where the postsynaptic acetylcholine receptors are located exactly opposite the active release sites for the neurotransmitter at the active zones (Fig. 5.9). This arrangement is likely to be optimal for rapid efficient detection of released neurotransmitter.

In the brain, information on the arrangement of postsynaptic receptors is much less clear but it seems that at many synapses in the brain, active zones are seen; it is therefore likely that there will be a preferential localization of receptors in the postsynaptic density of the active zone. This has been demonstrated for receptors for the neurotransmitter GABA (Wu and Siekewitz 1988). This in turn implies some kind of interaction between the receptor and the protein elements of the postsynaptic membrane or associated cytoskeleton.

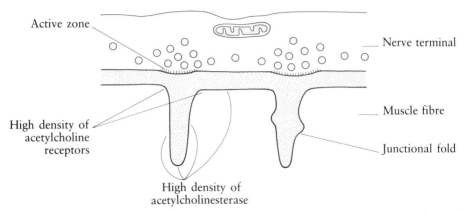

Figure 5.9   The location of receptors for the neurotransmitter acetylcholine at the neuromuscular junction. The diagram shows a vertical section through the neuromuscular junction with the junctional folds, active zones, and clusters of synaptic vesicles containing acetylcholine. Nicotinic acetylcholine receptors are found on the crests of the folds opposite the active zone release sites for acetylcholine. The degradative enzyme for acetylcholine, acetylcholinesterase, is found on the other parts of the postsynaptic membrane, including the troughs of the junctional folds. For further details see Fertuck and Saltpeter (1976) and Heuser and Reese (1981).

Exogenous application of the neurotransmitter mimics the normal action of released neurotransmitter on the postsynaptic membrane

For a number of reasons, some of which will be outlined below, it is frequently very difficult in the brain to mimic the postsynaptic action of neurotransmitter released upon stimulation of the presynaptic neurone by exogenous application of the neurotransmitter. This has, however, been very effectively carried out at the neuromuscular junction. At the neuromuscular junction acetylcholine is the neurotransmitter and in the absence of presynaptic neuronal stimulation, spontaneous small depolarizations (about 1 mV) are observed in the postsynaptic membrane (muscle end plate). These are thought to be due to the random spontaneous release of acetylcholine, each depolarization corresponding to the contents of one vesicle (several thousand acetylcholine molecules). These 'miniature end plate potentials' as they are called could be mimicked precisely by the iontophoretic application of acetylcholine from a very fine pipette. A similar correspondence is seen between the depolarization in the end plate due to electrical stimulation of the presynaptic neurone and exogenous application of acetylcholine (in larger amounts than for the miniature end plate potential).

  In the brain, however, synapses are less clearly defined physically than those in the neuromuscular junction and the complexity of circuitry in the brain and the close apposition of different neurones makes it very difficult to define the cell body and corresponding nerve terminal and synapse for one particular neurone. Some measure of synaptic actions may, however, be obtained electrophysiologically. For example for dopamine this has been obtained by recording electrical activity in cells in the caudate nucleus and putamen (target areas of the mesostriatal neurones) in the awake monkey. Iontophoretic application of dopamine reduces the spontaneous firing rate of these cells by about 50 per cent and this must reflect the normal synaptic release of dopamine (Rolls *et al*. 1984).

Indirect measures of the synaptic actions of dopamine have, however, been developed and one area of considerable activity has been these same mesostriatal dopamine cells that link the substantia nigra and neostriatum (caudate nucleus/putamen). Two models have been developed for synaptic actions of dopamine in the striatum. In the first, rats are given a high dose of amphetamine (which releases dopamine from synaptic stores) or L-DOPA (which is converted to dopamine in the brain). The animals then perform 'stereotyped behaviour' consisting of continuous sniffing, licking, or biting. This is considered to be due to the action of dopamine on receptors in the striatum (Janssen and Van Beren, 1978) and this has been established from the blockade of the behaviour by a series of dopamine antagonists (see next section).

The second model consists of the injection of dopamine into the striatum on one side of the brain of a rat. The rats then perform a turning motion away from the injected side (Pycock 1980). This contralateral turning can also be elicited by electrical activation of the substantia nigra on one side of the brain which activates the mesostriatal dopamine neurones leading to dopamine release into the striatum; in either case the movement is thought to be due to activation of striatal dopamine receptors on one side of the brain leading to an imbalance in the motor output pathways (see Chapter 10). Again dopamine antagonists block the behaviour, providing evidence for the involvement of dopamine receptors.

In both models other compounds have been recognized that mimic the actions of dopamine and are thus considered to act as agonists at central dopamine receptors, e.g. apomorphine, and 6,7-dihydroxyaminotetralin (ADTN). Although both models are indirect indications of the synaptic actions of dopamine, they have been extremely valuable in the discovery of dopamine receptor directed drugs (see next section).

The data obtained using the more direct and less direct models have also been corroborated by the *in vitro* test systems for dopamine receptors such as ligand-binding assays and activation of second messenger systems. Discussion of these will be reserved until Chapter 6.

The action of the released neurotransmitter can be blocked by specific antagonists

The models for neurotransmitter action at the synapse described in the previous section can be used for testing different substances as antagonists to block the action of the released neurotransmitter. Existence of specific antagonists is further evidence for the action of the neurotransmitter at specific sites which are the receptors which have the nature of proteins with recognition capability. The models described above for testing neurotransmitter action at receptors on neurones in the brain have certain deficiencies. The testing of antagonists at these receptors poses similar difficulties, particularly with respect of demonstrating specific action at the synapse. Nevertheless, the use of a range of models based on electrophysiology, behavioural studies, and *in vitro* biochemical approaches has led to the recognition of substances with the specific ability to block or antagonize the actions of neurotransmitters at the receptors (Table 5.3). In the case of dopamine a large number of compounds of different chemical classes (Tables 5.3 and 5.4) are recognized as dopamine antagonists and, more recently, selective antagonists of the two dopamine receptor subclasses have been developed. Many of these compounds are useful drugs and are used for example to treat schizophrenia (Chapter 13).

Termination of the action of the released neurotransmitter

In order to provide a satisfactory, rapidly responding signalling system at synapses, it is necessary for the neurotransmitter to be released, have its action, and then cease its action. This is partly achieved by providing a means for removal of the neurotransmitter from the synapse. Broadly speaking there are two mechanisms for this based on uptake of the neurotransmitter from the synapse into surrounding cells or destruction of the neurotransmitter in the synapse (Fig. 5.10).

   For dopamine and the other catecholamines the released neurotransmitter is removed from the synapse by a high affinity (K_m 0.4 μM) active transport process. These processes are generally dependent on Na^+ ions and are present in the membrane of the nerve terminal releasing the neurotransmitter. There are also lower affinity uptake mechanisms in surrounding neuroglial cells that may be important for subsequent metabolism of the neurotransmitter. Selective inhibitors are available to block the uptake of particular substances. For example, dopamine uptake into nerve terminals is blocked by benztropine and nomifensine (although this also inhibits noradrenaline reuptake). Many antidepressant drugs (see Chapter 14) are potent and selective inhibitors of the reuptake process for either noradrenaline or 5-hydroxytryptamine or both of these substances. The uptake of the catecholamine neurotransmitters terminates their action at the receptor and once inside the nerve terminal it can either be stored again in synaptic

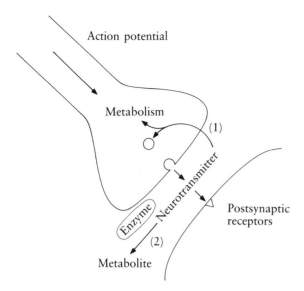

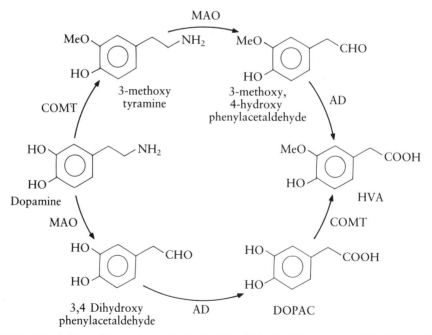

Figure 5.10 Termination of the action of a neurotransmitter. The diagram shows the principal means for the rapid termination of neurotransmitter action: (1) Active transport back in to the nerve terminal where the neurotransmitter may be either metabolized or repackaged into synaptic vesicles. The monoamine neurotransmitters e.g. noradrenaline, dopamine, and 5-hydroxytryptamine, are good examples. (2) Enzymic destruction by an enzyme present in the synaptic cleft. Good examples here are acetylcholine (acetylcholinesterase, see Fig. 5.9) and neuropeptides (neuropeptidases). The two processes are shown on one neurone for clarity but will not normally be present as such.

Figure 5.11 Metabolism of dopamine in the brain. AD, aldehyde dehydrogenase; COMT, catechol-O-methyl transferase; DOPAC, 3,4 dihydroxy phenylacetic acid; HVA, homovanillic acid; MAO, monoamine oxidase.

vesicles or metabolized. Some catecholamine does not get taken up and is metabolized in cells other than neurones.

Metabolism depends on three enzymes, monoamine oxidase, catechol-*O*-methyl transferase and aldehyde dehydrogenase whose catalytic actions are outlined in Fig. 5.11. Dopamine is metabolized principally to homovanillic acid (HVA) and dihydroxyphenylacetic acid (DOPAC) in the brain. The levels of these metabolites have been used as indices of the level of metabolic activity in the dopamine neurone population under study. The advantage of this is that it may be possible to obtain an indication of overall dopamine turnover in the brain from measurements of metabolites, e.g. homovanillic acid appearing in either cerebrospinal fluid or plasma. This in principle offers the possibility of obtaining an index of brain neuronal metabolism from measurements of body fluids (although see Chapter 9 for more consideration of the practical use of these techniques). For example, in Parkinson's disease, where there is a loss of the mesostriatal dopamine pathway (Chapter 10), homovanillic acid levels in cerebrospinal fluid are reduced. It should be realized, however, that measurements of neurotransmitter metabolism do not necessarily reflect the synaptic release of neurotransmitter. The rate of synthesis of a neurotransmitter can be altered without this necessarily affecting neurotransmitter release rates.

Monoamine oxidase is a membrane-bound enzyme found in the outer membrane of mitochondria in neurones and other cells. The neuronal enzyme is important for catecholamine metabolism so that it will act on free catecholamine that has been taken up after release and not restored in vesicles. The combined action of monoamine oxidase and aldehyde dehydrogenase, which is also found in the mitochondria, yields DOPAC which is an important metabolite of dopamine in the brain.

Monoamine oxidase is found in two forms, monoamine oxidases A and B, which are homologous but different proteins with different specificities and sensitivities to inhibitors. The properties of the two forms of the enzymes are given in Table 5.5 and both

Table 5.5 Different forms of monoamine oxidase

Monoamine oxidase form	Substrates		Inhibitors	
	Specific	Non-specific	Specific	Non-specific
A	5-hydroxytryptamine; noradrenaline		clorgyline	
		dopamine; tryptamine; tyramine;		iproniazid; nialamide; tranylcypromine
B	benzylamine; β-phenylethylamine		deprenyl	

oxidize dopamine. Both forms are present in human brain although the B form predominates. The relative importance and physiological significance of the two forms of the enzyme are not fully established but recent work (Westlund *et al*. 1988; Hsu *et al*. 1989) indicates a preferential localization of the A form in catecholamine neurones and the B form in 5-hydroxytryptamine neurones. Both forms are also found in other neurones and neuroglial cells. This may imply that in catecholamine and 5-hydroxytryptamine neurones, the enzymes are effecting some kind of protection of a neurone against uptake of the incorrect neurotransmitter. Since the specificities are not absolute this does not rule the enzymes out as primary metabolic sites as well.

Inhibitors of monoamine oxidase have been used as antidepressant drugs (see Chapter 14), underlining the importance of metabolism of catecholamines and indolamines for overall brain activity and function. Monoamine oxidase B in astrocytes is thought to be important for activation of the neurotoxin MPTP which has given a valuable model of Parkinson's disease (Chapter 10).

Catechol-O-methyl transferase is present in the cytoplasm of cells in many tissues including neurones and neuroglial cells in the brain, although it is considered that for metabolism of catecholamines this extraneuronal action is predominant. Therefore catechol-O-methyl transferase will act on DOPAC made available by neuronal metabolism to yield HVA and on dopamine taken up extraneuronally.

In summary, the action of dopamine is terminated by reuptake in to the nerve terminal where the catecholamine may be restored or metabolized. Dopamine that is not taken back into the nerve terminal is taken up extraneuronally and metabolized. A number of other neurotransmitters have their action terminated by reuptake, for example 5-hydroxytryptamine, GABA, and glutamate.

Whereas the metabolic pathway for degradation of catecholamines is rather slow and the removal of the substances from the synapse by uptake constitutes the rapid inactivation step, for other neurotransmitters there is a rapid metabolic inactivation within the synapse. For example, acetylcholine action is terminated by the esteratic cleavage of acetylcholine by acetylcholinesterase located on the extracellular basal lamina between the pre- and postsynaptic membranes at the neuromuscular junction. Neuropeptides are degraded by specific peptidase enzymes which are largely extracellular but membrane-bound proteins presumably located at the synapse (Kenny and Maroux 1982). Following degradation at least some of the products are retrieved, for example a high affinity choline transport system is found in the presynaptic membrane at cholinergic synapses to take back the choline product of acetylcholine hydrolysis.

Although removal of the neurotransmitter will terminate the stimulus to the postsynaptic receptors, there must also be mechanisms at the receptor level for terminating the intracellular responses. These will be outlined in Chapter 6.

Control of neurotransmitter release by presynaptic receptors

Many neurotransmitters, including dopamine, are known to exert effects at presynaptic receptors located on the nerve terminal. The principal effect of this interaction is to modulate release of neurotransmitter frequently in an inhibitory manner. This mechanism can be seen as a means whereby neurotransmitter release is regulated by a form of feedback inhibition by the released neurotransmitter itself and will maintain neurotransmitter release at a particular level. Therefore there is a self-regulation of release by a neurotransmitter at a nerve terminal releasing that neurotransmitter. The presynaptic receptors that allow this self-regulation of release have been termed autoreceptors (Fig. 5.12). Autoreceptors have been described for dopamine on the nerve terminals of mesostriatal dopamine neurones and these may be important in maintaining a tonic level of released dopamine.

An alternative situation has been frequently described where release of one neurotransmitter from an isolated nerve ending preparation is modulated (either positively or negatively) by another neurotransmitter (Fig. 5.12). It is presumed that this is due to interaction of one neurotransmitter with receptors on the nerve terminal releasing another neurotransmitter; this would then constitute presynaptic receptor modulation of release but not via autoreceptors. These presynaptic receptors are sometimes called heteroreceptors. This in turn requires that there be either an axo-axonic synapse responsible for the effect or diffusion of a released neurotransmitter some distance from

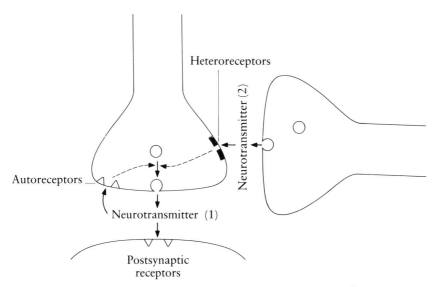

Figure 5.12 Presynaptic receptor control of neurotransmitter release. Control of neurotransmitter release is shown by the neurotransmitter itself acting at presynaptic receptors (autoreceptors) or via a second neurotransmitter acting at receptors that are presynaptic for the first neurone (heteroreceptors).

its release site to the presynaptic receptors. Neither of these mechanisms is well established at the cellular level in the brain. As an illustration of this second kind of presynaptic modulation, the release of acetylcholine from nerve endings in the striatum is inhibited by dopamine and this is thought to be via presynaptic receptors. The functional relevance of such presynaptic inhibition if it occurs at an axo-axonic synapse must be to enable an input from one part of the brain to influence activity (neuro-transmitter release) in another part. It should then be seen as part of the circuitry of the brain rather than a local modulatory effect as is the case of autoreceptor modulation.

The mechanism of action of presynaptic inhibition whether by autoreceptors or other-wise is not fully understood, but given that neurotransmitter release depends on Ca^{2+} ions, then effects of presynaptic receptors to reduce Ca^{2+} availability would provide a possible mechanism. One way this can be achieved is by presynaptic receptor inhibition of Ca^{2+} channels (Lipscombe *et al.* 1989). As indicated earlier, Ca^{2+} may induce release via stimulating phosphorylation of the synaptic vesicle protein synapsin and also by acting on a second, as yet undefined release trigger site. Both of these actions will be reduced by reductions in Ca^{2+}. It is also thought that presynaptic receptors may reduce the general excitability of the membrane via hyperpolarizing the membrane following modulation of K^+ channels (Miller 1990). This would also reduce neurotransmitter release by limiting the effects of the action potential arriving at the nerve terminal.

Overall the effects of presynaptic modulation will be initially to alter neurotransmitter release. In the case of catecholamine neurones, this will affect synthesis of the neuro-transmitter indirectly via feedback effects on tyrosine hydroxylase. In some dopamine neurones there also seems to be a direct effect of the dopamine autoreceptors on tyrosine hydroxylase activity, inhibition of enzyme activity occurring if the receptors are occu-pied. This adds a further layer of complexity to the modulation of neurotransmitter action at dopamine synapses. Thus the processes involved in dopamine synthesis and release from dopamine nerve terminals can be controlled acutely by four mechanisms: feedback control of tyrosine hydroxylase, phosphorylation of tyrosine hydroxylase upon nerve terminal depolarization, presynaptic receptor control of release, and presynaptic receptor control of tyrosine hydroxylase. This emphasizes the importance of tyrosine hydroxylase in the control of catecholamine synthesis and suggests that the control of the level of released dopamine has a great significance.

There is some evidence to suggest that presynaptic receptors for certain neuro-transmitters have different properties from their postsynaptic counterparts. Activation of dopamine autoreceptors is achieved at much lower concentrations of dopamine agonists than those required to activate postsynaptic dopamine receptors. Similar observations have been made for noradrenergic neurones although for these neurones a pharmaco-logically different adrenergic receptor may be present pre- and postsynaptically. In the case of the dopamine system, the presynaptic autoreceptor has the antagonist pharmaco-logical profile of a D_2 dopamine receptor but with an increased sensitivity to the agonist relative to a postsynaptic D_2 receptor. A simple explanation of this would be that at the presynaptic receptor fewer receptors need to be occupied to achieve a response than with the postsynaptic receptors but that the receptor protein involved is identical. Thus the presynaptic receptors would appear to be more sensitive to agonists than the postsynaptic ones. There is some experimental support for this suggestion (Meller *et al.* 1987) and mechanisms for these differences will be considered in Chapter 6.

Teleologically, the higher sensitivity of the autoreceptor might allow modulation of neurotransmitter release to occur despite some dilution of the neurotransmitter after diffusion away from its release site. The greater sensitivity of autoreceptors has been exploited in the administration of low doses of agonists to experimental animals in order to activate selectively the autoreceptors. This approach has also been considered for therapeutic intervention. For example, it has been suggested that dopamine neuronal activity in schizophrenia (Chapter 13) might be reduced by selective autoreceptor activation with a low dose of a dopamine agonist. Where there is a pharmacologically different receptor presynaptically then selective antagonist intervention might be feasible in order to increase neurotransmitter release; this idea has been considered in the treatment of Alzheimer's disease (Chapter 11) in order to increase acetylcholine release.

There are a number of problems with such approaches, one of which is knowing whether all neurones of a particular class have autoreceptors. If we consider the major classes of long dopamine neurones, i.e. the mesostriatal and mesocortical neurones, the mesostriatal neurones have autoreceptors at the nerve terminal that control dopamine release and synthesis and they also possess a second kind of autoreceptor on the cell body. This second kind of autoreceptor detects dopamine released from the dendrites when the cell fires and combination of dopamine with this autoreceptor reduces the cell firing rate. Whereas all mesocortical neurones have nerve terminal autoreceptors that regulate dopamine release, only those projecting to the piriform cortex also have cell body autoreceptors and nerve terminal autoreceptors that regulate dopamine synthesis (Wolf and Roth 1987). Mesocortical cells projecting to the cingulate and prefrontal cortices do not have cell body autoreceptors that control firing rate or nerve terminal autoreceptors that regulate dopamine synthesis. In consequence, these latter neurones show greater basal firing rates and also a lower responsiveness to exogenously administered dopamine agonists. This has considerable practical implications for the use of dopamine agonists and antagonists as drugs and I shall return to this point in the discussion of drugs for treating schizophrenia (Chapter 13).

I have concentrated so far on the effects of presynaptic receptors to inhibit neurotransmitter release. Stimulation of release has, however, been described after agonist occupancy of a presynaptic receptor although this does not refer to autoreceptors. For example, dopamine release in the striatum, presumably from nerve terminals of the mesostriatal dopamine neurones, is stimulated by acetylcholine acting via presynaptic receptors on the dopamine nerve terminals. This provides another means whereby one neuronal system can modulate another. In this case acetylcholine seems to stimulate dopamine release via the two classes of acetylcholine receptor, muscarinic and nicotinic, both presynaptically. The presence of both slow and fast acetylcholine receptors may provide flexibility in the time course of the control.

Synaptic sites of drug action—an overview

It should have become clear from the preceding discussion that there are many sites in the synapse where drugs can act to modify synaptic action and hence brain activity. Not only are there discrete sites within the synapse where drugs may be targeted but also different classes of synapse are defined by their neurotransmitter and this offers further selectivity in terms of chemical differences. As we shall see in later chapters, modulation of synaptic action and in particular modulation of chemically defined synapses is the principal way whereby therapeutic agents are derived for selective therapy in brain disease. This will be exemplified in more detail later but it is of use at this point to outline some of the key classes of drugs acting at synapses. This is done by means of a diagram (Fig. 5.13).

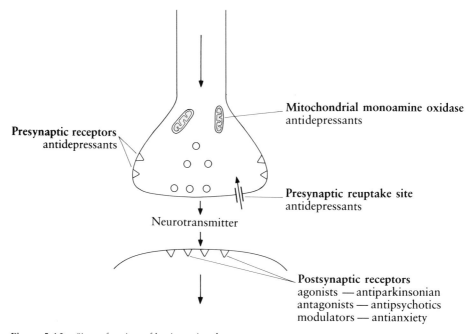

Figure 5.13   Sites of action of brain-active drugs.

Recommended reading

Boarder, M. R. (1989). Presynaptic aspects of cotransmission: relationship between vesicles and neuro-transmitters. *Journal of Neurochemistry*, **53**, 1–11.

Bradford, H. F. (1986). *Chemical neurobiology*. W. H. Freeman, New York.

Burgoyne, R. D. (1984). Mechanisms of secretion from adrenal chromaffin cells. *Biochemica et Biophysica Acta*, **779**, 201–16.

Carmichael, S. W. and Winkler, H. (1985). The adrenal chromafin cell. *Scientific American*, **253**(2), 30–9.

Chesselet, M. F. (1984). Presynaptic regulation of neurotransmitter release in the brain. *Neuroscience*, **12**, 347–75.

Cooper, J. R., Bloom, F. E., and Roth, R. H. (1986). *The biochemical basis of neuropharmacology*. Oxford University Press.

Guldberg, H. C. and Marsden, C. A. (1975). Catechol-*O*-methyltransferase: pharmacological aspects and physiological role. *Pharmacological Reviews*, **27**, 135–206.

Hokfelt, T., Johansson, O., Ljungdahl, A., Lundberg, J. M., and Schultzberg, M. (1980). Peptidergic neurones. *Nature*, **284**, 515–21.

Illes, P. (1986). Mechanisms of receptor mediated modulation of transmitter release in noradrenergic cholinergic and sensory neurones. *Neuroscience*, **17**, 909–28.

Iversen, L. L. (1974). Uptake mechanisms for neurotransmitter amines. *Biochemical Pharmacology*, **23**, 1927–35.

Klein, R. L. and Thureson-Klein, A. K. (1984). Noradrenergic vesicles: molecular organisation and function. *Handbook of Neurochemistry*, **7**, 71–109.

Kuffler, S. W., Nicholls, J. G., and Martin, A. R. (1984). *From neuron to brain*. (2nd edn.) Sinauer Associates Inc., Sunderland, MA.

McGeer, P. L., Eccles, J., and McGeer, E. G. (1987). *Molecular neurobiology of the mammalian brain*. Plenum Press, New York.

Molinoff, P. B. and Axelrod, J. (1971). Biochemistry of catecholamines. *Annual Review of Biochemistry*, **40**, 465–500.

Starke, K. (1981). Presynaptic receptors. *Annual Review of Pharmacology and Toxicology*, **21**, 7–30.

Walker, J. H. and Agoston, D. V. (1987). The synaptic vesicle and the cytoskeleton. *Biochemical Journal*, **247**, 249–58.

Whittaker, V. P. (1984). The structure and function of cholinergic synaptic vesicles. *Biochemical Society Transactions*, **12**, 561–5.

6   Receptors and receptor mechanisms

This chapter will concentrate on the structure, properties, and mechanisms of action of neurotransmitter receptors in the central nervous system. This emphasis on one component of the synapse reflects the importance of receptors as regulators of synaptic action, and as sites of drug action (Fig. 5.13) and the current detailed knowledge about receptors.

The idea of a receptor was first suggested in 1905 by Langley and for many years the term receptor implied an ill defined entity that conferred responsiveness to a particular substance on a tissue. Nowadays our view of receptors is much more sophisticated and at least in the case of neurotransmitter receptors we envisage the receptor as a protein containing a binding site for a neurotransmitter (at which specific antagonists may compete) and signalling across the membrane to elicit a change within the cell concerned.

It is important to emphasize that whereas in this chapter the focus is almost exclusively on receptors for neurotransmitters involved in the dynamic function of synapses, the brain does also contain receptors for growth factors and hormones that are important for more long term processes. In addition, some of the information considered here derives from studies of receptors in tissues other than brain but it is assumed that this information is applicable to brain receptors.

Assays for receptors

For many years receptors could be assessed only from the responses of intact cellular systems. More recently, *in vitro* biochemical assays for receptors have been introduced and have expanded greatly our knowledge of receptors and given them a reality in biochemical terms.

Functional studies of receptors in whole cell systems

A large body of information exists about receptors derived from studies on whole cell systems. For example, the electrophysiological response of a neurone following the application of a neurotransmitter gives some measure of receptor action. Similarly, behavioural responses to administered neurotransmitters in experimental animals can give information on receptor properties. Examples of such tests for dopamine receptors are given in Chapter 5. Although these kinds of tests can only give overall information about receptors and their final responses, they have served to provide a comprehensive classification of receptor types and their pharmacological properties, as well as acting as screening systems for drug discovery.

These tests have also emphasized the role of receptors as functional entities designed not only to recognize and bind the neurotransmitter but also to cause a response in the relevant cell. In terms of understanding the structure and function of receptors, however, *in vitro* biochemical assays are required but they must always be referred back to the whole cell system for validation.

In vitro *biochemical assays for receptors*

The *in vitro* assay systems for receptors that have been developed are based either on the ability of a substance (neurotransmitter (agonist) or a corresponding antagonist) to bind to a receptor or the ability of a neurotransmitter to stimulate a response following receptor binding. These two forms of *in vitro* biochemical assay can be understood by reference to the general equation for receptor action (Fig. 6.1).

$$R + L \rightleftharpoons RL \rightarrow X \rightarrow \text{RESPONSE}$$

Figure 6.1 General equation for receptor action. A ligand (L) is shown binding to a receptor (R) and producing a response in the tissue via an intervening event (X). This scheme will hold if the ligand (L) is an agonist (neurotransmitter) whereas for an antagonist the equations will proceed only as far as RL and tissue responses to agonist ligands will be prevented. If the receptor affects the opening of ion channels then the event (X) and the response are synonymous whereas for other receptors the event may represent a change in a second messenger, e.g. cyclic AMP or inositol trisphosphate, which subsequently leads to the tissue response.

First, it should be possible to detect the binding of a neurotransmitter or its antagonist (the ligand) to receptors in a suitable receptor-containing tissue. Normally the binding of the ligand is detected by using a ligand radiolabelled to a high specific activity, the assays are then termed *ligand-binding assays*. These assays have been very widely used to determine the number of receptors and the properties of receptors in brain and other tissues. For a detailed discussion of the practical and theoretical aspects see the reviews listed at the end of this chapter.

As an example of the use of ligand binding assays, D_2 dopamine receptors may be assayed by the binding of the radiolabelled drug [^{3}H]spiperone; this has been used on D_2 dopamine receptors in their native membrane-bound state, after solubilization from

Table 6.1 Receptors for neurotransmitters and neuromodulators

Receptor	Response	Radioligand
Fast ion channel linked		
Acetylcholine (nicotinic)	Na^+/K^+	$[^3H]/[^{125}I]$ α-bungarotoxin
$GABA_A$	Cl^-	$[^3H]$ muscimol; $[^3H]$ flunitrazepam (for benzodiazepine site)
Glutamate (aspartate)	Na^+/K^+	
—NMDA		$[^3H]AP5$; $[^3H]MK801$; $[^3H]CGP39653$
—AMPA		$[^3H]AMPA$; $[^3H]CNQX$
—KA		$[^3H]$kainic acid
Glycine	Cl^-	$[^3H]$strychnine
5-Hydroxytryptamine ($5\text{-}HT_3$)	Na^+/K^+	$[^3H]$quipazine; $[^3H]GR65630$
G-protein linked		
Non-peptide		
Acetylcholine (muscarinic) M_{1-3}	PLC (M_1, M_3) AC↓(M_2)K⁺↑(M_2)	$[^3H]N$-methylscopolamine (M_{1-3}); $[^3H]$pirenzepine (M_1)
Adenosine A_1	AC↓; K⁺↑; Ca^{2+}↓	$[^3H]$cyclopentyl-1,3-dipropylxanthine
A_2	AC↑	$[^3H]NECA$ (A_1occluded); $[^3H]CGS21680$
Adrenergic α_1	PLC	$[^3H]$prazosin; $[^{125}I]HEAT$
α_2	AC↓; K⁺↑; Ca^{2+}↓	$[^3H]$rauwolscine
β_1/β_2	AC↑	$[^3H]$dihydroalprenolol; $[^{125}I]$iodocyanopindolol;$[^3H]CGP12177$; $[^3H]$bisoprolol (β_1); $[^3H]ICI11851$ (β_2)
$GABA_B$	AC↓; K⁺↑; Ca^{2+}↓	$[^3H]$baclofen
Glutamate (ACPD) (metabotropic)	PLC	
Dopamine D_1	AC↑; PLC	$[^3H]SCH23390$; $[^{125}I]SCH23982$
D_2	AC↓; K⁺↑; Ca^{2+}↓	$[^3H]$domperidone; $[^3H]$spiperone (occluding α_1, $5\text{-}HT_2$); $[^3H]YM091512$
Histamine H_1	PLC	$[^3H]$pyrilamine
H_2	AC↑	$[^3H]$tiotidine
H_3	—	$[^3H]N$-methylhistamine
5-Hydroxytryptamine $5\text{-}HT_{1A}$	AC↓; K⁺↑	$[^3H]8OH$-DPAT
$5\text{-}HT_{1B}$	AC↓	$[^{125}I]$iodocyanopindolol
$5\text{-}HT_{1C}$	PLC*	$[^{125}I]LSD$ ($5\text{-}HT_2$ occluded)

Receptor	Response	Radioligand
5-HT$_{1D}$	AC↓	[³H]5-hydroxytryptamine (5-HT$_{1A,B,C}$ occluded)
5-HT$_2$	PLC	[³H]ketanserin
Peptide		
Angiotensin II	PLC; AC↓	[³H]angiotensin
Bradykinin (B$_1$, B$_2$, B$_3$)	PLC	[³H]bradykinin
Cholecystokinin (CCK B)	PLC	[³H]CCK8 (3,6MeNle)
Corticotropin (ACTH)	AC↑	[¹²⁵I]ACTH
Neurotensin	PLC; AC↓	[³H]neurotensin
Neuropeptide Y	PLC; AC↓	[³H]neuropeptide Y
Opiate		
μ	AC↓; K↑↑	[³H-Tyr]‖[**D**-Ala²,N methylPhe⁴, glycol⁵]enkephalin
κ	AC↓; Ca²⁺↓	[³H]bremazocine (μ,δ occluded); [³H]U69593
δ	AC↓; K↑↑; Ca²⁺↓	D-pen², D-pen⁵ [tyrosyl-³H]enkephalin
σ	—	[³H]di(2-tolyl)guanidine
Somatostatin	AC↓; K↑↑; Ca²⁺↓	[¹²⁵I]somatostatin-14
Substance P (tachykinin)		
NK1	PLC	[³H]substance P, (9-Sar,11-Met-(O₂))
NK2	PLC	[³H]neurokinin A
NK3	PLC; AC↓	[³H]senktide
Thyrotrophin releasing hormone (TRH)	PLC	[³H]3-methyl-His-TRH
Vasopressin V$_1$	PLC; AC↓	(d(CH₂)₅-Tyr-Me-[³H]arginine vasopressin
V$_2$	AC↑	[phenylalanyl-3,4,5,-³H] vasopressin
VIP	AC↑	[¹²⁵I]VIP

A list of the principal receptors and their responses is given together with typically used radioligands for ligand-binding assays. Receptors are categorized firstly as fast ion channel linked or G-protein linked, then within these groups according to the neurotransmitter involved; for each neurotransmitter, the receptor subtypes that are well defined from pharmacological studies are shown. The multiple isoforms of receptors uncovered by gene cloning are not shown. Under 'Responses', Na⁺, K⁺, Ca²⁺, and Cl⁻ refer to channels specific for the ion involved, AC is adenylyl cyclase, PLC is phospholipase C. The classification is based on Watson and Abbott (1992) to which the reader should refer for more information.

Abbreviations: AMPA, α-amino-3-hydroxy-5-methyl-isoxazole-4-propionate; CGS19755, 4-phosphomethyl-2-piperidine carboxylic acid; CNQX, 6-cyano-7-nitro-quinoxaline-2,3-dione; HEAT, 2-[β-(4-hydroxy-3-iodophenyl) ethylaminomethyl]-tetralone; ICI11851, erythro-DL-1-(7-methylindan-4-yloxy)3-isopropylaminobutane-2-o1; NECA, 5′-N-ethylcarboxamidoadenosine; 8OH-DPAT, 8-hydroxy-2-(dipropyl) amino tetralin; YM09512, *cis-N*-(1-benzyl-2-methyl pyrrolidin-3-yl)-5-chloro-2-methoxy-4-methylaminobenzamide.

membranes with detergent and after purification to homogeneity (see Strange 1987*a,b* for reviews) as well as in brain samples derived *post mortem* from patients suffering from a variety of brain diseases (see for example Seeman 1987 and also Chapter 13). Table 6.1 lists some commonly used radioligands used in ligand binding assays for brain receptors.

Secondly, the immediate post-receptor event can be used to assay the receptors; such assays are termed *functional in vitro assays*. For example for the nicotinic acetylcholine receptor, where the receptor is closely coupled to an ion channel (Na^+/K^+ channel), the receptor may be assayed *in vitro* by effects on the transport of $^{22}Na^+$, $^{86}Rb^+$, or Tl^+ (see Conti-Tronconi and Raftery 1982). Alternatively for many receptors, occupancy of receptors leads to alteration in the activity of an enzyme in the cell e.g. adenylyl cyclase or phospholipase C. Thus receptors of this kind can be assayed functionally by changes in the activities of one of these enzymes. For example, muscarinic acetylcholine receptors may be assayed by their effects on either phospholipase C (stimulatory) or adenylyl cyclase (inhibitory) (see Table 6.1 for functional assays for other receptors).

These two classes of assay (ligand-binding and functional) are both *in vitro* assays and particularly in the case of the ligand-binding assay measure only a part of the overall function of a receptor. Therefore they must be very carefully validated and a set of criteria may be laid down based on the properties of the receptor studied *in vivo* which should be satisfied by the *in vitro* assay if it is to be a valid measure of physiologically relevant receptors. These criteria are:

1. The distribution of *in vitro* ligand binding or functional receptor activity in various tissues should parallel the known distribution of receptors derived from *in vivo* studies.
2. The *in vitro* ligand binding or functional receptor activity should show 'saturation' at high ligand concentrations when all the receptors are occupied.
3. The *in vitro* ligand binding or functional receptor activity should show the same specificity that is associated with the relevant receptor from *in vivo* assays when a variety of ligands are tested.
4. As an extension of criterion 3 there should be a good quantitative correlation between the potencies of substances in the *in vitro* and corresponding *in vivo* assays or responses.

If these criteria can be reasonably satisfied for the *in vitro* assay then the assay may be taken as a good measure of *in vivo* receptors.

Molecular genetics applied to receptors

In the 1980s the study of receptors was revolutionized by the application of molecular genetics (gene cloning) to receptors of the nervous system. The results of these studies have been important for several reasons. First, isolation of the DNA sequences coding for receptors has allowed amino acid sequences to be determined and hydropathy analysis of these amino acid sequences has allowed models of the receptors to be proposed (see below). Hydropathy analysis entails examination of the amino acid sequence for runs of hydrophobic amino acids long enough to form membrane-spanning α-helices. Conventional biochemical studies would not have been able to give this information easily. Secondly, cloning of receptor genes has shown that there exists considerably more diversity of structure than had hitherto been considered. Several isoforms of individual receptor subunits exist in some cases and distinct receptor subtypes which had only been hinted at from pharmacological studies have now been recognized. Thirdly, the ability to express cloned receptor genes at high levels facilitates the study of receptors at the protein level using biophysical techniques.

In the discussion below data from all these different approaches to receptors will be considered.

The concept of two classes of neurotransmitter receptor

The results of *in vivo* tests for receptors showed that two broad classes of receptor could be discerned based on the speed of response. One class, e.g. nicotinic acetylcholine, gave responses within milliseconds whereas the other class, e.g. muscarinic acetylcholine, gave much slower responses (hundreds of milliseconds to seconds to minutes). Subsequent physiological and biochemical work confirmed this division, showing that the former class of receptor was associated with a rapid change in the excitability of the membrane. Where their structure has been examined, members of this class of receptor have each been found to consist of several subunits (usually five) which form an oligomeric protein that contains the receptor binding site and an ion channel (Fig. 6.2). This class of receptor will be fast acting as the receptor and ion channel are closely coupled. The second class of receptor was found to be associated frequently with alterations in adenylyl cyclase or phospholipase C and their associated second messengers. This class of receptor has usually been found to be a monomer containing the receptor binding site and to be part of a more loosely coupled system involving the receptor, a guanine nucleotide binding protein (G-protein) and a molecule responsible for effecting a change within the cell termed the effector (Fig. 6.3). This will be a slower acting system as several proteins need to associate to produce a response. The differential time courses of the two classes of receptor can thus be given a biochemical basis. More recent molecular biology studies have confirmed this division and showed that within each group the proteins are highly homologous related species (see below). The two groups of receptor have been termed class I and class II receptors (Strange 1988) or ionotropic and metabotropic (McGeer *et al.* 1987*a*), but neither of these nomenclatures is entirely satisfactory. In subsequent discussion I shall call the two groups of receptors 'fast ion

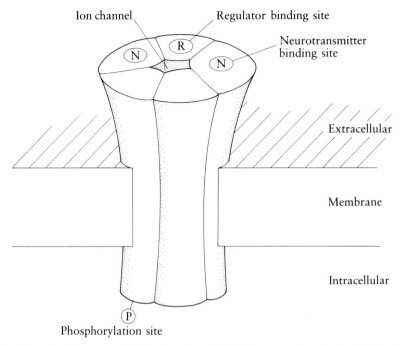

Figure 6.2 Generalized structure of a fast ion channel linked receptor showing the binding sites for the neurotransmitter, binding sites for regulators, and the ion channel contained on one pentameric structure. Examples of this receptor class are given in Table 6.1.

channel linked receptors' and 'G-protein linked receptors' as this nomenclature captures the essential mechanistic distinction between the two groups. Table 6.1 lists receptors according to this classification. I have previously subdivided neurotransmitters as fast and slow (Table 5.1)—their designation as fast and slow derives from actions on the two groups of receptor. In Chapter 7 the importance of this classification in the function of synapses in the brain and how it leads to a division of neural circuitry will be discussed.

The concept of two classes of receptor in the brain is important for the dynamic function of synapses but there are, as noted earlier, receptors for other substances in the brain such as hormones and growth factors. These are structurally and functionally distinct from the two classes of receptor outlined above. For example, the brain contains receptors for hormones such as insulin and for growth factors such as nerve growth factor and epidermal growth factor. These function by different mechanisms from those outlined above and in some cases the mechanisms depend on activation of a protein tyrosine kinase (see for example Carpenter 1987). Also, the brain is subject to the influence of a variety of hormones of the steroid hormone class, e.g. glucocorticoids. In general these hormones function to alter protein synthesis via binding to soluble receptor

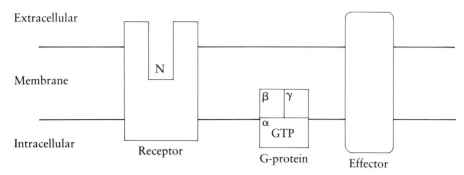

Figure 6.3 Generalized structure of a G-protein linked receptor showing the single subunit containing the binding site for the neurotransmitter N. Also shown are the G-protein and effector molecule, e.g. adenylyl cyclase, phospholipase C, or ion channel making up the transmembrane signalling unit. Examples of this kind of receptor are given in Table 6.1.

proteins within the cell that may be attached within the nucleus (see for example, McEwen *et al.* 1986).

Detailed structural and functional analysis of receptors
Fast ion channel linked receptors

The best characterized of this group are the nicotinic acetylcholine, GABA$_A$, and glycine receptors, but also included here are the several kinds of glutamate receptor and the 5-HT$_3$ subtype of 5-hydroxytryptamine receptor. Biochemical analysis, where this has been carried out, has established that these receptors consist of five subunits which are glycosylated integral membrane proteins. These combine to form an oligomeric protein array containing the receptor binding site(s), a central ion channel, and various additional binding sites for modulatory molecules. For example, the nicotinic acetylcholine receptor is modulated by compounds such as phencyclidine, histrionicotoxin, and local anaesthetics. The GABA$_A$ receptor is modulated by benzodiazepines, steroids, barbiturates, and picrotoxin (see Chapter 15), and the NMDA class of glutamate receptor is modulated by glycine and phencyclidine related compounds. It is assumed that modulatory sites exist for each of these different compounds.

The amino acid sequences of the subunits have been determined by gene cloning (Barnard *et al.* 1987; Olsen and Tobin 1990; Betz 1990; Boulter *et al.* 1990). Within a receptor the different subunits are highly homologous and there is also structural homology between subunits from some of the different receptors. In particular the predicted three-dimensional structures of each subunit based on hydropathy analyses show a common structural motif of four membrane-spanning α-helices which are then packed together (Fig. 6.4). The ligand-binding site is thought to be formed from the extracellular amino-terminal segment, which also bears oligosaccharide chains. The ion channel is thought to be formed from the second membrane-spanning segment of each subunit. Phosphorylation sites have been identified on the large intracellular loop and phosphorylation at these sites may be involved in regulating the rate of desensitization (see later).

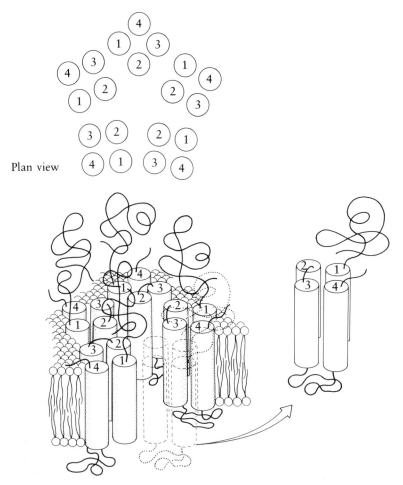

Figure 6.4   Predicted structure of a fast ion channel linked receptor derived from hydropathy analysis of the amino acid sequence. The structure is based on that proposed for the GABA$_A$ receptor (Olsen and Tobin 1990) but analogous structures are likely for the other fast receptors. Each subunit is predicted to be composed of four transmembrane α-helices linked by loops of varying length. The extracellular amino-terminal sections of each subunit contain consensus sequences for glycosylation and the intracellular loop linking the third and fourth transmembrane regions contains in different subunit isoforms potential sites for phosphorylation by protein kinase A or C or tyrosine protein kinase. Five subunits are shown packing together to form an oligomeric array with a central pore which would form the ion channel. The binding sites for ligands and regulators may be formed by the extracellular amino-terminal section. Redrawn from Olsen and Tobin (1990) with permission.

Multiple isoforms of each subunit have been described which are coded by different genes. Differential expression of different isoforms in different tissues may provide receptors with subtle differences in their pharmacological properties.

G-protein linked receptors

Biochemical analyses have established that there is a group of receptors which are integral membrane glycoproteins containing a receptor-binding site. Where analysed, they were found to be monomeric. They are linked via a second family of proteins, G-proteins, to their effectors, adenylyl cyclase and phospholipase C (specific for phosphatidylinositol bis phosphate), and as more recently discovered, ion channels selective for K^+ and Ca^{2+}. There may also be a linkage to phospholipase C and D (specific for phosphatidylcholine) (Billah and Anthes 1990) but the systems are not well characterized yet. Linkage to phospholipase A_2 has been described in the periphery and may yet be found in the brain.

The application of gene cloning techniques to these receptor proteins has shown that they are more homologous than had been expected. Each consists of a protein core of 40–70 kDa increased by glycosylation by a further 20–30 kDa. The homology is particularly striking when the amino acid sequences are used to predict a structure for the proteins (Lefkowitz and Caron 1988). For each receptor that has been analysed in this way, a structure containing seven transmembrane α-helices is predicted (Fig. 6.5); this has been found for all the G-protein linked receptors analysed so far. Thus it seems that receptors linked to G-proteins form a family of proteins with homologous structures. The amino acid sequences also show homologies between receptors for different neurotransmitters. For example, the muscarinic acetylcholine (M_1) and β_2- adrenergic receptors show about 25 per cent overall amino acid homology; this rises to 32 per cent in the transmembrane regions which seem to show striking conservation between different receptors. For example, the D_2 dopamine receptor shows considerable identity (up to 40 per cent) in these regions with the α_2- and β_2-adrenergic receptors and the 5-hydroxytryptamine 5-HT_{1A} receptor. The seven transmembrane α-helix model is given further support from similar observations on the visual pigment rhodopsin which functions to harvest light and transduces its signal across the membrane via a G-protein (transducin). Rhodopsin also shows the motif of seven transmembrane α-helices when a structure prediction is carried out. Perhaps the most compelling evidence that this model is correct comes from structural studies on the bacterial light-harvesting pigment, bacteriorhodopsin, which has been shown by cryo-electron microscopy to contain seven transmembrane α-helices (Caspar 1990; Henderson *et al*. 1990). This is a real structure rather than a predicted structure but the same motif is seen (see Findlay and Pappin (1986) for a discussion of the structure of rhodopsin).

The structures of these kinds of receptor are beginning to be understood in some detail

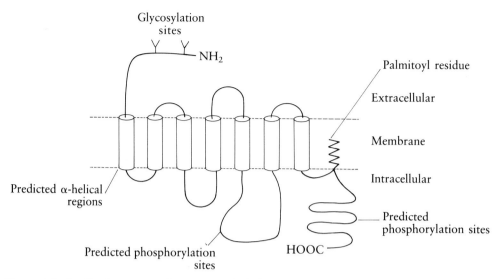

Figure 6.5 Predicted structure of a G-protein linked receptor derived from the amino acid sequence. Hydropathy analysis of the amino acid sequence predicts seven transmembrane α-helices linked by extra-membrane loops of varying length. Also found in the sequence are several consensus glycosylation sequences in the extracellular amino-terminal section, phosphorylation sites in the third intracellular loop and carboxy-terminal tail, and a palmitoylation site in the carboxy-terminal tail which may form a fourth intracellular loop.

using a combination of protein chemistry and molecular biology techniques. Analysis of the amino acid sequences predicts sites for glycosylation near the extracellular amino terminus of the proteins whereas sites for phosphorylation have been identified in the third intracellular loop and in the cytoplasmic carboxyterminal region for the β-adrenergic receptor. These phosphorylation sites may be important in short term desensitization of the receptor (Bouvier *et al.* 1989; Clark *et al.* 1989); this will be discussed in more detail later.

The receptor-binding site appears to be formed from the membrane-spanning α-helices, the extracellular loops and tails not being of major importance for this. The model depicted in Fig. 6.5 is, however, misleading in considering the formation of the receptor-binding site: the helices are not laid out in a line as shown in the figure but are likely to be folded around on to one another to form a bundle of helices which is secured by a disulphide bond. This is the arrangement of helices in bacteriorhodopsin and the structure of rhodopsin can be fitted quite well to this model (Findlay and Pappin 1986). It seems likely, therefore, that this will also be the case for the G-protein linked receptors—the kind of structure envisaged is shown in Fig. 6.6. This provides a cavity within the membrane into which the ligand may bind. Although the cavity is largely formed from hydrophobic amino acids, there are certain hydrophilic amino acids present

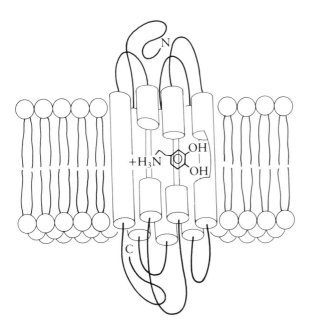

Figure 6.6 Three-dimensional model of a G-protein linked receptor. The seven transmembrane α-helices are shown in a bundle by analogy with the model of rhodopsin of Findlay and Pappin (1986) in turn derived from the structure of bacteriorhodopsin. The cavity formed by bundling of the transmembrane spanning regions forms the receptor-binding site and a ligand, in this case dopamine, is shown. N, amino terminus; C, carboxy terminus.

that must form critical contacts with the hydrophilic ligands influencing binding and specificity. For example, an aspartic acid residue in α-helix 3 has been identified as the counterion for the positive charge of dopamine, noradrenaline, and acetylcholine in their respective receptors.

The site for interaction with G-proteins has also been located and seems to depend on parts of the second and third cytoplasmic loops and the carboxy-terminal tail (Wong *et al.* 1990; Liggett *et al.* 1991). These must be close together in the folded structure. There are only a limited number of G-proteins (see below) and several receptors are known to interact with the same G-protein subtype. It might then be expected that common structural motifs might be recognized in the G-protein interaction regions of certain receptors; such motifs are beginning to be identified.

These kinds of detailed structural analyses of receptors must eventually lead to the unravelling of the mechanisms of action of these receptors at the detailed structural level. They may also enable prediction of drug structures that will fit receptor sites.

G-proteins

The importance of these proteins was first inferred from the requirement for GTP as a cofactor in the stimulation of adenylyl cyclase by certain receptors (Rodbell 1980). Subsequently it was realized that GTP-binding proteins or guanine nucleotide regulatory proteins (G-proteins) were essential for coupling certain receptors to their effectors. These are the receptors described in the previous section. The G-proteins involved in the function of these kinds of receptor are heterotrimeric proteins consisting of α, β, and γ subunits. From protein chemistry and molecular biology studies it is now clear that G-proteins are a family of proteins with different α subunits but more similar β and γ subunits.

Table 6.2 lists the G-proteins known at present together with some indication of their functional importance. The nomenclature of the G-proteins is now rather confusing. G_s was originally found as the G protein linked to adenylyl cyclase stimulation but it is now also known to be able to regulate Ca^{2+} channels (Yatani *et al.* 1987). The G protein involved in inhibition of adenylyl cyclase was originally termed G_i but gene cloning has detected three G_i species and protein isolation a further G_o protein whose function is not well defined. A group of G-proteins termed G_q have been isolated and are thought to be important for coupling to phospholipase C (Strathmann and Simon 1990). An additional species G_z also of unknown function has been isolated recently (Casey *et al.* 1990). G_{i1-3} and G_o are related in that they are all substrates for the bacterial toxin, pertussis toxin, which inactivates them. G_s on the other hand is a substrate for cholera toxin which permanently activates this G-protein; G_q and G_z are substrates for neither toxin.

A point of some importance which will be considered again later is the possible specificity of interaction between G-proteins and effectors. For example, does a particular G-protein interact with a particular effector *in vivo* or is interaction more general but limited by cellular populations of proteins? One approach to this is to reconstitute the interaction by adding a pure G-protein to a system; this has shown that

Table 6.2 G-protein subunits

G protein	Molecular weight	Function
$G_{s\alpha}$	44.5–46 (four variants)	AC$\uparrow$; $Ca^{2+}\uparrow$
$G_{i\alpha}$	40.4–40.5 (three variants, $G_{i1,2,3}$)	AC$\downarrow$($G_{i\alpha2}$)
$G_{o\alpha}$	39.9 (two variants)	$Ca^{2+}\downarrow$; $K^+\uparrow$
$G_{q\alpha}$	41.4 (three variants)	PLC
$G_{z\alpha}$	40.9	?
β	37.4 (four variants)	—
γ	8–10 (four variants)	—

The currently known G protein subunits are shown together with their molecular weights (calculated from their amino acid sequences derived from cloned genes) and some postulated functions. G_s exists in four forms derived by alternative splicing of a single gene, whereas there are three genes encoding $G_{i\alpha1,2,3}$. $G_{z\alpha}$ is a recently discovered protein of unknown function. G_β exists in four forms derived from at least two separate genes whereas there are four variants of G_γ (Birnbaumer 1990). Some functions that have been associated with the different G-protein α subunits are indicated but these are discussed in more detail in the text. G_0 has also been shown to play a role in neurite outgrowth (Strittmatter *et al.* 1990). AC refers to adenylyl cyclase, Ca^{2+} and K^+ to ion channels and PLC is phospholipase C.

receptor regulation of central neuronal K^+ channels is via G_o whereas in the peripheral nervous system G_{i1}, G_{i2}, and G_{i3} can regulate K^+ channels (Brown and Birnbaumer 1990). This reconstitution approach may not reflect the true situation *in vivo* and an alternative approach is to use G-protein specific antibodies to interfere with G-protein–effector interaction and block responses. These studies have provided evidence for specific linkage of G_s to adenylyl cyclase (stimulation), G_{i2} to inhibition of adenylyl cyclase, and G_o to attenuation of Ca^{2+} channels (Simonds *et al.* 1989; McKenzie and Milligan 1990). The information in Table 6.2 contains data from both approaches.

The structures of these G-proteins are outlined in Table 6.2. Each consists of an α subunit which contains the GTP-binding site and is involved in signalling to the effector; this subunit is the most variable component of the system. The α subunit is attached to a complex of β and γ subunits which show less variation in structure between different G-proteins and may act as a membrane anchor for the hetrotrimeric G-protein. In some cases (G_i, G_o, and G_z), the α subunit is acylated with myristic acid which may provide for further linkage to the membrane or assist in interaction with other proteins (Buss *et al.* 1987; Mumby *et al.* 1990*a*). Similarly the γ subunits may be isoprenylated (Mumby *et al.* 1990*b*; Yamane *et al.* 1990) accounting for the linkage of the $\beta\gamma$ complex to the membrane. As well as being able to bind GTP, G-proteins possess a GTP-hydrolysing activity (GTPase). This is important because as we shall see later the GTP-bound form of the G-protein is the active species and the GTP-hydrolysing activity deactivates the G-protein, terminating the activation of the effector.

Of some wider interest but related to G-proteins is the observation that Li^+ can inhibit certain receptor-linked responses such as stimulation of adenylyl cyclase and inositol phospholipid metabolism. This has been localized to an effect on the G-protein involved (Avissar *et al.* 1988) and is a possible candidate mechanism to account for the therapeutic effects of Li^+ in depression (Chapter 14). An alternative site of action of Li^+ is given below.

A distinct class of G-proteins of lower molecular weight has been discovered recently in several tissues including brain. These have at least one subunit with M_r about 25 000 which in some cases is modified by a botulinum neurotoxin (Aktories and Frevert 1987; Kawata *et al.* 1988). The function of these novel G-proteins is not clear at present but they may be involved in the regulation of vesicle transport within cells (Balch 1990).

Effector molecules of G-protein linked receptors
Adenylyl cyclase
This enzyme converts ATP into cyclic AMP and pyrophosphate and can be either activated or inhibited by G-protein linked receptors. Thus the receptor signals an increase or decrease within the cell of the classical second messenger, cyclic AMP. Adenylyl cyclase enzymes are a family of integral membrane glycoproteins consisting of a single subunit (M_r approximately 120 000) (Krupinski *et al.* 1989; Bakalyar and Reed

1990). The mechanism of regulation has been the subject of much research and speculation.

Although it is not universally accepted, a widely held scheme for the activation of adenylyl cyclase has been proposed (Gilman 1987; Freissmuth *et al*. 1989; Birnbaumer 1990) and is shown in Fig. 6.7. The active form of adenylyl cyclase is the complex with the α-subunit of G_s bearing GTP and Mg^{2+}. The α subunit dissociates from $\beta\gamma$ upon binding GTP. Inactivation of adenylyl cyclase is driven by hydrolysis of GTP to GDP by the GTPase activity of the G-protein α subunit. The receptor bearing its activating ligand (agonist; neurotransmitter) facilitates exchange of GDP for GTP and uptake of Mg^{2+} on the α subunit. Thus a cycle is set up with the liganded receptor performing a catalytic function to activate several G-protein α subunits.

Inhibition of adenylyl cyclase is much less well understood. It is thought that a species of G_i, G_{i2} in some systems, is involved in inhibition of adenylyl cyclase and GTP promotes dissociation to the α subunit (bearing GTP) and $\beta\gamma$ subunits. Again GTPase action converts GTP into GDP and the inhibitory receptor promotes exchange of GDP

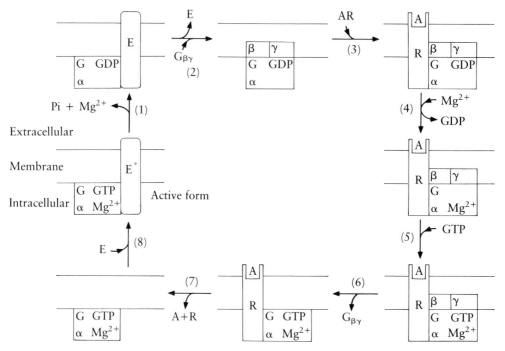

Figure 6.7 A generalized version of the G-protein activation and deactivation cycle (from Freissmuth *et al*. 1989 and Birnbaumer 1990). Key steps in the cycle are: (1) hydrolysis of GTP by the intrinsic GTPase of the G-protein; (2) dissociation of G_α from an effector (E) and recombination with $G_{\beta\gamma}$; (3–5) combination with the agonist–receptor complex (AR) which facilitates GDP/GTP exchange and Mg^{2+} uptake; (6) dissociation away from $G_{\beta\gamma}$; (7) dissociation of AR; (8) combination with the effector (E) to give the activated species $E^* \cdot G_\alpha \cdot GTP \cdot Mg^{2+}$.

for GTP. The precise role of $G_{i\alpha}$–GTP is not clear, however. In some studies it has been shown to inhibit adenylyl cyclase directly (see for example Wong *et al.* 1991), while other studies have suggested that inhibition is due to the $\beta\gamma$ subunits released upon dissociation which by mass action drive the reassociation of $G_{s\alpha}$ and $\beta\gamma$ to deactivate adenylyl cyclase. These possibilities are outlined in Fig. 6.8.

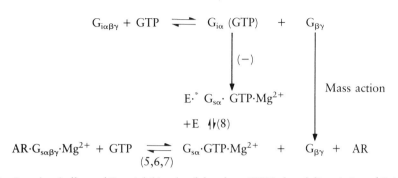

Figure 6.8 Postulated effects of G_i to inhibit adenylyl cyclase. GTP induced dissociation of G_i is shown to $G_{i\alpha}$(GTP) (which may inhibit adenylyl cyclase (E) directly) and $\beta\gamma$ which may drive reassociation of $G_{s\alpha}$ and $G_{\beta\gamma}$ thereby deactivating adenylyl cyclase (E). The generally greater quantities of G_i than G_s in cells drives the reassociation in the direction shown by mass action effects. The numbers refer to the steps of Fig. 6.7 used here. AR is a stimulatory agonist-receptor complex as in Fig. 6.7. The inhibitory receptor complexed with its agonist (not shown) would facilitate exchange of GDP and GTP on G_i leading to dissociation of $G_{i\alpha}$ (GTP) and $\beta\gamma$.

What is also unclear at present is what happens to the activated α subunits within the cell. It might be expected that they would be free in the cytosol once they have separated from $\beta\gamma$ which is held in the membrane; a theory has been proposed by Rodbell (1985) based on this. This may be the case for $G_{s\alpha}$ but some α subunits ($G_{o\alpha}$, $G_{i\alpha}$, and $G_{z\alpha}$) are covalently modified with a myristic acid which may serve to keep the α subunits of these G-proteins attached to the membrane even after they have separated from $\beta\gamma$ (Mumby *et al.* 1990*a*).

Also important for regulation of cyclic AMP levels within cells is the enzyme phosphodiesterase. This hydrolyses cyclic AMP to AMP and so will reduce cyclic AMP levels within a cell once a stimulatory signal has finished. The cyclic AMP signal within a cell activates a cyclic AMP dependent protein kinase (protein kinase A). This then leads to phosphorylation of proteins within the cell. The identities of these proteins are only beginning to be understood but effects have been described on receptors (both fast ion channel linked and G-protein linked), ion channels, G-proteins, enzymes involved in neurotransmitter biosynthesis, and a variety of other proteins whose function is as yet unclear.

Phospholipase C

This enzyme hydrolyses the minor membrane phospholipid, phosphatidyinositol bis phosphate (PIP_2), to inositol trisphosphate (IP_3) and diacylglycerol (DAG) (Fig. 6.9). The enzyme can be activated by a group of G-protein linked receptors via their G-proteins, leading to increases within the cell of IP_3 and DAG, both of which are second messengers. This cell signalling system is less well understood than the adenylyl cyclase system. The phospholipase C enzyme has not been fully characterized but recently a family of enzymes of different molecular sizes has been isolated and their amino acid sequences obtained (Rhee *et al*. 1989; Meldrum *et al*. 1991). The mechanism of activation is not known at present. G-proteins are known to participate to link receptor and phospholipase C and in some cases the family of G_q proteins is involved. It seems likely that the mechanism of activation will prove to be similar to that of adenylyl cyclase but this remains to be shown. Stimulation of phospholipase C is the commonly observed response but recently a minority of receptors have been shown to inhibit the enzyme (e.g. adenosine A_1 and dopamine D_2) which therefore shows the same spectrum of regulation as adenylyl cyclase. The mechanism of inhibition is not understood (Linden and Delahunty 1989).

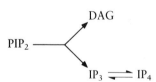

Figure 6.9 Hydrolysis by phospholipase C of the membrane phospholipid phosphatidylinositol bisphosphate (PIP_2) yields diacylglycerol (DAG) and inositol trisphosphate (IP_3) which can be converted to inositol tetrakisphosphate (IP_4).

The two second messengers (IP_3 and DAG) are associated with different cellular effects. IP_3 releases Ca^{2+} from the endoplasmic reticulum giving a transient cytosolic Ca^{2+} signal. Some IP_3 is phosphorylated to inositol tetrakisphosphate (IP_4) which may be involved in altering Ca^{2+} distribution between intracellular stores providing sustained Ca^{2+} responses. The Ca^{2+} binds to calmodulin which can activate a number of enzymes including Ca^{2+}/calmodulin dependent protein kinase. DAG activates a separate Ca^{2+} dependent protein kinase C. The two arms (IP_3/Ca^{2+} and DAG/protein kinase C) of this second messenger system can interact. For example, protein kinase C activation inhibits PIP_2 hydrolysis and activates Ca^{2+} pumping and will tend to reduce the Ca^{2+} signal from the IP_3/Ca^{2+} arm. The rise in Ca^{2+} caused by IP_3 activates the protein kinase C. These interactions can give rise to oscillations in intracellular Ca^{2+} which may be important in setting rhythms in cells. The precise effects of the two second messengers in the nervous system are unclear but effects of protein kinase C have been described on receptors (both groups mentioned above), ion channels, enzymes, G-proteins, and other cellular proteins. Effects of Ca^{2+}/calmodulin dependent protein kinase have been also described on a variety of proteins including synapsin I and tyrosine hydroxylase. A role for this kinase in laying down of memory has been proposed (Kennedy 1988).

The metabolism of inositol phosphates has taken on added interest because of the effects of Li^+ to inhibit breakdown of inositol monophosphate by inhibition of the inositol monophosphatase. This site of action is one of the best candidates for a site of action of Li^+ in exerting its therapeutic effect in manic depressive illness (Chapter 14) although effects on G-proteins have also been described above. It has been speculated that as the brain relies on *de novo* synthesis of inositol from glucose (via inositol monophosphate) for its supply of inositol, then chronic Li^+ therapy might lead to sequestration of inositol in the inositol phosphates, thus depleting the inositol phospholipids and leading to functional inactivation (via substrate depletion) of receptors linked to phospholipase C in certain parts of the brain. It will be the receptors that are specially active at which Li^+ will exert the maximal effect.

Ion channels

Indications have been given above of the ability of G-protein linked receptors, via second messengers such as cAMP, DAG, and IP_3, to regulate ion channels via phosphorylation. G-protein linked receptors may regulate ion channels more directly via G-proteins without the intervention of second messengers.

A number of receptors e.g. α_2-adrenergic, muscarinic acetylcholine, D_2 dopamine, $GABA_B$, opiate, and 5-HT_{1A} 5-hydroxytryptamine (North *et al*. 1987) can regulate certain K^+ channels via G-proteins, leading to a hyperpolarization of the cell. It is thought that the α subunit of G_o regulates the K^+ channel in the brain although in other tissues such as the heart all three G_i species will perform this function. Similarly, effects of receptors via G-proteins to regulate Ca^{2+} channels have been described e.g. $GABA_B$, muscarinic acetylcholine, and opiate receptors have been shown to inhibit Ca^{2+} channels in nervous tissue and G_o is thought to be important here (Brown and Birnbaumer 1990). Effects of receptors to stimulate Ca^{2+} channels via this route have been described in the periphery (Rosenthal *et al*. 1988) and G_s is directly responsible without the involvement of adenylyl cyclase (Brown and Birnbaumer 1990).

The speed of these G-protein linked ion channel responses is intermediate between the enzyme linked G-protein responses and the fast ion channel linked receptor responses and has been reported to be of the order of hundreds of milliseconds or longer. This must be a reflection of the interactions of the three protein species.

Organization of G-protein linked receptor signalling systems

It should be apparent that G-protein linked receptors signal to the interior of the cell via systems consisting of two additional components, a G-protein and an effector. For some neurotransmitters the receptors are able to influence multiple effectors, potentially producing a multiplicity of cellular responses. For example, adrenergic receptors taken as a group can stimulate and inhibit adenylyl cyclase, stimulate phospholipase C, open K^+ channels and inhibit Ca^{2+} channels, whereas dopamine receptors stimulate and inhibit adenylyl cyclase and open K^+ channels, may stimulate phospholipase C and may regulate Ca^{2+} channels. These kinds of multiple effects of neurotransmitters have implications for the multiplicity of the individual components in the system.

An important question is whether for each effector (E) response a separate receptor (R) and G protein subtype will be found so that the lines of signalling could be described as:

$$R_1 \rightarrow G_1 \rightarrow E_1$$
$$R_2 \rightarrow G_2 \rightarrow E_2$$
$$\vdots \qquad \vdots \qquad \vdots$$
$$R_n \rightarrow G_n \rightarrow E_n$$

At present the information on this is not clear; this is partly due to the rapid development of the field. It seems possible that when all the receptor and G-protein isoforms have been described using gene cloning techniques, then for every effector response to a neurotransmitter one or more distinct receptor isoforms and a specific G-protein will be associated with that response. The receptor isoforms may be pharmacologically highly distinct or they may differ only at the receptor–G-protein coupling site.

In Tables 6.1 and 6.2 some of the currently known specificities are outlined. However, the information in these tables also shows some lack of specificity. One possible reason for this lack of specificity may be that at present not all the species are recognized. Therefore examples where one apparently distinct receptor or G-protein is linked to different effectors may eventually be resolved by the isolation of new isoforms. For example the G-protein G_s apparently performs the dual function of activating adenylyl cyclase and Ca^{2+} channels. This may be functionally important in tissues like the heart where one receptor (β-adrenergic) can provide a rapid Ca^{2+} signal (via Ca^{2+} channel activation) and a slower Ca^{2+} signal (via adenylyl cyclase activation with the cAMP in turn activating Ca^{2+} channels through protein kinase A) (Yatani and Brown 1990). Nevertheless, even in this case, given that there are four G_s isoforms available, separate isoforms could be specifically linked to each of the two effector responses. Another reason for apparent lack of specificity may be that these apparently multiple effects reflect the *in vitro* test system and cellular constraints, for example interactions with the cytoskeleton may place restrictions on receptor/G-protein/effector arrays *in vivo*.

The relative numbers of the receptor/G-protein/effector components may also be important. Different receptor:G-protein or G-protein:effector ratios in different cells will mean that different proportions of the total receptor population will need to be occupied to achieve maximal activation of the effector. This will result in different apparent abilities of the same agonist to activate the effector in different tissues. This could be the origin of the apparent differences in agonist sensitivities at presynaptic and postsynaptic receptors (Chapter 5). Differences in receptor : G-protein : effector ratios in different tissues could also provide a biochemical rationalization for variation in the pharmacological concept of 'spare receptors'. Pharmacologically a tissue has been defined as having 'spare receptors' for a response when a full response to receptor activation is achieved by occupancy of only part of that receptor population. This could well reflect a large receptor : G-protein or G-protein : effector ratio.

I have argued here for segregated lines of signalling from one receptor to its effector and hence to the cellular response. The protein kinase activities associated with one system can, however, alter the activities of another. For example, activation of phospholipase C leads to activation of protein kinase C which can phosphorylate receptors, G-proteins, adenylyl cyclase, and ion channels, altering their activity whereas activation of the adenylyl cyclase signalling pathway raises cAMP levels which in turn raise the activity of protein kinase A which can phosphorylate phospholipase C (inhibiting it) so that there can be considerable 'cross-talk' between the different lines of signalling. This provides for a high degree of complexity in intracellular signalling.

Summary of physiological consequences of receptor activation

An extremely complex picture of receptor activation is now emerging and it is necessary to attempt to present an overview of the physiological consequences. For fast ion channel linked receptors, activation leads to a very rapid (millisecond) alteration in the electrical properties of the cell membrane (depolarizing or hyperpolarizing) and in Chapter 3 the consequences of such changes in cell excitability for action potential generation were considered. For G-protein linked receptors, receptor activation has a wider range of consequences. For some of these kinds of receptor linked to ion channels this is a slow (hundreds of milliseconds) change in the permeability of the membrane to either K^+ (via channel opening) or Ca^{2+} (via closure of previously open channels), leading to a slow electrical change in the membrane. In functional terms this can be important: a slow change in K^+ permeability will produce a long lasting hyperpolarization of the membrane and may limit action potential generation in that membrane. Inhibition of Ca^{2+} flux or activation of K^+ flux by receptors may underlie the inhibition of neurotransmitter release by presynaptic receptors (Chapter 5).

For other G-protein linked receptors associated with either adenylyl cyclase or phospholipase C there will be changes in the phosphorylation states of proteins via the different protein kinases. If these proteins are ion channels there will be a very slow (seconds to minutes) change in the electrical properties of the membrane. For example noradrenaline (via β-adrenergic receptors, cAMP, and protein kinase A) has been shown to inhibit a slow Ca^{2+} dependent K^+ channel that normally hyperpolarizes hippocampal pyramidal cells and limits action potential firing by the axon hillock region of the neurone in response to sustained depolarizations. Action potential firing in these cells occurs more freely in the presence of noradrenaline as this brake on the cell membrane excitability has been removed (see Chapter 7 for more details).

A second example of this kind of effect is afforded by a cultured cell line that responds to application of bradykinin by sequential slow hyperpolarization (approximate duration 10 s) and depolarization (approximate duration 100 s). This sequence of events, which provides quite complex control of the membrane excitability, can be accounted for by bradykinin stimulation of phospholipase C, the IP_3 signal leading to the hyperpolarization (via a Ca^{2+} dependent K^+ channel) and the DAG signal causing the depolarization via protein kinase C catalysed phosphorylation (inhibition) of a second class of K^+ channel, the M channel (Higashida and Brown 1986).

Alternatively, G-protein linked receptor activation may lead via phosphorylation to changes in the activities of other synaptic proteins, e.g. proteins involved in neuro-transmitter synthesis and release. As will be described in the next section this can be important in regulating receptor desensitization but it is also likely to be important for longer term regulatory events in the brain such as in the laying down of short term memory. As also indicated, phosphorylation allows cross-talk between different G-protein linked receptor systems and between fast ion channel linked and G-protein linked receptor systems.

Regulation of receptor activity

Receptors are responsible for highly selective signalling at synapses but their activity is also capable of regulation. Two kinds of receptor regulation may be distinguished according to their time courses. The first, desensitization, is a rapid event and is observed as the loss of responsiveness to an agonist in a tissue following a strong acute stimulation of that tissue. It involves events at the receptor itself and varies according to the proper-ties of the receptor. The physiological significance of desensitization at brain receptors is not clear but it may provide a mechanism to prevent over-stimulation at synapses by excess released neurotransmitter.

The second regulation mechanism is slower and is frequently observed when tissues are challenged chronically with an agonist. The number of receptors in the cell is reduced and this is often referred to as 'down-regulation'. Such regulation may not have any physiological significance under normal conditions but as discussed below may be a reflection of the mechanisms associated with synthesis and degradation of receptors at the cell membrane. If perturbed, however, as in the case of drug treatment, the regulation may have great significance. Each mechanism will be considered in turn.

Desensitization

For fast ion channel linked receptors such as the nicotinic acetylcholine receptor, desensitization is observed upon exposure to acetylcholine for tens of milliseconds or
longer. Desensitization involves a switch via a conformational change in the receptor
protein from an active state bearing agonist and with the ion channel open to desensitized states with closed ion channels. The agonist binding affinity also increases
upon desensitization. Phosphorylation of these kinds of receptor in peripheral tissues
accelerates the rate of desensitization but desensitization can occur independently of
phosphorylation. Phosphorylation can be mediated by protein kinase A, protein kinase
C, and protein tyrosine kinases thus allowing for cross-talk between G-protein linked
and fast ion channel linked receptor systems. For neuronal fast ion channel linked
receptors, phosphorylation may enhance desensitization but there may be differences
between central and peripheral systems in their response to phosphorylation (Berg *et al.*
1989; Browning *et al.* 1990).

For a G-protein linked receptor such as the β-adrenergic receptor, activation of the
receptor is slower and desensitization slower still, taking tens of minutes to reach a
maximum. Desensitization involves a fairly rapid uncoupling of receptor from G-protein
and effector followed by sequestration of the receptor into a light membrane fraction
which is separate from the plasma membrane but may be a vesicular compartment
associated with it. Desensitization of this kind is triggered by phosphorylation of the
receptor on its carboxy-terminal tail; there is a specific β-adrenergic receptor kinase (β-
ARK) (Benovic *et al.* 1989) which phosphorylates the receptor when it is occupied by
agonist and a regulatory protein, β-arrestin then interferes with receptor–G-protein
interaction (Lohse *et al.* 1990). Sequestration seems then to promote dephosphorylation
and the receptor may be recycled back to the plasma membrane. This gives a mechanism
for homologous desensitization, i.e. desensitization of a response to a particular agent
caused by that agent. Homologous desensitization is also contributed to by receptor
phosphorylation by protein kinase A via the receptor-mediated cAMP signal, but the site
of phosphorylation is different being on the third intracellular loop (Bouvier *et al.* 1989;
Clark *et al.* 1989; Hausdorff *et al.* 1990).

Both the muscarinic acetylcholine and α_2-adrenergic receptors are also substrates for
the β-ARK (Kwatra *et al.* 1989) which may therefore act to phosphorylate several
receptors in their activated forms. This would then constitute a general mechanism for
homologous desensitization.

Heterologous desensitization of receptors can also be observed whereby responses to
several receptors are desensitized by activation of one system. For example, in certain
cloned cell lines, prolonged incubation with either noradrenergic agonists or prosta-
glandins, both of which raise cAMP levels, leads to desensitization of responses to both
agents. In this case activation of protein kinase A must lead to phosphorylation of

components of both signalling systems, e.g. receptors and G-proteins, inhibiting their function. Since protein kinase A can also affect phospholipase C linked receptor systems and protein kinase C can affect adenylyl cyclase linked systems also at the level of receptors and G-proteins, there is considerable scope for heterologous desensitization.

Down-regulation

Whereas short term stimulation of several receptors can lead to desensitization, longer term stimulation of many receptors leads to alterations in the numbers of receptors at cell surfaces. Where there is a reduction in receptor number this is often termed 'down-regulation'. This is a result of alterations in the rates of receptor turnover at the cell surface. A general scheme for receptor turnover, derived mainly from studies on peripheral tissues, is shown in Fig. 6.10 and depicts the mechanisms involved in regulating the number of receptors at the surface of a cell. A critical event is the clustering of receptors at regions of the cell surface called coated pits where coated vesicles bud off into the cell interior. There they lose their coat to become smooth vesicles. The relation of these smooth vesicles to those sequestering the G-protein linked receptors when they undergo desensitization is not clear at present. The smooth vesicles then fuse with endosomes and from here the receptors can either recycle back to the plasma membrane or be degraded in lysosomes leading to receptor degradation. Elements of the Golgi complex may be involved here. There is also new synthesis of receptors in the endoplasmic reticulum and the newly synthesized receptors are contained in vesicles which ultimately fuse with the plasma membrane after passage through the Golgi complex. The balance of the degradation and replacement rates determines the level of receptors at the cell surface (see Schimke (1973) for more details of the quantification) and it is likely that the contributions of the two rates have differential importance for different receptor types.

This general scheme is suitable for a neuroglial cell or for receptors on the cell body of a neurone (postsynaptic receptors). For receptors at the nerve terminal (presynaptic receptors), the receptors removed from the cell membrane must be cycled back to the cell body for degradation and new receptors must be synthesized within the cell body and dispatched to the terminal by axonal transport (Chapter 3).

The balance between synthesis and degradation can be disturbed by altering the level of receptor stimulation. This has been most clearly described for G-protein linked receptors, e.g. the β-adrenergic receptor. Chronic stimulation by agonist accelerates removal of receptor from the cell membrane without affecting the replacement rate so that the net result is a reduction in cell surface receptor number (down-regulation).

In vivo, such regulation may be important where an agonist drug is administered to a patient. For example, patients with Parkinson's disease (Chapter 10) are treated with a precursor of dopamine (L-DOPA). These patients have been found in some studies to have an increased number of dopamine receptors (up regulation) as a result of loss of

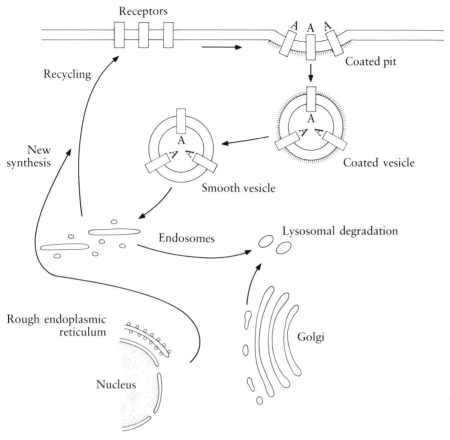

Figure 6.10 Receptor cycling mechanisms to and from the plasma membrane. Clustering of ligand (agonist)–receptor (AR) complexes in areas of the cell called coated pits leads to internalization of coated vesicles containing AR. The coated vesicles lose their coat and progress to the endosomal compartment (endosomes) which appears as smooth vesicles and tubules. The acidic environment of the endosomal compartment will ensure ligand dissociation. From here receptors may be recycled on vesicles back to the plasma membrane or degraded by lysosomes; Golgi elements may be involved. There will also be new synthesis of receptors which will be directed to the plasma membrane via Golgi elements. If the receptors are at the nerve terminal, both degradation and new synthesis will require axonal transport (Chapter 3). The figure is not in proportion.

brain dopamine. Treatment with L-DOPA reduces the number of receptors (down-regulation) by replenishing the dopamine stimulation. See Chapter 10 for more information on receptors in Parkinson's disease.

Alternatively, administration of a drug which is an antagonist will effectively reduce the agonist stimulation and lead to an increase in the number of receptors at the cell surface (up-regulation). Many psychoactive drugs are antagonists of G-protein linked receptors and it is thought that as part of their therapeutic effect they may alter receptor number (see Chapters 13 and 14 for examples of this). G-protein linked receptors have also been reported to be regulated by steroid hormones, e.g. androgens and gluco-corticoids. This is generally seen as a stimulation of receptor synthesis and steroid receptor responsive elements have been recognized on certain G-protein linked receptor genes.

The balance of degradation and synthesis of fast ion channel linked receptors differs from that described for G-protein linked receptors. Although fast receptors, e.g. nicotinic acetylcholine receptors, participate in a synthesis/degradation cycle similar to that described in Fig. 6.10, the effects of denervation of a tissue on receptor number are different from that seen in G-protein linked systems. For neuronal nicotinic acetylcholine receptors, denervation leads to receptor loss and corresponding innervation leads to receptor induction. This may reflect the production by the nerve terminal of a receptor inducing factor (Berg *et al.* 1989) or a fundamental difference in receptor regulation where the agonist induces rather than down-regulates receptors (Wonnacott 1990).

Recommended reading

Benovic, J. L., Bouvier, M., Caron, M. G., and Lefkowitz, R. J. (1988). Regulation of adenylyl cyclase coupled β-adrenergic receptors. *Annual Review of Cell Biology*, **4**, 405–28.

Berridge, M. J. (1987). Inositol trisphosphate and diacylglycerol: two interacting second messengers. *Annual Review of Biochemistry*, **56**, 159–93.

Berridge, M. J. and Irvine, R. F. (1989). Inositol phosphates and cell signalling. *Nature*, **341**, 197–205.

Blackshear, P., Nairn, A. C., and Kuo, J. F. (1988). Protein kinases 1988: a current perspective. *FASEB Journal*, **2**, 2957–69.

Bourne, H. R., Sanders, D. A., and McCormick, F. (1990). The GTPase superfamily: a conserved switch for diverse cell functions. *Nature*, **348**, 125–32.

Changeux, J. P., Devillers-Thiery, A., and Chemovilli, P. (1984). Acetylcholine receptor: an allosteric protein. *Science*, **225**, 1335–45.

Colbran, R. J., Schworer, C. M., Hashimoto, Y., Fong, Y. L., Rich, D. P., Smith, M. K., and Soderling, T. R. (1989). Calcium/calmodulin dependent protein kinase II. *Biochemical Journal*, **258**, 313–25.

Downes, C. P. and Macphee, C. H. (1990). Myoinositol metabolites as cellular signals. *European Journal of Biochemistry*, **193**, 1–18.

Gilman, A. G. (1987). G proteins: transducers of receptor generated signals. *Annual Review of Biochemistry*, **56**, 615–49.

Goelet, P., Castelluci, V. F., Schacher, S., and Kandel, E. R. (1986). The long and the short of long term term memory—a molecular framework. *Nature*, **322**, 419–22.

Hanks, S. K., Quinn, A. M., and Hunter, T. (1988). The protein kinase family: conserved features and deduced phylogeny of the catalytic domain. *Science*, **241**, 41–52.

Hopfield, J. F., Tank, D. W., Greengard, P., and Huganir, R. L. (1988). Functional modulation of the nicotinic acetylcholine receptor by tyrosine phosphorylation. *Nature*, **336**, 677–80.

James, G. and Olsen, F. W. (1990). Fatty acylated proteins as components of intracellular signalling pathways. *Biochemistry*, **29**, 2623–34.

Kikkawa, U., Kishimoto, A., and Nishizuka, Y. (1989). The protein kinase C family: heterogeneity and its implications. *Annual Review of Biochemistry*, **58**, 31–44.

Lefkowitz, R. J. and Caron, M. G. (1988). The adrenergic receptors: models for the study of receptors coupled to guanine nucleotide regulatory proteins. *Journal of Biological Chemistry*, **263**, 4993–6.

Levitzki, A. (1988). From epinephrine to cyclic AMP. *Science*, **241**, 800–6.

Lochrie, M. A. and Simon, M. I. (1988). G protein multiplicity in eukaryotic signal transduction systems. *Biochemistry*, **27**, 4957–65.

McGeer, P. L., Eccles, J. C., and McGeer, E. G. (1987). *Molecular neurobiology of the mammalian brain*. Plenum Press, New York.

Molinoff, P. B., Wolfe, B. B., and Weiland, G. A. (1981). Quantitative analysis of drug–receptor interactions: II Determination of the properties of receptor subtypes. *Life Sciences*, **29**, 427–33.

Nahorski, S. R. (1988). Inositol polyphosphates and neuronal calcium homeostasis. *Trends in Neurosciences*, **11**, 444–8.

Nairn, A. C., Hemmings, H. C., and Greengard, P. (1985). Protein kinases in the brain. *Annual Review of Biochemistry*, **54**, 931–76.

Neer, E. J. and Clapham, D. E. (1988). Roles of G protein subunits in transmembrane signalling. *Nature*, **333**, 129–34.

Nicoll, R. A. (1988). The coupling of neurotransmitter receptors to ion channels in the brain. *Science*, **241**, 545–51.

Rosenthal, W., Hescheler, J., Trautwein, W., and Schultz, G. (1988). Control of voltage dependent Ca^{2+} channels by G protein coupled receptors. *FASEB Journal*, **2**, 2784–90.

Simon, M. I., Strathmann, M. P., and Gautan, N. (1991). Diversity of G proteins in signal transduction. *Science*, **252**, 802–8.

Strange, P. G. (1988). The structure and mechanism of neurotransmitter receptors. Implications for the structure and function of the central nervous system. *Biochemical Journal*, **249**, 309–18.

Strange, P. G. (1988). The use of radiochemicals for studying receptors. In *Radiochemicals in biomedical research* (ed. E. A. Evans and K. G. Oldham) Critical Reports on Applied Chemistry, Vol. 24, pp. 56–93. Wiley, Chichester.

Weiland, G. A. and Molinoff, P. B. (1981). Quantitative analysis of drug–receptor interactions: I. Determination of kinetic and equilibrium properties. *Life Sciences*, **29**, 313–30.

Wileman, T. L., Harding, C., and Stahl, P. (1985). Receptor mediated endocytosis. *Biochemical Journal*, **232**, 1–14.

7 *Functional properties of neurones*

In the preceding chapters the properties and functional characteristics of individual neurones have been described in some detail. Neurones do not, however, function in isolation—the brain is composed of an enormously complex array of neurones organized in pathways, networks, and other regular groupings. It is this overall, organized set of neurones that gives the brain its tremendous power.

Given the present level of knowledge and technology it is not possible to provide anything other than very sketchy models of how groups of neurones might function together. Therefore this chapter presents a number of principles of neuronal organization that transcend studies on individual neurones. I hope that the reader can then begin to see how these principles might be employed in producing the overall activity of the brain. In Chapter 8 an attempt will be made to relate back from the known functions mediated by the brain to these organizational principles. In most cases in this chapter the organized systems of neurones are not described in great detail; the reader is referred to the general references at the end of the chapter for more detail. In a few cases, however, some detail is given so that other principles of neuronal function may emerge.

Networks and pathways formed by neurones

Two simple organizational principles can be stated based on the properties of neurones as already outlined. Neurones communicate with one another at synapses where chemical neurotransmission occurs. Thus the brain must contain networks of neurones communicating with one another. Within the networks, divergence can be seen when a neurone has a branching axon that can influence more than one postsynaptic cell at synapses. Alternatively, convergence can occur with more than one nerve terminal influencing one postsynaptic cell. These very simple ideas are illustrated in Fig. 7.1.

It is an oversimplification to imply, as Fig. 7.1 does, that the networks are formed by single neurones—generally there will be groups of neurones with similar organization. A set of neurones linking one part of the brain with another is often referred to as a neuronal pathway. This has already been illustrated in the case of dopamine neurones and dopamine pathways (Chapter 5). The pathways, the neurones they innervate, and

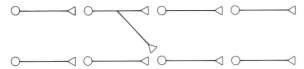

Figure 7.1 Simple networks formed by neurones. Neurones are shown forming synapses with adjacent cell bodies of other neurones. One neurone is shown with a branching axon so that it can affect two other neurones (divergence). One neuronal cell body is shown receiving two synaptic inputs (convergence). These synaptic inputs need not be the same sign so integration of signals occurs here (see Chapter 4 and discussion later in this chapter). The diagram is a gross over-simplification as neurones generally receive many hundreds of synaptic inputs (see Chapter 3) and neurones are often organized into pathways containing many similar neurones.

any interneurones involved in local processing must underlie the overall neuronal networks.

Regular groupings of neurones

Another organizational principle within the brain is that there are repeated regular groupings of neurones which are functionally important. These are apparent in certain brain areas such as the cerebral cortex, cerebellum, and striatum. The principles and their implications will be outlined below.

Microscopic examination of the cerebral cortex has shown that the neurones and nerve terminals contained in these brain regions are found in distinct layers (Fig. 7.2). Six layers are usually distinguished, labelled I–VI starting from the outside. On the whole, the layering is preserved throughout the cerebral cortex, and the cell types of the cerebral cortex (pyramidal and the group of cells collectively called stellate cells, Chapter 3) show similar distributions in the different layers. Pyramidal cell bodies are found in abundance in layers II, III, V, and VI, whereas stellate cells are found in all layers, but only in large numbers in layer IV. Different cortical regions, however, show different relative abundances of the different cell types so that the layering thicknesses differ and the over-all thickness and appearance of the cortical regions are different (Fig. 7.3). This is the basis for the divisions of the cerebral cortex defined by Brodmann (Chapter 2).

The basic cellular connectivity pattern of the cerebral cortex may be summarized as follows (Fig. 7.4). Inputs to the cerebral cortex arise from the thalamus (which acts as a kind of gateway for incoming sensory information) and from other parts of the cerebral cortex (cortico-cortical association fibres). Within the cerebral cortex are interneurones (the group of cells termed non-pyramidal or stellate cells with dendrites, cell bodies, and axons remaining in the cortex) which contribute to the local processing of information. The output pathways arise from pyramidal cells projecting their axons to either the thalamus, or to other parts of the cerebral cortex (association fibres), or to non-thalamic,

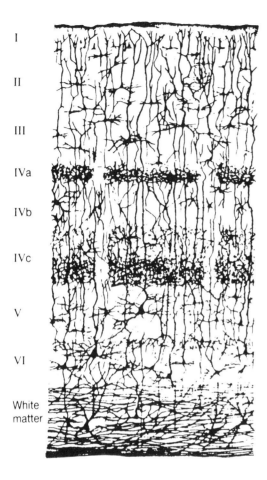

Figure 7.2 Cellular layering patterns in the cerebral cortex. The diagram shows the six layers of the cerebral cortex that are typically defined. Prominent stellate cells are seen in layer IV which is further subdivided; pyramidal cell bodies are seen in layers II, III, V, and VI. Taken from Rakic (1979) with permission.

non-cortical parts of the central nervous system (e.g. neostriatum (caudate nucleus, and putamen) and spinal cord). Inputs and outputs are segregated to certain layers. Thalamic inputs terminate mostly on stellate cells in layer IV, whereas inputs from other cortical regions terminate in several layers. Pyramidal cells in layers II and III provide cortico-cortical association outputs, whereas those in layer V provide non-thalamic, non-cortical outputs, and those in layer VI provide thalamic outputs.

The different layering patterns of different cerebral cortical regions (Fig. 7.3) can then be understood in the light of the function of the different regions. Sensory areas of the cerebral cortex, that is those receiving incoming sensory information, receive a large input from the thalamus terminating on the stellate cells in layer IV. Hence sensory areas such as the primary visual cortex have prominent stellate cells and layer IV is particularly prominent. The abundant stellate cell (granule cell) layer is responsible for the term 'granular cortex' applied to such a region.

In contrast, the primary motor cortex is involved in sending out information from the

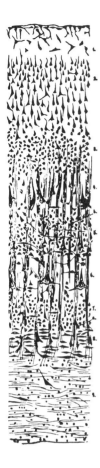
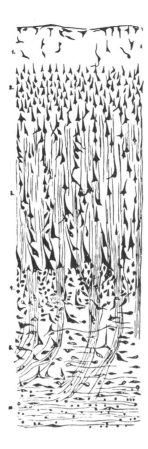

Figure 7.3 Cellular layering patterns in different regions of the cerebral cortex. On the left is shown a section through the visual cortex, a sensory region, showing the prominent stellate cells in layer IV. On the right is shown a section through the motor cortex with prominent pyramidal cells. Taken from Changeux (1985) with permission.

cerebral cortex and pyramidal cell layers including layer V (with large pyramidal cells projecting axons to the spinal cord) are particularly prominent, whereas the stellate cells (layer IV) are much less prominent. Association regions of the cerebral cortex, involved in linking information from different cortical regions, receive many inputs from other cortical regions and send many outputs to other cortical regions, and the layering pattern is intermediate between the two extreme examples cited above.

Therefore, whereas the layering and the distribution of cell types between the layers is a constant feature of all cerebral cortical regions, it is the thickness of the layers and the relative numbers of the cell types that differ from region to region. The number of each cell type in each layer is therefore determined by the function of the region concerned and the input and output requirements. Therefore, it is not the cell types themselves but their arrangements that determine and are determined by the function of the cortical region.

The existence of functionally different cortical regions is one example of the mapping of function in the brain, and as shown in Chapter 2, within a given cortical region there is even more discrete mapping of the body surface on to a particular cortical region, e.g.

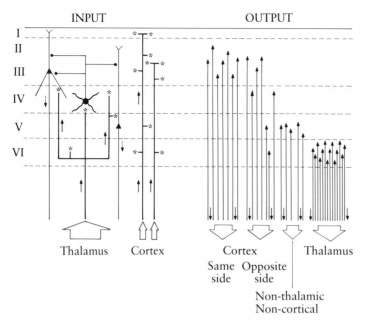

Figure 7.4 Principal inputs and outputs of the cerebral cortex. The diagram on the left shows the inputs from the thalamus terminating mainly on stellate cells in layer IV and inputs from other cortical regions terminating in several layers. On the right pyramidal cell outputs are shown from layers II and III to other cortical regions, from layer V to non-thalamic, non-cortical targets and from layer VI to the thalamus.

motor cortex or somatosensory cortex. This mapping is subdivided even further. Experiments with microelectrodes examining the cerebral cortex for more discrete functions have localized these functions to small units (Fig. 7.5). In the primary visual cortex, vertical slabs of cortex (0.25–0.5 mm wide) have been recognized to be associated with preference for one eye (ocular dominance) and along a slab, divisions about 50 μm wide have been recognized which are associated with the axis of the visual field. This corresponds to the angular orientation of bars or object edges to which the cells respond best. Within one vertical column all the neurones in the different cortical layers are associated with preference for one eye and one axis of visual field. The idea has evolved, therefore, that the cerebral cortex, as well as being organized into layers, is also organized into columns or modules; within each module the neurones are dedicated to a particular discrete function determined by the input or output pattern of that module. Similar columnar organization has been inferred in other cortical regions, for example in the somatosensory cortex (the region of the cerebral cortex involved in receiving sensory information from different parts of the body).

These columns of cells would then represent the basic processing unit of the cerebral cortex and would determine the smallest unit of information that can be received by the brain and hence sensed from the periphery. The columns will receive information from sensory organs via the thalamus, columns will be linked together via cortico-cortical association fibres, and there will be outputs from columns, for example to the thalamus. Although the cellular composition of columns will differ from region to region the

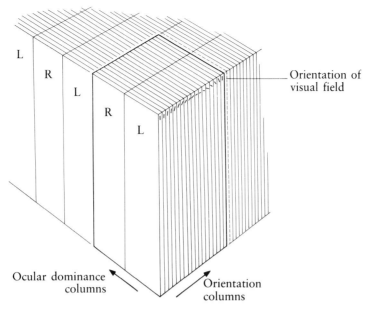

L

R

L

R

L

Orientation of
visual field

Ocular dominance
columns

Orientation
columns

Figure 7.5 Organization of the cerebral cortex into columns or modules. The diagram shows a small section of primary visual cortex and is based on information in Hubel and Wiesel (1979) and Kuffler *et al.* (1984). Along one coordinate axis there are alternating bands of cortex that respond to information from the right (R) or left (L) eye (ocular dominance columns). Along the other coordinate axis orientation columns are seen which respond to different orientations of the visual field. The actual patterns in the cerebral cortex are not as regular as this diagram implies but the general principles hold.

column can still be considered as the basic processing unit. In Chapter 8 a theory of consciousness is presented based on the function and linked circuits of these columns. Others have presented more complex theories of the arrangements of cortical neurones, see for example Changeux (1985). It has also been argued that the columnar arrangement does not exist throughout the cerebral cortex and the organization of neurones is more diverse, reflecting the diversity of function in the cortex (Swindale 1990).

An analogous but simpler layered structure is seen in part of the cerebellum, the cerebellar cortex, which forms the outer layer of the cerebellar hemispheres. Three principal layers can be discerned (Fig. 7.6). The outer layer is called the molecular layer, the intermediate layer the Purkinje cell layer, and the inner layer the granular layer. There is only one major output cell type, the Purkinje cell, which can be likened to the pyramidal cell in the cerebral cortex. The Purkinje cell has its cell body in the Purkinje cell layer and a widely branching dendritic tree in the molecular layer. Its dendritic tree is in one plane at right angles to the main axis of the cortex.

The granular cell layer is dominated by a very large number (about 10^{11}) of densely packed small neurones, mostly granule cells, although there are a few larger neurones

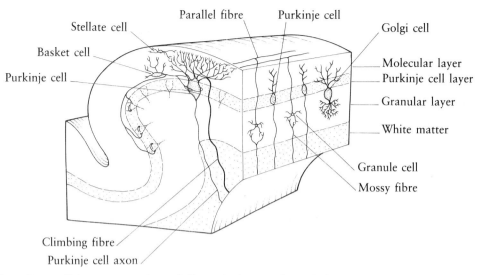

Figure 7.6 Cellular patterns in the cerebellum. The diagram shows the layering patterns in a section of the cerebellar cortex. The three layers (molecular, Purkinje, granular) are shown. The principal output cell is the Purkinje cell with its cell body in the Purkinje layer and its dendrites in one plane in the molecular layer. The granular layer has many granule cells and a few Golgi cells; granule cell axons are shown rising into the molecular layer to produce parallel fibres at right angles to the Purkinje cell dendrites and contacting them. The interneurones in the molecular layer are termed stellate and basket cells. Inputs to the cerebellar cortex are termed mossy fibres (terminating on granule cells) and climbing fibres (terminating on Purkinje cells).

called Golgi cells. Whereas the granule cell bodies are in the granular layer, their axons rise into the molecular layer where they produce extensions termed parallel fibres. These fibres run parallel to the axis of the cerebellar cortex and therefore have the ability to contact the dendrites of Purkinje cells. Although parallel fibres and Purkinje cell dendrites dominate the molecular layer, there are also a few interneurons called basket cells and stellate cells. Inputs to the cerebellar cortex are termed mossy and climbing fibres. Mossy fibres terminate on granule cells which in turn via their parallel fibres influence the activity of sets of Purkinje cells. Climbing fibres terminate on groups of Purkinje cells whose activity they control.

Thus in terms of their overall organization the cerebellar and cerebral cortices are similar in that they possess interneurones, input cells, and output cells, and the inputs and outputs are highly segregated to particular layers. Whether there is a modular organization in the cerebellar cortex is not clear, but the Purkinje cell bodies are found in regular repeating arrays so that this could be the case. It has been suggested that functionally distinct microzones, analogous to cerebral cortical columns, exist in the cerebellum (Ito 1984).

Another but different example of a regular arrangement of neurones is afforded by the neostriatum (caudate nucleus/putamen). The principal neuronal cell type, representing 95 per cent of the striatal neurones, is termed the medium spiny neurone because of its size and spiny dendrites (Fig. 7.7). These cells have a large dendritic tree and receive the majority of striatal inputs from the cerebral cortex (glutamate-containing cells), from the thalamus, from the substantia nigra (dopamine cells), and the raphe (5-hydroxy-tryptamine cells), and they also receive input from intrinsic striatal cells (Fig. 7.8). The medium spiny cells are also the output cells sending axons to the pallidal complex (globus pallidus) and substantia nigra (see Chapters 5, 10, and 11 for more discussion of this). There are also a number of intrinsic neurones (interneurones) within the striatum including a class of large aspiny cells that use acetylcholine as neurotransmitter. The neurotransmitter within the medium spiny cells is thought to be GABA though as will be described later, different populations of medium spiny cell exist with different peptide cotransmitters. Thus the striatal neurones follow the same overall organization as for the cerebral cortex and cerebellum, i.e. input cells, interneurones, and output cells. Given the large preponderance of medium spiny cells it should be clear that the function of the striatum will be dominated by these cells and later in this chapter I shall speculate about how these cells might function.

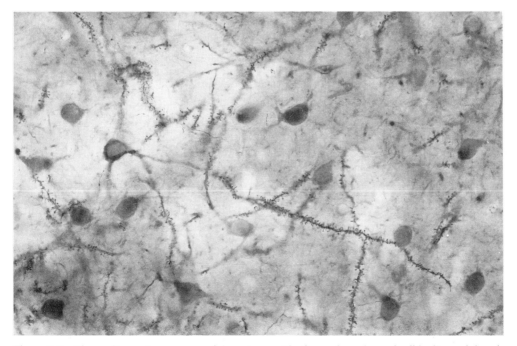

Figure 7.7   The medium spiny neurone of the striatum. The figure shows several cell bodies and densely spiny dendrites of medium spiny neurones in the caudate nucleus of the cat. By courtesy of Dr J. P. Bolam, University of Oxford.

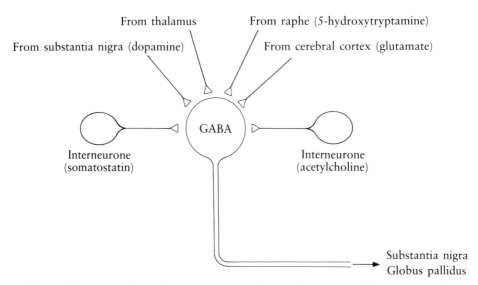

Figure 7.8 Cellular composition of the neostriatum (caudate nucleus/putamen). The principal cell type of the striatum is the medium spiny neurone (Fig. 7.7) which is characterized by the neurotransmitter GABA and a number of neuropeptides. The medium spiny cells are the main projection neurones of the striatum and receive inputs from extrinsic neurones as well as interneurones such as the aspiny cholinergic and somatostatin neurones. The diagram only shows the input and output relationships of the medium spiny cell—the dendrites have been omitted. Also omitted are inputs from axon collaterals of neighbouring medium spiny cells (see the text of this chapter for discussion of this and Chapters 10 and 11 for more details of the function of these neurones).

Domains have been found within the striatum termed striosomes and the extra-striosomal matrix (see also Chapter 5). These are somewhat irregular histochemically and neurochemically distinct compartments arranged in a three-dimensional array within the striatum. The striosomes are 100–500 μm across and are embedded in the much larger matrix (White 1989; Gerfen 1989; Graybiel 1990). Separate populations of medium spiny cells are found within each domain; each domain receives segregated inputs from different parts of the brain and sends outputs to different parts. Thus there are segregated parallel neuronal systems based on domain organization in the striatum. How this relates to the actual regularity of packing of cells, if at all, remains to be determined.

The striatum has an important role in controlling motor function. This will be considered further in the chapters on the movement disorders of Huntington's disease (Chapter 11) and Parkinson's disease (Chapter 10). Part of the information received from the cerebral cortex by the striatum is on the movements of different parts of the body. The innervation from the cerebral cortex to the striatum, which presumably carries this information on movement, is topographically organized and it has been shown that in the striatum groups of neurones may be recognized that are associated with the movement of particular parts of the body (Alexander and DeLong 1985). These groups of neurones may correspond to certain postulated subdivisions of the matrix (matrisomes, Graybiel (1990)) so that this would be a way of mapping the body on to the striatum. This mapping of the body on the striatum is reminiscent of the mapping already described for other brain regions and the striosome/matrix (and perhaps the matrisome) organization is reminiscent of the cortical column arrangement so that certain general principles of brain organization should be apparent.

Information flow within neuronal circuitry

Coding of information in neurones

In Chapter 3 it was shown that neurones possessed the unique property of electrical excitability and could propagate action potentials from the cell body along the axon to the nerve terminal. The action potential is the form in which information is transferred in the nervous system. It is, however, limited in its information content as it is an all or none signal, there being no possibility of fractions of an action potential. Therefore if quantitative information is to be coded in some way—and all kinds of quantitative information are required to be coded from different sensory organs and within the brain—then the quantitative information is coded in terms of the frequency of action potential propagation. This can be seen very easily for a peripheral system, the stretch receptor of a muscle spindle. These stretch receptors report the degree of stretch in muscle spindles and are important for the control of posture. Sensory axons from the stretch receptors relay information to the spinal cord (in terms of action potentials) and increasing stretch in the muscle spindle gives rise to greater frequencies of action potential propagation down the sensory axon. Similar principles hold in the central nervous system but we need to remember that most central neurones have a spontaneous level of firing impulses (action potentials) (Chapter 4) which can either be increased or decreased according to the inputs received by the neurone. Here the ability of neurones to integrate different inputs needs to be taken into account.

Integration by neurones

Individual neurones may receive hundreds or thousands of synaptic inputs from nerve terminals. Each of these inputs will have some effect on the target neurone; an integration of the input strengths takes place at the neuronal cell body and the frequency of action potential firing at the axon hillock is modulated accordingly (Chapter 4). It is possible to discern four qualities of the inputs to a neurone that can affect the input strength (Fig. 7.9).

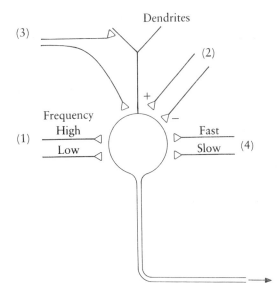

Figure 7.9 Different kinds of input to neurones and their integration. The diagram illustrates the different qualities of the inputs that may affect a single neurone. (1) Firing frequency in the synaptic input may vary and the amount of neurotransmitter released will vary accordingly. (2) The signs of the synaptic inputs may be different. (3) The inputs to the neurone may be spatially different—axodendritic or axosomatic. (4) The neurotransmitter may be fast or slow acting. The neurone then integrates these inputs over time (1 and 4), by sign (2), and spatially according to the membrane properties of the cell (3) and action potentials are fired by the neurone according to the membrane potential at the axon hillock.

1. The *frequency* of action potential firing in synaptic inputs may differ. Although the arrival of a single action potential may lead to the release of a small amount of neurotransmitter and hence a small postsynaptic electrical change, repetitive firing of action potentials will lead to the release of more neurotransmitter and hence give rise to a more substantial postsynaptic effect. The greater the frequency of action potential firing in the input neurone the greater will be the neurotransmitter release and postsynaptic effect. Action potentials arriving at a presynaptic terminal will therefore tend to have a cumulative effect on the membrane potential of the postsynaptic cell. Hence a temporal summation is made of the activity due to a single nerve terminal and also the electrical activity due to the many inputs impinging on a single neurone.

2. The *signs* of inputs may be different. The different nerve terminals impinging on a neurone may release excitatory neurotransmitters which will tend to depolarize the neuronal membrane or inhibitory neurotransmitters which will counteract the depolarization. A summation of the signs of the inputs to a neurone will therefore be made.

3. The inputs to a neurone may be *spatially* different. Inputs to a neurone may be on the dendrites (axo-dendritic) or directly to the cell body (axo-somatic). Both these kinds of inputs are spatially separate from the part of the neurone where new impulses are generated. This is the axon hillock (Chapter 4) which is especially susceptible to firing action potentials. The axon hillock will fire action potentials at a particular basal rate when its membrane is depolarized below the threshold. The influences that will alter its depolarization state and hence its firing rate will be the inputs, excitatory and inhibitory, to the neurone. A single excitatory input to the cell body will cause a small depolarization that will spread some distance from the synapse by setting up local circuit currents

(Chapter 4) dying away as it does. Several excitatory inputs will reinforce one another and the depolarization may spread sufficiently to alter the membrane potential and hence the firing rate of the axon hillock. It can be seen that an excitatory input to a dendrite may be much less effective than one to the cell body as it will have further to spread. Inputs to the dendrites may be boosted by special dendritic trigger zones which are locally excitable regions of the dendritic tree that can boost the spread of a depolarization by firing action potentials. These behave in much the same way as the nodes of Ranvier on a myelinated axon (Chapter 4).

For inhibitory inputs, spatial considerations again are important. Inhibitory inputs to the cell body are more effective at controlling axon hillock activity than those to the dendrite for the same reasons discussed above. In fact, as noted in Chapter 3, many inhibitory synapses are axo-somatic. An axo-dendritic inhibitory synapse may, however, be particularly suited for influencing a nearby excitatory axo-dendritic input. These interactions between different inputs to a dendrite may frequently occur on dendritic spines which could be considered as local processing units of the dendritic tree (Fig. 7.10). Whether an excitatory input to a spine gains access to the main dendritic tree and hence the cell body, will depend on the presence and activity of a local inhibitory input. We shall see examples of this later in this chapter when the function of the cells in the striatum are discussed. Thus at the level of the whole cell body and at the level of the spine, a spatial summation of the inputs occurs.

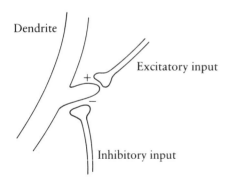

Dendrite

Excitatory input

Inhibitory input

Figure 7.10 Dendritic spines as integrators of neuronal activity. A dendritic spine is shown receiving an excitatory input to the spine head and an inhibitory input to the spine neck. The inhibitory input is well placed to control access of the excitatory input to the main dendritic tree. Clear examples of this kind of arrangement are seen in the striatum (see also Fig. 7.15) where the excitatory input is glutamatergic and the inhibitory input is dopaminergic or GABAergic and in the cerebral cortex where dopamine inhibits an undefined excitatory input to spines (Freund *et al*. 1984; Goldman-Rakic *et al*. 1989).

4. The *time courses* of the post-synaptic effect of the neurotransmitter from different inputs may be different. This discussion has so far neglected a further feature of neuronal responses, considered in more detail in the next section, namely the response times for different neurotransmitters. All the types of integration described above have referred to interactions between fast excitatory and inhibitory neurotransmitters. There will also be influences from slow neurotransmitter based systems and these are likely to have a more global excitatory, inhibitory, or modulatory effect on large numbers of fast synaptic inputs.

In summary then, integration of all these different inputs occurs and the membrane of the axon hillock senses the resultant net membrane potential (postsynaptic potential) and fires action potentials accordingly. Three aspects of the integration can be stressed. First there is integration of the excitatory and inhibitory influences. Secondly there is spatial integration dependent on the position of the input on the neurone. Thirdly there is temporal integration dependent on the frequency of inputs and their duration. These factors determine the frequency of action potential firing from the axon hillock. Some of these points will be exemplified in the discussion of circuitry below.

Neuronal circuits within the brain

In Chapter 6 the properties of receptors were discussed in some detail. A clear structural and functional division was made into fast (fast ion channel linked) and slow (G-protein linked) receptors. Although the speed and efficiency of synaptic transmission must depend upon a number of factors, a critical event is the combination of neurotransmitter and receptor with the outcome that synapses dependent on slow receptors are likely to act more slowly than those dependent on fast receptors. The former synapses are therefore likely to be involved in longer term effects. A helpful distinction can therefore be made between fast circuits based on fast synapses and fast receptors and slow circuits based on slow synapses and slow receptors. There is some support for such a distinction from functional and anatomical considerations and the properties of the two types of circuitry will be outlined below.

Fast circuits

These are neuronal circuits based on synapses with fast ion channel linked receptors. In the mammalian brain they do not show great complexity in terms of the neurotransmitters involved. The principal fast excitatory neurotransmitter is glutamate (or aspartate) and the principal fast inhibitory neurotransmitter is GABA. Acetylcholine (acting at nicotinic receptors) and glycine play only minor rather circumscribed roles. Within the cerebral cortex there is evidence that the neurotransmitter used by pyramidal cells is glutamate whereas many interneurones (stellate cells) use GABA—it has been estimated that up to 30 per cent of the total neuronal population in the cerebral cortex is GABAergic. Similarly in the striatum the main input to the principal cell type, the medium spiny cell, is from glutamate neurones in the cortex and the medium spiny output cells themselves use GABA as a neurotransmitter.

Therefore we can envisage a major network of fast circuits within the mammalian brain based on glutamate (excitatory) and GABA (inhibitory). Although this is chemically rather simple it is anatomically very complex and the functional power must derive from the anatomical complexity. These fast circuits cooperate with and are modulated by slower circuits (Fig. 7.11). Although there are long axoned GABA neurones many GABA neurones are interneurones and participate in feedback loops of various kinds; an example of this principle is shown in Fig. 7.12.

Slow circuits

These are neuronal circuits based on synapses with slow (G-protein linked) receptors and are chemically much more complex than fast circuits owing to the large number of neurotransmitters acting via this type of receptor. The slower time course of these circuits means that they are likely to be involved in longer term modulatory events: an example of this is given in Chapter 6 for the modulation of the excitability of the hippocampal pyramidal cell. Depolarization of these cells leads to opening of voltage-sensitive Ca^{2+} channels in the axon hillock region and the consequent rise in intracellular Ca^{2+} concentration has two effects. Firstly, it leads to opening of fast voltage and Ca^{2+} dependent K^+ channels that are important for membrane repolarization after the action potential (Chapter 4). Secondly the Ca^{2+} leads to opening of slow Ca^{2+} dependent K^+ channels that are important for hyperpolarizing the membrane and limiting action

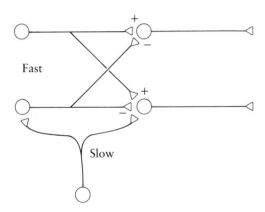

Figure 7.11 Fast and slow circuitry in the mammalian central nervous system. The diagram shows fast circuits based on excitatory (largely glutamate) and inhibitory (largely GABA) neurones modulated by a slow neurone. The circuitry depicted is in an idealized form for illustrative purposes only.

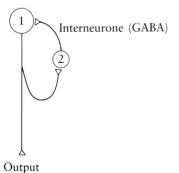

Figure 7.12 Role of GABA-containing neurones in feedback inhibition. Firing in neurone 1 will lead to output along its axon as well as a self-limiting feedback inhibition via the axon collateral and the inhibitory GABA interneurone 2. This is a simplified version of interrelationships in the hippocampus where neurone 1 is a pyramidal cell and neurone 2 a basket cell.

potential firing in response to sustained depolarizations. Stimulation of slow acting receptors on the same cells, for example adrenergic receptors that raise cAMP levels, leads to phosphorylation and inhibition of the slow Ca^{2+} dependent K^+ channels. The membrane is not hyperpolarized and a brake is taken off action potential firing (Nicoll 1988).

Later in this chapter a further example of modulation by slow circuitry will be considered in which the neurotransmitter dopamine suppresses the basal firing rate of a neurone so that it can be more responsive to its inputs. This can be seen as an enhancement of the 'signal-to-noise ratio' in the system. Noradrenaline is thought to act in a similar manner in some systems, as are other slow neurotransmitters (Foote and Morrison 1987; Robbins and Everitt 1987; McCormick 1989).

These are examples of modulation of the electrical excitability of cells. There are other possibilities for slow modulation including alteration of the amount of neurotransmitter released from one nerve cell by a slow modulation from a second terminal via pre-synaptic receptors at an axo-axonic synapse. The effects of the slow neurone could also be to cause changes in receptor phosphorylation and hence the rate of desensitization (see Chapter 6). These possibilities are outlined in Fig. 7.13. Longer term alterations in synaptic function are likely to be important for the mechanisms of laying down of memory.

If the distinction between fast and slow circuits is to hold, then it is important that in fast circuits the conduction time of impulses, which in turn is dependent on the conduction velocity and axonal length, does not limit the performance of the system. In general it seems that the properties of the neurones in fast systems guarantee conduction

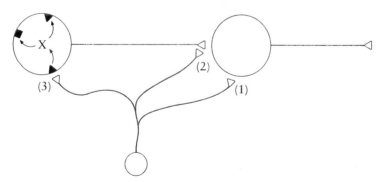

Figure 7.13 Possible effects of slow neurotransmitters. A neurone depending on a slow neurotransmitter is shown having effects on other neurones. The effects may be (1) to alter the membrane potential of a neurone so that its firing rate is altered; (2) to alter the amount of neurotransmitter released from a nerve terminal via an axoaxonic synapse (via heteroreceptors—see Chapter 5); (3) to alter the concentration of a second messenger (X) within the cell body which will in turn alter the phosphorylation state of other proteins such as receptors, affecting their rate of desensitization or turnover, or ion channels, affecting the membrane potential and the cell firing rate (as in 1).

times less than or comparable to the neurotransmitter–receptor delays, that is in the region of a few milliseconds. This is achieved by having unmyelinated axons that conduct sufficiently rapidly over a short distance or myelinated fibres that conduct very rapidly over longer distances. For example, in the rat corticostriatal glutamate pathway, the unmyelinated fibres conduct at about 10 m s^{-1} with a conduction time of a few milliseconds (Jinnai and Matsuda 1979; Wilson 1986; Bauswein *et al*. 1989) whereas in longer pathways, e.g. the pyramidal tract, axons of these glutamate neurones are myelinated and conduction occurs at much higher velocities (30–50 m s^{-1} (Bauswein *et al*. 1989)).

By contrast, conduction velocity may not be as important for the slower circuits as these will be limited in their performance by the neurotransmitter–receptor delay. There are indeed examples of neurones containing the neurotransmitters acetylcholine, dopamine, noradrenaline, and 5-hydroxytryptamine where the axons are thin and often unmyelinated with conduction velocities of the order of 0.5 m s^{-1} that lead to conduction times in the rat of the order of 50 ms (Guyenet and Aghajanian 1978; Foote *et al*. 1983; Foote and Morrison 1987; Moore and Bloom 1978). In other, larger species, however, the greater axon length demanded by the larger brain may require higher conduction velocities if axonal conduction time is not to limit the performance of the neurone. Indeed in species such as the monkey there is a tendency for neurones to be myelinated, these same neurones being unmyelinated in the rat (Azmitia and Gannon 1983; Aston-Jones *et al*. 1985). In one study of the same noradrenergic neuronal population in rat and monkey, conduction velocities were about 0.5 m s^{-1} in rat but 1 m s^{-1} in monkey (Aston Jones *et al*. 1985). The result of these differences is that the conduction time in the two species is very similar despite the longer distances to be travelled by impulses in the larger species. This suggests that at least in this pathway the conduction time is important for the functioning of the animal and it is conserved among species by modification of the neuronal properties. In summary, the properties of the neurones are adjusted to fulfil their function be it fast or slow transmission.

The speed of the release process for the neurotransmitter is unlikely to limit the performance of either fast or slow circuits. Where this has been measured (see Chapter 5), it occurs in a few milliseconds. There are, however, suggestions that release of neurotransmitters, presumably mostly neuropeptides, from large synaptic vesicles is slower than that from small vesicles (see Chapter 5) (De Camilli and Jahn 1990). Whether this will limit the function of the, already, slower system is unclear.

Some slow circuits have also been shown to exhibit anatomical features not seen in fast circuits. These slow circuits arise from localized groups of neuronal cell bodies which send axons to reach targets some distance away and there is extensive divergence (branching) so that a relatively small group of cell bodies can affect a much larger target area. Although there are well defined nerve terminals and synapses, the branching axons sometimes have varicosities containing neurotransmitter within their target area. Thus there is some resemblance to the postganglionic autonomic neurons of the periphery although in the brain conventional synapses are formed by both the terminals and varicosities and the terminals are often topographically organized in a precise fashion rather than being randomly distributed.

Extreme examples of this arrangement are provided by the monoamine neuro-transmitters noradrenaline and 5-hydroxytryptamine (Fig. 7.14). Neurones containing these neurotransmitters form localized groups of cell bodies that produce widely branch-ing axons that fan out to affect very large and diverse areas of brain. They are thus ideally suited to modulate function in large areas of brain and it is thought that noradrenergic and 5-hydroxytryptamine systems may play a role in the control of arousal and attention (Robbins and Everitt 1987) (see also Chapters 14 and 15 for a discussion of the role of these systems in the actions of certain psychoactive drugs). Despite the widely branching nature of the axons, it has been shown that the nerve terminals are not randomly distributed—for example in the cerebral cortex they are found only in certain of the cellular layers (Foote and Morrison 1987; Parnevalas and Papadopoulos 1989). As indi-cated above, it is currently thought that wherever there is a nerve terminal or varicosity, this forms a conventional synapse. This point has been discussed earlier in Chapter 5 in relation to dopamine neurones. For 5-hydroxytryptamine neurones there are some reports of terminals or varicosities without synapses (Herve *et al.* 1987; Soghomonian *et al.* 1988; Seguela *et al.* 1989) although in other studies, synapses are routinely found (see for example Parnevalas and Papadopoulos 1987). It seems best at present to assume that wherever there is a terminal or varicosity there will be a synapse but a further question here concerns the possible leakage of neurotransmitter from the synapse to receptors not located at that synapse. I have discussed this before and will return to it later in relation to Parkinson's disease (Chapter 10).

Dopamine neurones are also located in restricted groups of cell bodies and have

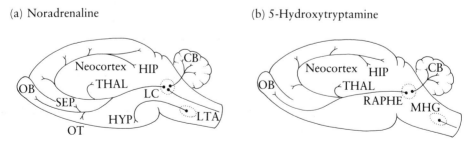

(a) Noradrenaline   (b) 5-Hydroxytryptamine

Figure 7.14 Principal neuronal populations containing the neurotransmitters noradrenaline and 5-hydroxytryptamine. The diagrams illustrate the widely branching nature of these neuronal systems. (See also Fig. 12.7). CB, cerebellum; HIP, hippocampus; HYP, hypothalamus; LC, locus coeruleus; LTA, lateral tegmental area; OB, olfactory bulb; OT, olfactory tubercle; MHG, medullary 5-hydroxytryptamine group; SEP, septum; THAL, thalamus.

branching axons, but the terminal fields are more restricted than for the other mono-amines and there is a topographical arrangement between the groups of cell bodies and their target areas (see Chapter 5). For cholinergic neurones that innervate the cerebral cortex, there is also innervation of large areas of the cerebral cortex from a fairly restricted part of the lower brain (see Chapter 12 for more discussion of this). Again there is a topographical relation between groups of cell bodies and their terminal fields (Foote and Morrison 1987) with little evidence of the multiple branching seen in adrenergic and 5-hydroxytryptamine neurones. For other slow neurotransmitters the information on pathways is less complete but there is evidence of multiple branching systems in some cases, e.g. histamine and some neuropeptides.

As well as being very diverse chemically, based on large numbers of slow acting neuro-transmitters, the slower circuits also show some diversity in their time courses. This is partly due to differences in the receptor mechanisms; it has been shown in Chapter 6 that whereas all these receptors are linked via G-proteins to their effectors, if the effector is an ion channel then the response occurs in a few hundred milliseconds whereas for an enzyme effector (e.g. adenylyl cyclase, or phospholipase C) the response is much slower (seconds to minutes). Also, however, the duration of the signal produced may be dependent on the speed of removal of the neurotransmitter from the synapse. For peptides this seems to be quite slow, so peptide responses can last longer than classical monoamine responses. These time courses should all be compared with those of the fast (class I) linked systems where the response occurs in a few milliseconds.

The large differences in time scale between the fast and slow circuits seems likely to mean that on the whole, processing of information can occur in the fast circuits independently of the slow circuits which then modulate the fast circuits. If information processing depended on a mixture of fast circuits and slow circuits, the performance of the overall network would be reduced to the speed of the slow circuits. The slow circuits dependent on ion channel linked receptors could, however, participate in some form of processing alongside the fast circuits as their time courses do not differ as radically.

In the later chapters on brain diseases, an important issue will be the ability to treat the disease by altering neurotransmitter action. Where there is a clear deficit of a neuro-transmitter, e.g. in Parkinson's disease (Chapter 10), then replacement of the deficient neurotransmitter is a possible strategy for drug therapy. Owing to the different functional properties of slow (modulatory) and fast (phasic and strictly time dependent) circuitry this is likely to be a viable course of action only for the slow circuitry. For the slow circuits a fixed level of agonist provided by the therapy may be satisfactory whereas for fast circuits this can never provide the rapid time dependent pulses of agonist necessary. This may account for the success of this approach for Parkinson's disease where a slow neurotransmitter (dopamine) deficit occurs (Chapter 10). For Alzheimer's disease (Chapter 12), where both cortical glutamate (fast) circuits and cholinergic (slow) circuits are deficient, it seems less likely that replacement will be possible.

The situation may be rather different where there is no actual loss of neurones, rather there is some kind of subtle functional alteration. In these cases, a drug that modulates either a fast circuit (e.g. antianxiety drugs) (Chapter 15) or slow circuit (e.g. antidepressant) (Chapter 14) may be useful.

Details of an electrical circuit in the central nervous system

Earlier in this chapter some of the cell types and cellular interactions for neurones in the cerebral cortex, cerebellum, and striatum were outlined. Although some of the details of cellular behaviour in these brain areas are becoming clearer, it is not yet possible to draw complete circuit diagrams owing to the cellular complexity. This must, however, be a goal of future studies. For the striatum, however, we can make a reasonable start as it is dominated by a single type of cell.

The principal neuronal cell type of the striatum, as discussed earlier, is defined by its morphology and is termed the medium spiny neurone owing to the size of its cell body (10–20 μm) and the abundant dendritic spines (Fig. 7.7). The medium spiny cells have been estimated to represent 95 per cent of the striatal cells and have a large dendritic tree (250–300 μm in diameter) and an axon projecting from the striatum forming the major output pathway. The axon also gives rise to local branches that contact other medium spiny cells (axon collaterals). Although medium spiny cells are morphologically rather homogeneous they may not be chemically so. The principal neurotransmitter expressed by the cells is GABA but it is likely that different peptides are coexpressed, e.g. substance P, enkephalin. It has recently been shown that there are separate populations of neurones containing GABA/substance P or GABA/enkephalin (Anderson and Reiner 1990). This chemical heterogeneity is not important for our present discussion but emphasizes the organization of the striatum into separate compartments as discussed earlier. In Chapter 11 it will be shown how a knowledge of these different populations of striatal neurones may be important for understanding the neuropathology of Huntington's disease.

The major input to the medium spiny cells (Fig. 7.8) comes from the cerebral cortex (glutamate containing cells); this input is topographically organized and rapidly conducting. In addition there is an important input from the substantia nigra (dopamine mesostriatal pathway). There are other inputs to the medium spiny cells that are less well characterized, including those derived from the thalamus and some interneurones (see Fig. 7.8). Cortical inputs primarily form asymmetric (type I) synapses on to dendritic spines whereas mesostriatal dopamine inputs are by symmetric synapses (type II) on to both dendritic spines and interspine shafts with a few inputs on to cell bodies (Figure 7.15). There are many instances of dendritic spines receiving both of these inputs with the cortical input to the spine head and the mesostriatal input to the spine neck. This arrangement suggests some kind of local interaction (see Fig. 7.10).

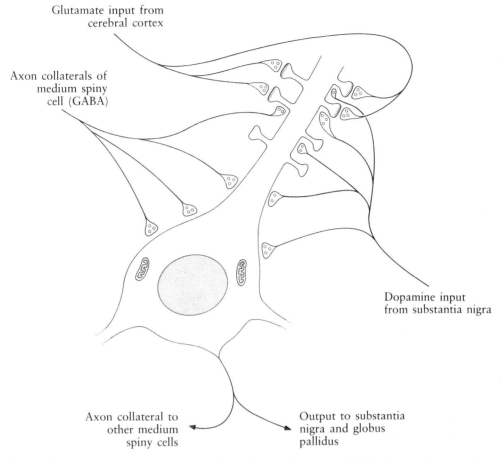

Glutamate input from
cerebral cortex

Axon collaterals of
medium spiny
cell (GABA)

Dopamine input
from substantia nigra

Axon collateral to
other medium
spiny cells

Output to substantia
nigra and globus
pallidus

Figure 7.15 Detailed neuronal connections for a striatal medium spiny cell. The diagram shows a medium spiny cell with its spiny dendrites, cell body, and output axon with axon collateral. Inputs from the cerebral cortex (glutamate, excitatory), axon collaterals (GABA, inhibitory), and substantia nigra (dopamine) are shown. The interactions of cortical inputs and nigral or axon collateral inputs to dendritic spines (Fig. 7.10) and neighbouring regions are shown. .

Local axon collaterals make symmetric synapses, also on to dendritic spines and interspine shafts but increasingly on proximal regions of the neurones, that is on or near the cell body. Again there are many examples of dendritic spines receiving inputs from the cerebral cortex and a local axon collateral and the arrangement of the two inputs is similar to that outlined above with the cortical input to the spine head and the collateral input to the spine neck. Thalamic inputs are via asymmetric synapses on to dendritic shafts and it is thought that thalamic and cortical inputs are on to separate populations of medium spiny cells that may nevertheless communicate via their overlapping dendritic fields or via axon collaterals. The relation of this form of heterogeneity in the medium spiny cell population to other forms of heterogeneity described earlier is unknown.

Having outlined the circuitry we may begin to make some suggestions about the function of the circuitry; this discussion will be restricted to the cortical inputs. These cortical inputs are excitatory, being dependent on glutamate as neurotransmitter, and lead to rapid depolarization of the medium spiny neurones. The excitation causes medium spiny neurones to fire action potentials which in turn leads to an inhibitory output (because GABA is their neurotransmitter). Action potentials firing in local axon collaterals will inhibit neighbouring medium spiny cells which will have the effect of focusing information patterns from the cerebral cortex. Thus a more diffuse input pattern from the cerebral cortex will tend to be sharpened by the collateral inhibition, with the stronger parts of the input pattern diminishing the weaker parts. The inhibition by axon collaterals will occur at the level of the cell body, interspine shafts, and spine necks. In the latter case it will have a particularly potent effect on the cortical input, effectively controlling access of the cortical signal to the dendritic tree.

The dopamine input will have a different functional consequence as it is a slow system and so is likely to perform some modulatory role over the essentially fast actions of glutamate. It has been suggested that an important role of the dopamine input is to reduce the basal firing rate of the medium spiny neurones so that when they are excited this excitation may be distinguished as a larger increase in firing rate; the 'signal-to-noise ratio' is increased. There are dopamine synapses on medium spiny neurone cell bodies and dendritic shafts consistent with this idea. The large number of synapses on to the necks of dendritic spines that also receive a cortical input to the head means that the mesostriatal dopamine innervation can have a selective control on the cortical input regulating (inhibiting) its influence on the cell excitability. The fact that some cortical inputs are on to spines that do not receive a dopamine input suggests that the meso-striatal dopamine pathway may control the pattern of cortical input to the striatum, selectively suppressing certain parts of it. Therefore dopamine may have a selective effect on cortical input via synapses on to dendrites and a more general effect via synapses on to cell bodies and dendritic shafts. A similar interaction between a symmetric dopamine synapse and an as yet uncharacterized asymmetric synapse on to dendritic spines has been described in the cerebral cortex (Goldman-Rakic *et al.* 1989) suggesting that this arrangement may be a general means for dopamine to control excitatory inputs to neurones.

Thus dopamine can have two broad effects on the medium spiny cells of the striatum. It may facilitate signal transmission through the cells by altering the 'signal-to-noise ratio' for excitatory inputs and it may very selectively inhibit inputs on to dendritic spines. Also there appear to be different subclasses of dopamine receptor (D_1, D_2) on different populations of striatal medium spiny cells (Gerfen *et al.* 1990). These ideas can account for the stimulatory and inhibitory effects of dopamine that have been described functionally on different cell populations in the striatum (Albin *et al.* 1989). This point will be discussed further in Chapters 9 and 10.

Although we only have a rather rudimentary idea of the circuitry involved, this discussion has highlighted important principles of brain circuitry e.g. collateral inhibition of neighbouring cells, integration at the level of the spine, and modulation to improve signal detection, and we can begin to see how a neuronal network might function.

The overall flow of information in the brain and within the regions of the cerebral cortex

In previous sections it has been established that within the cerebral cortex, distinct regions may be discerned associated with discrete functions and having different cellular layering patterns but basically similar structures overall, for example the primary somatosensory cortex, which receives primary body sensory information, the visual cortex, and the motor cortex. Within these regions the body surface is mapped, often several times, reflecting the neurones projecting to or from the cortical region (Chapter 2). This mapping of the body surface may be traced to columns or slabs of neurones in the cortex as discussed above. Whereas for many cerebral cortical regions a clear function can be assigned, there are three broad regions of the cerebral cortex to which no simple function can be attached. It was thought that these were involved in associating information from the sensory areas and so they have been termed 'association' cortices. I shall now attempt to sketch the flows of information into the cerebral cortex and out again and the key role of association regions (Fig. 7.16).

Information from the sensory organs such as the eyes, ears, and nose about our environment is sent to the cerebral cortex via the thalamus which acts as a kind of relay station. There are also maps of the body surface in the thalamus similar to those described earlier in the cerebral cortex so that incoming sensory information is topographically organized. The neurones for one particular sense terminate in one or more primary cerebral cortical regions, e.g. primary somatosensory cortex or primary visual cortex. These primary cortical regions in turn project to one or more higher order cortical regions which may also receive their own projections from the thalamus directly, e.g. secondary somatosensory cortex and posterior parietal cortex (sensory). The information in the higher order cortical regions is still associated with the particular sense but whereas in the primary area there is a fairly clear map of the body surface, in the higher order areas there is a more complex representation of the sensory information as processing has occurred in the primary region. An important principle should be apparent which is of separate parallel processing of information from the sensory organs via the thalamus to primary and thence to higher order cerebral cortical regions associated with that sense.

Sensory input

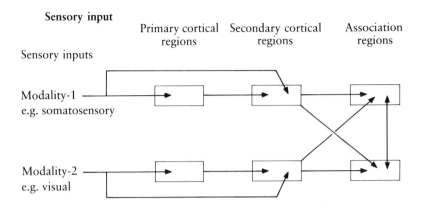

Motor function

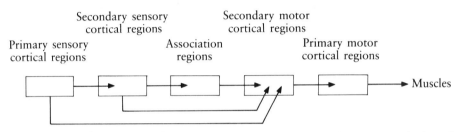

Figure 7.16   Flows of information within the cerebral cortex. For clarity the diagram omits 'backwards' connections between different regions. In the upper diagram, for each sensory modality there are separate primary and secondary cortical regions e.g. primary somatosensory cortex, secondary somatosensory cortex.

The higher order cerebral cortical regions then project neurones to the association areas of the cerebral cortex (Fig. 2.9). These are the prefrontal cortex, the parietal–temporal–occipital cortex, and the limbic cortex and are involved in our highest order brain functions. The prefrontal cortex is involved in cognitive function and motor planning, the parietal–temporal–occipital cortex is involved in higher sensory function and language, and the limbic cortex (which includes the cingulate and parahippocampal gyri, the tip of the temporal lobe (temporal pole or polar temporal cortex) and the orbital surface of the frontal lobe) is involved in emotion and memory. Parts of the limbic cortex will be important for later discussions of mental disorders (Chapters 13, 14, and 15). The three association cortices are also interconnected. The above discussion of association regions is a gross simplification of their functions and in subsequent chapters more specific aspects of their function will be highlighted. In a simplistic way, however, we can see that from the parallel sensory inputs to the brain a representation of the world around us is made, this will include the blending of sensory information in the association cortices. The actual representation of the sensory information will depend on the activities of large numbers of neurones in several sensory cortices and the association cortices. In Fig. 7.16 the principal flows of information in the somatosensory and visual pathways are outlined in order to illustrate the ideas outlined above.

Some experimental support for these proposals comes from studies on cerebral blood flow during various activities. Cerebral blood flow can be monitored by using a radio-tracer (xenon gas) (see Chapter 9 for more details of these measurements)—increases in blood flow in particular brain regions are thought to reflect increased neuronal activity in that brain region (Lassen *et al*. 1978). Figure 7.17 shows some of the experiments which show that for particular sensory inputs, the primary cortical regions associated with that sensory modality are especially activated, e.g. the auditory cortex for listening to speech, although there is always activity throughout the brain with a bias towards the frontal lobes. If the subject is asked to read silently, then several cortical regions including visual areas but also higher cortical regions are active. When the subject is asked to perform certain mental tasks, areas outside the primary sensory and motor cortices are activated. This includes some association regions, particularly the prefrontal cortex, which as

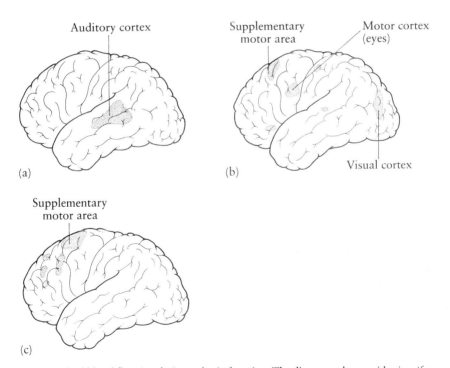

Figure 7.17 Cerebral blood flow in relation to brain function. The diagrams show a side view (front to the left) of the brain and the regional blood flow measured using radioactive xenon gas (Lassen *et al*. 1978). Shading indicates areas of increased bloodflow and presumed cortical activity. In (a) the subject listened to speech, in (b) the subject read silently and in (c) the subject performed a mental operation.

suggested above is important for cognitive function (Roland *et al.* 1987). It should be emphasized that these studies do not show that only the areas highlighted are active during the task. Many areas will be active but the highlighted areas will be especially so.

The sensory-association circuitry is also connected with sub-cortical brain regions and this is important for such functions as emotion in its cognitive and autonomic realization. Thus the limbic association cortex is connected with the hippocampal formation and the hypothalamus, the latter being particularly important for the central and peripheral realization of emotion.

As well as functioning to receive incoming sensory information, the cerebral cortex is important for initiating action, for example motor behaviour. Analogously to the organization of sensory cortices, both primary and higher order motor cortices have been recognized. Once the decision to perform a motor operation has been made—this presumably is a function of the association cortices—the execution of the movement requires the cooperation of three regions of the cortex, the higher order motor regions of the premotor and supplementary motor cortices (this latter region is important for planning of movement), and the posterior parietal cortex (which supplies important sensory information). These regions then project to the primary motor cortex which together with the higher order motor cortices instructs muscles appropriately. As well as this cerebral cortical control of movement there is important participation of subcortical structures. These are the cerebellum and the neostriatum (caudate nucleus/putamen). These structures have been referred to a number of times already and will be covered in more detail in the chapters on the two brain diseases of motor function, Parkinson's disease and Huntington's disease (Chapters 10 and 11).

The activities of brain areas during motor tasks have been examined using the cerebral blood flow technique outlined above; Fig. 7.18 shows some experimental data. In the study shown, the subject was asked to speak aloud, with the result that the mouth–tongue–larynx areas of the motor and somatosensory cortex, the auditory cortex, and the supplementary motor area showed increased activity. The auditory and somatosensory cortices are responding to sensory input, the motor cortex is involved in instructing muscles, and the supplementary motor area is important for planning movement.

It should be apparent that the motor control system in the cerebral cortex is organized similarly (albeit in reverse order) to the sensory systems with primary, higher order, and association regions in a hierarchical relationship. Fig. 7.16 summarizes the flows of information. Before leaving this discussion of the flow of information in the cerebral cortex it is important to make the point that as well as 'forward' connections there are also 'reverse' connections between different cortical areas and between the cerebral cortex and thalamus. These in principle allow for the backward flow of information and the comparison with input information. This feature will be taken up again in Chapter 8.

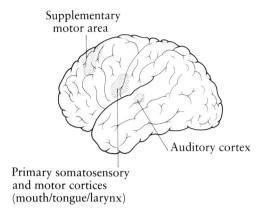

Supplementary
motor area

Auditory cortex

Primary somatosensory
and motor cortices
(mouth/tongue/larynx)

Figure 7.18 Cerebral blood flow in relation to brain function during motor tasks. The technique is the same as in Fig. 7.17. The subject was asked to speak aloud.

Artificial neural networks

The complexity of the connections within the brain is so great as to be overwhelming and may render it difficult ever to understand completely how neural circuitry functions. An alternative and fruitful approach is afforded by modelling of brain-like circuitry through computer simulation or hardware implementation in so called neural networks. I shall call these artificial neural networks to distinguish them from the biological (natural) neural networks which are the main subject of this chapter. A detailed discussion of artificial neural networks is beyond the scope of this book but it is hoped that the next few paragraphs will give the reader a sense of the kind of strategies that are being used and the information that can be obtained. For more details the reader should refer to the general references at the end of the chapter.

Artificial neural networks are composed of 'units' or 'neurones' modelled in hardware or software that are meant to represent neurones and do indeed assume many of the properties of biological neurones. The units are often organized into layers (Fig. 7.19) and units in each layer are connected to units in the next layer. Often every unit in one layer is connected to every unit in the next layer. Thus the networks are highly interconnected as in biological neural networks. The connections between units then represent axons and synapses and the input of one unit into another is given a 'strength' that represents an amalgam of some of the qualities of synaptic interactions described earlier, for example sign of input, or frequency of firing. Each unit then receives a number of inputs and an integration of these inputs takes place. The unit then generates an output ('firing rate') that is often a graded function of the integrated input. These operations are all expressed as defined mathematical functions of the inputs.

The strengths of the connections between units (the 'weights') can be altered in order to adapt or 'train' the network. In a 'supervised' learning scheme this can occur when an external operator (or 'teacher') adjusts the connection strengths in order to match more

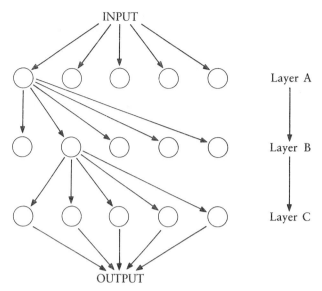

Figure 7.19   Artificial neural network. The network consists of units (circles) which represent neurones and have similar properties. The network is realized on a computer. Units are arranged in layers and units in one layer are connected to the units (often every unit) in the next layer: only some of these connections are shown in the diagram for clarity. Each input to a unit is given a 'strength' and each unit performs an integration of all its input strengths and then assumes an output activity ('firing rate') which is related to the integrated input strength. The connection strengths can be altered by the operator or according to a learning rule such as the Hebb rule described in the text.

closely the output of the overall network with a desired output (see below). This situation does not seem to be relevant to the brain, where learning occurs spontaneously with experience so that training can be said to be 'unsupervised'. Thus alternative 'unsupervised' schemes have been devised whereby the connection strengths alter according to a pre-specified rule. Frequently this depends on increasing the connection strength if an input and output to a unit correlate and decreasing the strength if these do not. This is termed a Hebb rule after the neuropsychologist Donald Hebb, who first suggested it as a learning principle in a slightly different form.

Therefore the artificial neural networks have many similarities to real neural networks and 'units' assume many of the properties of real neurones. Some key properties of real neurones are, however, sometimes ignored. For example, the spatial and temporal consequences of axo-dendritic versus axo-somatic inputs to a neurone are not usually considered. In some networks a branched output from a single unit can have positive and negative effects at its different 'terminals'. Despite these caveats, artificial neural networks can have striking capabilities and may give us insights into the real networks. This is a very active area of current research; some examples of what has been achieved, are given below.

Zipser and Andersen (1988) have developed a three-layered network that can be 'trained' to model the properties of certain cerebral cortical neurones (Fig. 7.20). The network models the behaviour of neurones in the posterior parietal cortex that represent the spatial location of objects using information on the retinal location of a visual stimulus and the position of the eyes when looking at the object, contained in separate populations of cortical neurones. The model network is trained by presenting retinal and eye position data to the first layer of units. This layer is connected to the second 'hidden' layer which in turn connects to the third outer (output) layer. The outer layer of units

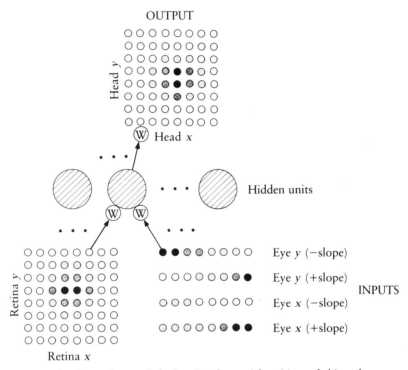

Figure 7.20 An artificial neural network for locating the spatial positions of objects from eye and retinal coordinates (Zipser and Andersen 1988). The network attempts to model the ability of certain neurones in the posterior parietal cortex to represent the position of objects in relation to the head of an animal given input information on the spatial position of the eye and on the coordinates of the object on the retina. In the artificial network there are two sets of input units, representing the coordinates (x and y) of the object in relation to the retina and the position of the eye. These feed in to a 'hidden layer' of units which are analogous to the neurones in the cerebral cortex that can represent spatial position. These hidden units in turn feed to output units that actually contain the representation of the coordinates of the object (x and y) in space relative to the animal's head. Each input and output unit connects to each 'hidden' unit. The network was 'trained' by giving it randomly selected pairs of input eye positions and retinal positions. The connection strengths or weights (w) of the different units are altered in order to match the desired output (spatial position of object) with the achieved output. The diagram is modified from Zipser and Andersen (1988) with permission.

contains a representation of the spatial location of the object. The actual and desired output are compared and the error is used to 'back-propagate' information to the hidden layer changing its properties (connection strengths). The data are presented to the first layer again and the properties of the hidden layer altered until an appropriate correspondence with the desired output is achieved. Two interesting conclusions emerge. First, the network can be used to model the performance of the cortical cells quite accurately. Secondly, the 'hidden' units in the second layer adopt properties, that is relative firing rates, similar to those seen in the cortical neurones. Thus there is a striking congruence between the natural and artificial neural networks. It must be said, however, that in the human brain, training of the network of neurones, i.e. learning, cannot take place by the method described here for the artificial network. There is no evidence for systems that compare desired and actual outputs in the human brain; instead learning seems to depend on the presentation of information and its retention in some form. This is an unsupervised process in that there is no external adjusting of connection strengths to achieve desired results; the real network learns independently. Recently it has been suggested that there may be error-detecting neurones in the brain that could participate in this learning process (Barinaga 1990).

Because of this fundamental difference between this type of artificial network, in which connection strengths are altered to achieve a desired output, and real neuronal networks, other kinds of 'unsupervised' networks have been examined. For example, Linsker (1988, 1990) has devised networks with multiple layers, each layer being richly interconnected with the next layer (Fig. 7.21). The network is not designed to implement any particular task, rather random information is presented to the first layer and then propagated through the different layers. With repeated presentations of information to the top layer of units, the connection strengths to deeper units alter spontaneously according to a Hebb rule: the connection strength is increased if the input and output of a unit correlate and decreased if they do not. With such a multilayered network and repeated presentation of information, the units in the third and subsequent layers gradually adopt organizational properties that are similar to the modular arrays of neurones in the mammalian visual system that were described earlier. If these results are of relevance to biological neural networks, they suggest that, given certain constraints, the network could 'self-organize'. This could have important implications for the development of regular neuronal patterns such as the cortical modules described earlier.

Furthermore, a network of this kind can 'learn' to recognize certain patterns of input activity and so could act as a pattern recognition device. The 'learning' would consist of repeated presentation of the pattern that is desired to be recognized, the connection strengths between units altering accordingly. Certain units in deep layers of the network will then be maximally activated by the learned pattern and the network will then be able to recognize it and distinguish it from other different patterns.

Rather different kinds of artificial network have been described which can actually

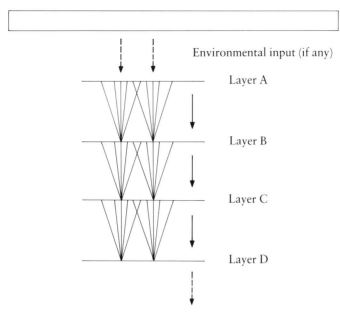

Figure 7.21 Self-organizing model neural network (after Linsker 1986*a*,*b*,*c*). The network contains several layers of units connected to units in the next layer in a feed-forward manner. In the diagram several units in one layer are shown connecting to one unit in the next but each unit in one layer also connects to several units in the next. Not all units are interconnected but a spatial restriction is placed on the extent of interconnectedness—in practice this means that one unit in for example layer A connects only to units in layer B in spatial proximity. A 'learning' rule applies in that input connection strength is increased if input and output activity to a unit correlate. Presentation of random information to layer A causes units in deep layers to organize in to particular patterns of activity as described in the text.

undergo unsupervised learning. These are called adaptive resonance theory (ART) networks (Carpenter and Grossberg 1988, 1990). The details of these are beyond the scope of this book but the networks are able to store patterns of activity related to inputs to the system. Subsequent presentation of new input patterns leads to a comparison being made between the input pattern and the stored patterns. If a match is detected between the input and a stored pattern then reinforcement (resonance) occurs. Such mechanisms are attractive for the function of recognition strategies in the human brain where a comparison may be made between the pattern of electrical activity due to the present input state and some pattern stored in memory (Chapter 8). In the model ART networks, an important role is assigned to so-called 'gain control' systems which could be model counterparts of the slow neuronal systems described earlier.

The main impetus for constructing artificial neural networks is their use as novel, powerful computational devices. Already, however, it seems that important information about the brain may be emerging from a study of these artificial neural networks so that the neuroscientist should not dismiss them as mathematical curiosities. As artificial networks are constructed with units that resemble more and more the properties of actual neurones, then increasingly useful information should emerge.

Recommended reading

Crick, F. (1989). The recent excitement about neural networks. *Nature*, **337**, 129–32.

Foote, S. L., Bloom, F. E., and Aston-Jones, G. (1983). Nucleus locus cereuleus: new evidence of anatomical and physiological specificity. *Physiological Reviews*, **63**, 844–914.

Gerfen, C. R. (1988). Synaptic organisation of the striatum. *Journal of Electron Microscopy Technique*, **10**, 265–81.

Goldman-Rakic, P. S. (1988). Topography of cognition: parallel distributed networks in primate association cortex. *Annual Review of Neuroscience*, **11**, 137–56.

Graybiel, A. M. (1990). Neurotransmitters and neuromodulators in the basal ganglia. *Trends in Neuroscience*, **13**, 244–54.

Hubel, D. H. and Wiesel, T. W. (1979). Brain mechanisms of vision. *Scientific American*, **241**(3), 130–44.

Iversen, L. L. (1984). Amino acids and peptides: fast and slow chemical signals in the nervous sytem? *Proceedings of the Royal Society of London B*, **221**, 245–60.

Jones, E. G. (1986). Neurotransmitters in the cerebral cortex. *Journal of Neurosurgery*, **65**, 135–53.

Kandel, E. R. and Schwartz, J. H. (1985). *Principles of neural science*. Elsevier, New York.

Linsker, R. (1990). Perceptual neural organisation: some approaches based on network models and information theory. *Annual Review of Neuroscience*, **13**, 257–81.

McGeer, P. L., Eccles, J., and McGeer, E. G. (1987). *Molecular neurobiology of the mammalian brain*. Plenum Press, New York.

Mountcastle, V. B. (1978). An organizing principle for cerebral function: the unit module and the distributed system. In *The mindful brain* (ed. G. M. Edelman and V. B Mountcastle), pp. 7–50. MIT Press, Cambridge.

Pandya, D. N. and Seltzer, B. (1982). Association areas of the cerebral cortex. *Trends in Neurosciences*, **5**, 386–90.

Rumelhart, D. E. and McClelland, J. L. (1986). *Parallel distributed processing: explorations in the microstructure of cognition*, Vol. 1. MIT Press, Cambridge, MA.

Shepherd, G. M. (1988). *Neurobiology*. Oxford University Press, New York.

Sjenowski, T. J., Koch, C., and Churchland, P. S. (1988). Computational neuroscience. *Science*, **241**, 1299–306.

Smith, A. D. and Bolam, J. P. (1990). The neural network of the basal ganglia as revealed by the study of synaptic connections of identified neurones. *Trends in Neurosciences*, **13**, 259–65.

Strange, P. G. (1988). The structure and mechanism of neurotransmitter receptors. *Biochemical Journal*, **249**, 309–18.

Strange, P. G. (1990). Role of the mesostriatal dopamine pathway. *Trends in Neuroscience*, **13**, 93–4.

Young, J. Z. (1987). *Philosophy and the brain*. Oxford University Press.

Zeidenberg, M. (1990). *Neural network models in artificial intelligence*. Ellis Horwood, Chichester.

8   *The mind–body problem*

Science explained people, but could not understand them. After long centuries among the bones and muscles it might be advancing to knowledge of the nerves but this would never give understanding.

E. M. Forster, *Howards End*

In this chapter the difficult issue of the mind–body problem is considered. This basically concerns the relationship between mental function and the physical brain. It is important to do this as several disorders of the brain will be discussed in subsequent chapters. In many of the disorders there are changes in mental function and it will be important to have a basic framework for rationalizing how it is possible to account for normal mental function in terms of the activities of neurones. In this way it will be possible to account for changes in mental function in terms of changes in neuronal function. Therefore this chapter stands at the interface between the descriptions of basic neuronal properties in the previous chapters and the subsequent descriptions of brain disorders.

So, what is the mind–body problem? Here again the role which the brain plays in bodily function needs to be considered. First, the brain performs a controlling role over bodily function, for example the control of muscle contraction, hormone secretion, metabolism, and many other basic functions. This can be considered in terms of a set of mechanistic regulatory biochemical mechanisms. Secondly, however, there are aspects of brain function, particularly well developed in humans, that do not fit so easily into these kinds of mechanistic descriptions, at least at first sight. These are aspects such as consciousness of self and surroundings, thinking, formulation of plans and intentions, feeling, emotion, memory, etc.; these are collectively referred to as our mind. The contrast between the 'mind' aspects of the brain and the more mechanistic description of brain function can generate a problem. The contrast between 'mind-type' descriptions and mechanistic or 'body-type' descriptions of the brain has taxed philosophers for thousands of years and has come to be called the mind–body problem. The reader should refer to the general references at the end of the chapter for other discussions of this problem.

The position of the author, which was outlined in Chapter 1, is that the functions of the brain, collectively termed the mind, derive from and may be equated with the overall function of the set of nerve cells in the brain as described in previous chapters. I shall attempt to provide a theory for this later in this chapter but first it will be necessary to give some historical background. Resolution of the mind–body problem is one of the greatest challenges to current science and the problem is also important for our subsequent discussions of brain disorders as outlined above.

Historical view of the mind–body problem

From the earliest speculations on the nature of man until the present day, one strongly held view is that the mind and body are separate, distinct entities. Hypotheses of this kind are termed dualist hypotheses of brain function and state that the body and in particular the physical brain can be viewed mechanistically but that the mind is some entity with different or undefined physical character which cannot be treated in the same way. In early theories the mind was seen as synonymous with the soul, forming an integral part of the prevailing religious culture. For example, Plato (about 400 BC) took a dualist view separating soul and body and in addition divided the soul into three parts, the intellectual, irascible, and concupiscable parts.

The most clear statement of a dualist hypothesis, however, comes from Descartes (Fig. 8.1) who in 1637 put forward ideas that have permeated philosophical views right up to the present day. He proposed that we have a physical body which behaves like a machine and a soul which is a totally separate kind of substance. For Descartes, the

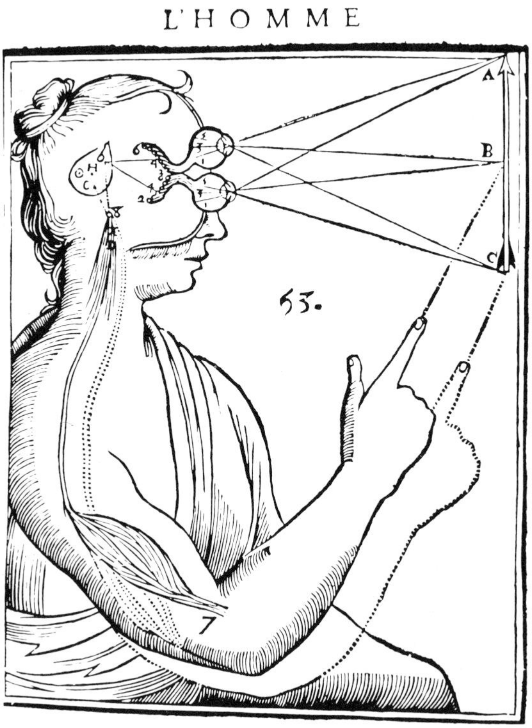

L'HOMME

Figure 8.1 The mind–body problem as seen by Descartes in his *Treatise of Man* (1664). Descartes proposed that the pineal gland (the pear shaped object in the centre of the head) was the site of interaction between the soul and the brain. Sensory information, here from the eyes, is conveyed to the brain and thence to the muscles by means of 'animal spirits' in nerves. The movement of animal spirits is also detected by and can be altered by the soul in the pineal gland. In this way the soul (mind) can influence muscular activity based on sensory information.

pineal gland in the brain was the site of interaction between the soul and the physical body, allowing the soul to exert control over the body. The separation of soul/mind from body was important at the time as it freed scientists to work on the mechanical body without violating the 'religious' soul. Subsequently others have propounded dualist ideas with the mind being associated with the brain; despite the inability to define the properties of the separate soul/mind in terms of known physical forces, dualistic hypotheses are still vehemently espoused. Sherrington, the eminent neurophysiologist, stated in the earlier part of this century 'that our being should consist of two fundamental elements offers I suppose no greater inherent improbability than that it should rest on one only' (Sherrington 1906). In the last few years the eminent philosopher, Popper, and the neuroscientist Eccles have maintained a strong dualist hypothesis (Popper and Eccles 1977). Their 'mind' is separate from the physical brain although it interacts with the brain and exerts control over it. No proper description is given of the physical properties of the 'mind', however. Nevertheless, it is clear that some individuals, including well respected scientists who have made major contributions to the understanding of basic brain function, have problems in reconciling the 'mind-type' aspects of brain function with the physical nature of the brain and so they have propounded dualist hypotheses of brain function.

As alternatives to these dualist ideas, a group of hypotheses termed monist hypotheses have been proposed. These propose that the only entity that exists is the physical brain and that its properties are sufficient to account for all the functions of the brain, both 'mind-type' and 'body-type'. There is therefore no need to split mind and body and no need to postulate a separate, nebulous entity to account for the mind. Some monist theories have gone so far as to deny the existence of 'mind-type' aspects of brain function but this is not a necessary prerequisite of monist theories. Rather, we can propose that the 'mind-type' activities of brain do exist and are an integral part of human existence but they derive from the total activity of the nerve cells in the brain which have been described in earlier chapters.

Monist theories can be found as early as the ancient Greeks, for example Democritus (about 400 BC) spoke in terms of psychic atoms responsible for thought. Hobbes (1651), writing in response to Descartes, proposed a monist philosophy of mind and body and with the increase in basic scientific knowledge about the brain, together with the advent of Darwinian ideas on natural selection (in the late nineteenth century), monist theories have gained in importance.

Extreme versions of monist philosophy have denied either the existence of the mind (stating that all 'mind-type' aspects of brain function are explicable in behavioural terms) or its importance (stating that the 'mind-type' aspects of brain function are a by-product of the function of the mechanistic brain). To deny the 'mind-type' aspects of the brain is, however, to deny a large part of human existence, for example creativity, thinking, emotion, and other specifically human attributes.

There are, though, modern monist theories that allow for the 'mind-type' aspects of the brain; these can be broadly termed 'identity' theories. These state that the 'mind-type' aspects are a reflection of the mechanistic aspects and a result of them. The total activity of the complex network of cells in the brain results in the 'mind-type' aspects of brain function. Therefore every 'mind-type' process must have a corresponding correlate in terms of nerve cell activity however complex that may be. In this way mechanistic and 'mind-type' descriptions of brain function are descriptions of the same neural activity but at different levels. This is the position taken by me and outlined in Chapter 1. These kinds of theories are satisfactory in that they explain all the aspects of brain function that have been outlined previously without invoking any mysterious entity with ill-defined properties. It is perhaps fair to say, however, that there is a major gulf in terms of properties between the 'mind-type' and mechanistic aspects. It is this gulf which supports and encourages dualist hypotheses. Those who subscribe to monist hypotheses, however, should only recognize the gulf and attempt to bridge it with theories that can show how the total activity of brain cells can give rise to the 'mind-type' aspects. I shall attempt to bridge this gulf later in this chapter.

There are three further important points that should be mentioned before concluding this section. The first point concerns a preoccupation of some philosophers over whether knowledge about the world around us is achieved only through our senses, as suggested by Hume and Locke, or whether knowledge can be obtained by thought alone as suggested by Leibnitz. The philosopher Kant took a middle path and postulated that the knowledge we have which structures our lives depends on our senses (sensibility) and our thoughts (understanding). By this view the sensory information we receive can be influenced by our thoughts so that our view of the world (as depicted by our sensory apparatus) is dependent on the way our thoughts operate on sensory information and thus on the way our brain processes are patterned. As will be shown, it is likely that the brain is designed to detect certain critical features in the environment and so we may be structuring our view of the environment around us on the basis of the apparatus detecting it. Therefore the 'reality' we perceive is very dependent on the structure and function of our brains.

The second point concerns the existence of the conscious and unconscious. Freud proposed that much of our existence depends on unconscious thoughts and drives. This implies that there is substantial brain activity that does not reach the level of conscious awareness but which nevertheless may have an important role in overall brain function and may influence conscious processes. The existence of the unconscious provides an extra dimension to the 'mind-type' aspects of brain function and should be taken into account in any all-embracing theories of brain function.

The third point concerns the relationship of the mind–body problem to approaches to brain disorders. Discussions of such philosophical ideas may seem very distant from both the previous descriptions of neurones and the clinical and neurochemical descriptions of brain disorders to follow. Nevertheless, the implicit or explicit stance of an individual over the mind–body problem can strongly influence their approach to brain disorders which are, after all, disorders of mind and body. A dualistic splitting of mind and body may lead to an unnecessary emphasis on either mind or body in theories and treatments of brain disorders. A monist approach that denies the importance of 'mind-type' brain functions is equally damaging and either approach has encouraged many western clinicians to rely heavily on psychoactive drugs in the treatment of brain disorders to the exclusion of other therapies. It seems to me that a proper account must be taken of both the mind and body aspects of brain function as derived from the total activity of the neurones in the brain in the description and treatment of brain disorders. I shall show how this is important in the subsequent chapters.

A hypothesis for mental function

This section presents a summary of a way to look at the functions of the human brain that is consistent with the general thinking in this book. The choice of the title of this section was deliberately 'a hypothesis for mental function' rather than 'a hypothesis for the mind' to emphasize that I am seeking to account for a series of functional properties rather than aiming to describe an entity or thing.

It is proposed that the brain functions in terms of the four descriptive levels presented in Chapter 1. Thus there is the overall physical brain containing an exceedingly complex network of nerve cells functioning chemically and electrically. The overall function of this, as well as controlling bodily homeostasis, is to give rise to brain functions such as consciousness, intentions, memories, etc. which together comprise mental function. Every mental state is in principle analysable in terms of, and equivalent to, a state of activity of the nerve cells. I see no convincing evidence for additional forces or properties that might suggest the existence of some other entity.

So, how do we put together a hypothesis to describe the totality of human brain function? How do we satisfy and eliminate dualist hypotheses of brain function and derive consciousness, thought, and memory out of a network of brain cells? The approach suggested is based on treatments of this problem provided by Edelman and Mountcastle (1978), Changeux (1985) and Edelman (1987).

The theory proposed here depends on the properties of neurones as outlined in the preceding chapters. Quite recently, Penrose (1989) has suggested that quantum mechanical (probabilistic) principles need to be applied to the functions of the overall neuronal network in the brain in order to understand the mental functions of the brain. He has proposed that a new theory of physics will eventually be required to understand brain function. Although I have treated neurones and neuronal interconnections as defined and definable entities, it seems likely that when there are so many inter-connections between neurones, some kind of probabilistic descriptions of their activities may be appropriate. For example, if a neurone receives hundreds or perhaps thousands of synaptic inputs, it seems likely that the functional output states of that neurone may be achieved by more than a single input configuration. If this argument is extended to the overall brain then it is suggested that brain function may have some probabilistic character.

A coded representation of the world

Our sensory systems, e.g. sight, hearing, and touch, function to transmit information via the thalamus to the primary regions of the cerebral cortex associated with each sensory modality. The information from each sense is processed and transformed within the primary cortical region and passed on to the other secondary cortical regions connected with that sense (see Chapter 7). Further processing and transformation occur and eventually information is passed on to the association areas of the cerebral cortex where it is integrated with all the other incoming sensory information. In this way we make a representation of the world around us in the activities of millions of neurones in the brain.

Our picture of the world around us is dependent on our senses and the way the sensory information is processed by the brain systems. In Chapter 2 it was shown how information coming from certain areas of the body is better represented on the sensory areas of cerebral cortex than information from other regions. Thus we may detect certain features of the world better than others. This is true for example in both vision and hearing where we can detect only certain wavelengths of light and only certain frequencies of sound. We may also have a special ability to detect specific aspects of the world, for example faces, and the structures of our brain may reflect this. As well as providing detection of specific features in the external world, the detailed structure of our brains is also likely to be important in the development of certain faculties. For example, Chomsky has suggested that we have a special ability to acquire language—if so then this must reflect brain structure, and the structures of languages that we develop must also reflect in some way this brain structure. Therefore our picture of the world is dependent both on our sensory apparatus and on the brain pathways that process the information outlined earlier. This very much parallels the ideas of Kant on sensibility and understanding. Fodor (1983) has argued recently that the brain contains separate parallel modular input systems for analysis of sensory information. These then feed in to what he calls central systems in which the parallel input channel architecture is lost. In terms of our discussion here and in Chapter 7, these input systems would correspond to the primary cerebral cortical regions associated with a sensory modality whereas the central systems would correspond to the association cortical regions.

It is important to emphasize that in interacting with the world we receive sensory information and form a representation of the world based on that sensory information. Because of the limitations of our sensory detection equipment and because the sensory information is transformed by our brains, whose structure will be dependent on our genetic character and our previous experience, the 'reality' that we perceive will be something we ourselves construct on the basis of sensory input but heavily dependent on brain processing.

The information derived from sensory input is contained in the electrical and chemical activities of millions of cells in the cerebral cortex. As described earlier (in Chapter 7), each region of the cerebral cortex is composed of modules or units of cells with many interconnections both within and between modules. Therefore our sensory image of the world is contained in an electrical/chemical pattern of activity in many cortical modules in different regions of the cerebral cortex. It seems likely that information from different sensory modalities is processed and passed from one cortical region to another with some information finally converging on the association areas. Therefore different regions of the cerebral cortex cooperate with one another and with the association areas and together contain some kind of coded representation of the sensory input and hence the world. Although there may be a funnelling of information, the actual information derives from and is dependent on very large proportions of the cerebral cortex. Although definitive experimental support for such a scheme cannot be provided, the results of mapping of brain function are not inconsistent with these ideas. Such experiments depend on determining cerebral blood flow as an index of cerebral (neuronal) activity; the results outlined in Chapter 7 show that large areas of brain are active at all times with particular areas especially active under certain circumstances. The results support the idea of separate modular sensory input systems and the activation of higher order brain areas, especially association areas, when more complex tasks are performed.

We may, therefore, view the brain as a highly sophisticated information processing device capable of making a coded representation of the world around us at any one time. It is important to realize that I am not suggesting that the brain contains a kind of snapshot of the external world, but that the brain contains some representation of the sensory input in electrical/chemical signals. This idea will now be used to account for consciousness, memory, thoughts, and emotions.

Learning and memory

The idea of the brain as simply an information processing device is not sufficient to explain all brain function, as learning and memory are both key features. Therefore the cortical modules must have the ability to be modified in such a way as to store information in a readily retrievable form. How this is done is not understood but presumably it involves an alteration in the strength of synaptic interaction between and within modules (the reader is referred to the recommended reading for further discussion).

I suggest, therefore, that from birth, and probably before birth, we receive information and learn to associate certain patterns in the cortical modules with certain features of the external world. These patterns can be stored in some way so that they can be recognized as familiar. For example, the faces of our mother and father must be entities that we see frequently from birth and must create specific patterns in the cortical modules which are then stored on a permanent basis. Thus we quickly begin to recognize them as familiar. The emotions associated with being fed or cherished will add extra emphasis to the storage of these patterns and their recognition. Also, as we learn language we are able to apply a label to the faces and the recognition of the stored pattern. In this way by learning from birth we are able to recognize external features of the world by virtue of the concordance of the cortical module pattern with stored ones.

The idea invoked above, that emotion may be important in the laying down of memory, will be elaborated later. What, however, is emotion, and how are emotional feelings generated? It is generally considered that the parts of the brain collectively referred to as the limbic system together with certain cerebral cortical regions (e.g. limbic association cortex, Chapter 7) are responsible for emotion. If we take an emotion such as pleasure, then it seems likely that at least in part this must result from the conjunction between the planned and the actual outcomes of events. Thus the cerebral cortex must be involved in planning a course of action (see below) and comparing this with the actual outcome. Conjunction must activate cortical–limbic pathways which then feed back to the cortex and generate a part of the feeling of pleasure. Activation of the limbic system will also lead to activation of the autonomic nervous system, giving the typical peripheral responses associated with emotions. An alternative example is anxiety, which seems to reflect the anticipation of some unpleasant, unwanted, or threatening situation. Recognition of these kinds of situation by the brain leads to the feeling of anxiety (realized via the limbic system) which is associated with peripheral signs such as increased heart rate, sweating, etc. as well as the central manifestation of the feeling of anxiety. In Chapter 15 anxiety will be discussed in more detail.

Consciousness of self and of the world

In attempting to provide a rationalization for consciousness in terms of the model proposed earlier, an additional property of the cortical modules will be invoked. As described in Chapter 7, the cortical modules have very rich forward and backward interconnections with one another and also with the thalamus. Thus there is extensive potential for the formation of looped circuits away from an individual cortical module and back to the cortex. This then provides the possibility for what has been termed re-entry. This refers to a process whereby the information contained in terms of electrical patterns in the cortical modules at a particular instant can be cycled and re-entered alongside the information pattern an instant later. This enables in principle some kind of comparison to be made between the present information pattern derived from present sensory inputs and the pattern obtained an instant previously.

Therefore, I am suggesting, as have others, that we are continually making a representation of the world in terms of a pattern of electrical activity in the cortical modules. The present pattern can be compared with that obtained an instant previously which has been placed in the cyclical looped pathway. Such a comparison between the present pattern and that seen an instant earlier might give a mechanism for generating consciousness of one's place in the world. If we then add to this the ability to store permanently and retrieve previous patterns of information which represent previous portions of our existence and the possibility that this stored material can be used by re-entry for comparison with present information, then consciousness of self might also be generated.

Thinking

On the whole, the kind of electrical patterns in the cortical modules that have been considered so far have been based largely on external sensory input. They are, as described, coded representations of the external world.

These cannot, however, be the only kinds of patterns that are possible as a major part of our brain activity seems to be in terms of ideas, imagination, thinking, and formulating plans. Although these functions may be based on previous sensory experience and may lead to generation of behaviour and interaction with the world, in themselves they usually have little actual sensory component.

These functions, therefore, must be associated with the patterns of information stored in the cortical modules and based on our previous experience. The generation of ideas, imagination, thoughts, etc. must entail the generation of new patterns of electrical activity in the cortical modules. It has been suggested that this occurs by selection of new patterns from large pre-existing subsets of patterns. If so then the new patterns generated or selected must be modelled on or dependent on previous patterns. These previous patterns will be stored ones which are in turn dependent on previous experience. In addition it seems likely that there may be intrinsic 'rules' for generating new patterns of information based on the way the brain is put together. This must be the case as our thoughts are frequently structured in a fairly productive way. Thinking is also an active process so there must be an active generation or selection of new patterns.

On this kind of hypothesis, early experience, which will correspond to periods of rapid brain development when remodelling of precise neuronal connections can occur, must be critical in the laying down of early memories and behaviour patterns. In particular it seems likely that the emotions associated with early experience will influence significantly the degree to which these early experiences are stored in memory. It is likely, however, that throughout our lives, events linked with strong emotions will be more strongly retained in our memories but this has particular significance during early experience while the brain connections are still being laid down.

This may mean, therefore, that events which occur early in our lives and which are associated with strong emotion may influence our subsequent behaviour patterns. We can rationalize this at a neuronal level by suggesting that specific patterns of electrical activity are stored strongly during an early phase of our lives. The generation or selection of new patterns of electrical activity within the cortical modules may then be influenced by these patterns stored at an early stage. Importantly, we are likely to be generally unaware of these (unconscious) influences. Thus our overt behaviour may be the result of external sensory input, conscious thought, and unconscious influences.

The end result of these processes is the generation of a new pattern of electrical activity in the cortical modules. This can remain as a pattern within the cerebral cortex, in which case it might be called a thought. The thought might then have consequences such as the funnelling out of electrical activity into the motor areas of the cortex so that actions can be initiated and a behavioural interaction with the world can occur.

Conclusion

The model presented here begins to show how, from a complex network of nerve cells organized into an information processing and storage system, we may generate the mental ('mind-type') aspects of brain function without recourse to dualism. The model provides a firm basis for the consideration in subsequent chapters of brain disorders where mental function is disturbed. In particular it provides a framework for the understanding of how individuals may vary in their personalities, their response to events around them, and their susceptibility to mental diseases. Individuals will differ at the level of brain architecture; these differences are likely to depend both on genetic factors influencing brain development and on experience which will also modify brain development. If brain architecture shows individual variation then all aspects of mental function must do the same; this point is returned to in subsequent chapters.

There still exists, however, a major gulf to bridge, in considering the model: how do we account for the enormous complexity of the information processing ability of the human brain? We can speak of patterns of electrical activity in cortical modules, but do we have any idea of how a set of modules might offer the vast complexity that must be inherent if the brain is to process, store and retrieve so much information?

This is beginning to be approached in the construction of artificial neural networks, as outlined in Chapter 7. These show at least how parallel arrays of neuronal 'units' can give greater processing ability than simple, serially connected units. Nevertheless, we must not forget that actual verification of hypotheses of the kind sketched above will be exceedingly difficult. It will require some kind of tool for monitoring human brain neuronal activity in such a way as to detect sufficient complexity. It seems likely that we may be able to postulate theories and simulate some aspects of brain function, but we may never be sure that we are correct because the system is too complex to monitor accurately.

Recommended reading

Blakemore, C. and Greenfield, S. (1987). *Mindwaves*. Blackwell, Oxford.

Blakemore, C. (1977). *Mechanics of the mind*. Cambridge University Press, London.

Brazier, M. A. B. (1979). Challengers from philosophers to neuroscientists. In *Brain and mind* (Ciba Foundation Symposium 69), pp. 5–29. Excerpta Medica, Amsterdam.

Bunge, M. (1980). *The mind–body problem*. Pergamon Press, Oxford.

Changeux, J. P. (1985). *Neuronal man*. Oxford University Press.

Churchland, P. S. (1988). The significance of neuroscience for philosophy. *Trends in Neurosciences*, **11**, 304–7.

Crick, F. (1989). Neural Darwinism. *Trends in Neurosciences*, **12**, 240–8.

Edelman, G. M. and Mountcastle, V. B. (1978). *The mindful brain*. MIT Press, Cambridge, MA.

Edelman, G. M. (1987). *Neural Darwinism*. Oxford University Press.

Fodor, J. A. (1983). *The modularity of mind*. MIT Press, Cambridge, MA.

Goodman, A. (1991). Organic unity theory: the mind body problem revisited. *American Journal of Psychiatry* **148**, 553–63.

Gregory, R. L. (ed.) (1987). *The Oxford companion to the mind*. Oxford University Press.

Kandel, E. R. and Schwartz, J. H. (1985). *Principles of neural science*. Elsevier, New York.

Penrose, R. (1989). *The emperor's new mind*. Oxford University Press.

Popper, K. R. and Eccles, J. C. (1977). *The self and its brain*. Springer International, Berlin.

Rose, S. (1976). *The conscious brain*. Pelican Books, Harmondsworth.

Scruton, R. (1982). *Kant*. Oxford University Press.

Searle, J. (1989). *Minds, brains and science*. Penguin Books, Harmondsworth.

9 *Disorders of human brain— a general introduction*

In the following chapters six disorders of human brain that present with specific groups of clinical symptoms—Parkinson's disease, Huntington's disease, Alzheimer's disease, schizophrenia, affective disorders, and anxiety—will be discussed. For each disorder a clinical description will be given, followed by a description of any neuropathological and neurochemical changes. Treatments for the disorders will then be considered. Following this, an attempt will be made to relate the neuropathological and neurochemical changes for each disorder, where relevant, to the clinical symptoms so that it may be possible to analyse the source of the brain dysfunction in the disease and the normal role that the dysfunctioning systems play in behaviour.

In each of the disorders considered, except Parkinson's disease, psychological disturbances are a prominent feature of the symptom pattern. Parkinson's disease, therefore, could be considered separately as, although it is a brain disorder with a clear neurological degeneration, it is primarily a disorder of movement. Nevertheless it is quite proper to consider it in a book like this as it has strong functional links with some of the more psychological disorders.

In considering the disorders with prominent psychological symptoms it is important to introduce some terms that have been used in the past in their classification. These terms will be referred to later and have implications for the way the disorders are approached. One division of psychological disorders has been into neuroses and psychoses. In a neurosis the normal mental reactions to the stressful situations of life become exaggerated but the symptoms reported, for example anxiety, are not qualitatively different from normal experience. Examples of neuroses considered here are the anxiety disorders and mild depressive illness.

By contrast in a psychosis, patients lose contact with reality and they experience life in a distorted way; this can be due to delusions, hallucinations, or misinterpretations. Psychoses are further subdivided by some into 'organic' and 'functional' groups. The organic psychoses are characterized by disturbances of consciousness and memory and it is a presumption that organic psychoses involve some (organic) degeneration of brain. Examples of organic psychoses are dementia and delirium; the behavioural changes in some cases of Alzheimer's disease and Huntington's disease patients also fit into this category.

Other psychoses have been termed 'functional', partly because their aetiology was unknown and there was no evidence of organic changes. Nevertheless, because of the prominent behavioural changes, there must be alterations in neuronal activity and these disorders have therefore been termed functional. Schizophrenia and affective disorders have in the past been considered as typical functional psychoses. This classification now seems rather outdated especially, when as will be shown in Chapter 13, there is evidence of organic changes in schizophrenia.

Although some of these terms, for example neuroses and psychoses, continue to be used, especially in everyday speech, it is not my intention to use them in any classificatory sense. Indeed, some of the modern classifications of mental disorders such as the *Diagnostic and statistical manual of mental disorders* (3rd edition, revised) (DSM III-R) of the American Psychiatric Association (1987) have ceased to use the term neurosis. I intend instead to deal with each disorder or group of disorders separately. Although the observed behavioural changes could be due to irreversible neuronal loss (previously described as 'organic') or reversible alterations in neuronal activity (previously described as 'functional'), I prefer to see these two extreme possibilities as part of a continuum of possible changes rather than as separate entities. Where issues of classification are encountered I shall follow the guidelines of DSM III-R of the American Psychiatric Association (1987) or the classifications suggested by Gelder *et al*. (1989).

In considering these six disorders of human brain which present specific changes in behaviour, the fundamental question that is being asked is, in a particular behaviour, what is happening in the brain normally to produce this behaviour and how is brain function disturbed in the disorder? It is useful therefore to consider the methods that can be used to probe human brain function and some of the strengths and limitations of these methods before proceeding to cover the disorders in detail.

Methods for the analysis of human brain function

Studies on body fluids and blood cells

It has been very popular to make measurements of neurotransmitters or their metabolites in accessible body fluids such as urine, plasma, or cerebrospinal fluid or to measure the levels of receptors or enzyme activities related to neurotransmitter metabolism in platelets or other blood cells. The intention of making such measurements is to gain some insight into central neurotransmitter activity, particularly in disorders, from accessible peripheral measurements.

Although it is relatively easy to make such measurements, it is not clear to what extent the levels of neurotransmitters or metabolites in urine, plasma, or cerebrospinal fluid do in fact reflect central activity. Urine levels of metabolites may be more a reflection of gut metabolism except in rather specific circumstances. For example, it is thought that a large proportion of the urine levels of the noradrenaline metabolite 3-methoxy-4-hydroxy-phenethyleneglycol may in primates reflect central metabolism. Plasma levels of metabolites are also likely to reflect peripheral rather than central metabolism of the neurotransmitter in most cases.

Cerebrospinal fluid is closer to the brain than urine or plasma but here again the levels of metabolites in cerebrospinal fluid will be strongly influenced by any spinal metabolism of the neurotransmitter if the spinal cord contains neurones dependent on the particular neurotransmitter. In some cases, however, the cerebrospinal fluid levels of metabolites do seem to reflect central metabolism; an example here is homovanillic acid, the metabolite of the neurotransmitter dopamine. The spinal cord does not contain many dopamine neurones so central metabolism is reflected in the cerebrospinal fluid concentration of this metabolite. For example, in Parkinson's disease (Chapter 10), where there is a major loss of dopamine neurones from the brain, homovanillic acid levels in cerebrospinal fluid are reduced.

Some workers have attempted to improve the sensitivity of cerebrospinal fluid measurements of catecholamine and indoleamine metabolites by blocking the exit of their acidic metabolites from the cerebrospinal fluid with the drug probenecid. For example, after probenecid treatment the accumulation of the 5-hydroxytryptamine metabolite, 5-hydroxy indole acetic acid in cerebrospinal fluid is reduced in some studies on patients suffering from depression relative to control patients. This suggests a reduction in brain 5-hydroxytryptamine synthesis in those patients. There are some questions, however, as to whether the 5-hydroxy indole acetic acid arises from brain or spinal metabolism of 5-hydroxytryptamine.

In summary then, measurements of neurotransmitters and metabolites in accessible body fluids must be considered with caution. Even if changes in a metabolite are seen under certain conditions then it is important to realize that this may be due to changes in neurotransmitter metabolism which are not necessarily reflected in functional changes at brain synapses. For example, for the indoleamine, 5-hydroxytryptamine, neurotransmitter release is very tightly controlled (see Chapter 5). Synthesis of the indoleamine, however, appears to be in excess of functional needs and a proportion of the synthesized indoleamine is metabolized intraneuronally without being released. Synthesis of 5-hydroxytryptamine can be increased by administration of L-tryptophan to experimental animals and this does not lead to increased 5-hydroxytryptamine release unless metabolic degradation is also blocked. Therefore rates of synthesis and metabolism, which would be reflected in cerebrospinal fluid metabolite levels, do not necessarily reflect changes in neurotransmitter release and function.

There has also been great interest in making measurements on blood platelets. This is partly due to their accessibility and partly because they possess several activities related to neurotransmitters and that are also found in neurones. The hope has been that measurements of these activities in platelets may give information on the analogous activities in central neurones and the common embryological origins of platelets and neurones has strengthened this feeling. Some workers have even suggested that the platelet, which contains 5-hydroxytryptamine, uptake systems for 5-hydroxy-tryptamine, monoamine oxidase (which could degrade 5-hydroxytryptamine), and 5-hydroxytryptamine receptors, could be used as a model for a 5-hydroxytryptamine neurone. The extent to which the corresponding neuronal and platelet activities are identical and under identical regulation is unclear, so although many results have been published on platelet neurotransmitter-related activities, the relevance of these data to central activities is uncertain.

In concluding this section, a further peripheral measurement will be mentioned. These are the neuroendocrine tests which attempt to probe central receptor activities from peripheral measurements of the effects of drugs on neuroendocrine function. These tests have been extensively used to probe receptor function in depression and a full discussion will be given in the chapter on affective disorders (Chapter 14).

Measurements on biopsy samples of human brain

It is very rare to perform a biopsy of human brain for obvious reasons. Occasionally, however, it is necessary to remove a small section of brain at neurosurgery to obtain access to a brain tumour or for diagnostic purposes. The availability of biopsy samples enables measurements to be made of brain activities that may be very sensitive to the integrity of the brain tissue. Such measurements might not be possible or might be uncertain in post-mortem brain tissue. To give one example, a comparison has been made of cerebral cortical acetylcholine synthesis and glucose metabolism in the brains of normal and Alzheimer's disease patients using biopsy samples. The control samples came from normal tissue from patients where tumours were being removed at neuro-surgery whereas the Alzheimer's disease samples were from diagnostic craniotomy. The results showed that acetylcholine synthesis in cerebral cortex was reduced in Alzheimer's disease patients relative to controls, presumably reflecting the loss of cholinergic neurones in this disease (Sims *et al*. 1981, 1983) (Chapter 12). By contrast, CO_2 production by metabolism of glucose was increased in the Alzheimer's disease patients, possibly reflecting increased metabolism in the remaining nerve terminals.

Measurements on post-mortem human brain

In principle, measurements of neurone number, neurotransmitters, metabolites, receptors, and metabolic enzymes and other indices of neuronal function in post-mortem samples of human brain should give some indication of the status of these parameters prior to death. Much useful information has indeed been obtained about brain disorders by studying post-mortem brain samples and some of the information will be considered in the subsequent chapters. These studies do, however, pose substantial problems because of the variable state of the tissues obtained and the variable stability of some of the indices of neuronal function. Some of these variables are discussed below.

There will be variation in the post-mortem delay in obtaining the brain tissue and different brain activities decline at different rates after death as the tissues lose their integrity. Whereas neurotransmitter receptors are relatively stable in post-mortem human brain tissue, the same cannot be said for activities more dependent on tissue integrity such as neurotransmitter uptake mechanisms. Nevertheless, if samples are suitably matched with normal controls for age, sex, and post-mortem delay, meaningful measurements can be obtained which can shed light on disease processes.

The state of the patient prior to death (agonal state) is also important: a slow or stuporous agonal state may lead to hypoxia and substantial tissue damage which may accelerate *post mortem* (Fig. 9.1). Also the patient may have been given drugs which could affect the measurements to be made if they remain in the tissues.

Studies with human tissues are further complicated by variability due to genetic differences and differences in diet between individuals. The manner in which the brain tissue is stored is also very important. It will usually be necessary to freeze tissue and it seems that if the tissue is frozen slowly in iso-osmotic solution at $-70°C$ and thawed rapidly, this yields a preparation which is functionally and metabolically active. Indeed, parameters such as neurotransmitter uptake, which is very sensitive to tissue integrity, can be measured in post-mortem brain samples frozen in this way. Other parameters

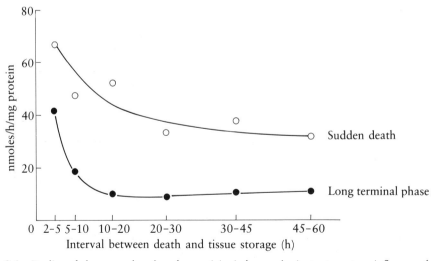

Figure 9.1 Decline of glutamate decarboxylase activity in human brain *post mortem*: influence of agonal state. The figure shows the glutamate decarboxylase activity in brain samples with different post-mortem delays from patients dying suddenly or after a long terminal phase. (From Dodd *et al.* 1988 with permission.) Enzyme activity is better preserved for patients dying suddenly.

such as the number and affinity of neurotransmitter receptors are less sensitive to the precise manner of freezing and thawing.

It seems therefore that a range of indices of neuronal function can be measured in suitably stored post-mortem brain tissue. In this way, if suitably matched control samples are also assessed, information about human brain diseases can be obtained. If changes are seen in the disease state it will be important to determine whether the change is due to a degenerative or developmental change—this distinction will be encountered later in the discussion of schizophrenia (Chapter 13).

Imaging techniques for examining living human brain

Whereas much useful information has been obtained from studies of human brain *post mortem*, it is desirable to be able to make measurements on living human brain so that patients may be diagnosed more clearly in life. This has become possible in recent years through the introduction of certain imaging techniques for examining the human brain in life.

In *computerized axial tomography* (CAT) or computerized tomography (CT) as it is sometimes called, X-rays are used to reveal the internal structure of the brain. Multiple narrow beams of X-rays are rotated around the head in a particular plane and are transmitted slightly differently by the different parts of the brain. From the many different readings taken of the X-ray transmission, a computerized analysis of the results (tomography) enables a picture to be constructed of a 'slice' through the brain. The resolution of the technique depends on the apparatus used but can be less than 1 mm. CAT has given excellent images of living human brain that correspond well with similar pictures obtained from post-mortem studies (Fig. 12.3). CAT has had a major impact on current concepts of schizophrenia, showing clearly that in this disorder there are structural changes in the brain, which are seen in CAT scans as an enlargement of the ventricles in schizophrenics relative to control patients. The results of these studies will be considered in more detail in the chapter on schizophrenia (Chapter 13).

Magnetic resonance imaging (MRI) exploits the different water contents of different parts of the brain. Water molecules provide strong magnetic resonance signals; using this technique and computer analyses similar to CAT, striking images of living human brain ('slices') can be obtained (Fig. 9.2) with resolution that can sometimes be comparable to that in fixed and sectioned anatomical material. The images are more detailed than those given by CAT scanning and avoid the small hazards of X-rays. MRI has been particularly useful in diagnosis of the demyelination of multiple sclerosis. Further examples of the use of the technique will be given in subsequent chapters.

Whereas CAT and MRI produce detailed but static images of living brain *positron emission tomography* (PET) allows dynamic functional images to be obtained. In PET a reporter substance labelled with a positron-emitting isotope, e.g. ^{11}C, ^{13}N, ^{15}O, or ^{18}F, is

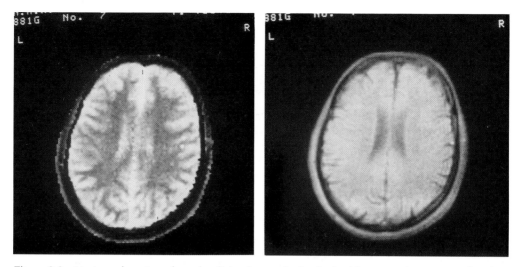

Figure 9.2 Horizontal sections through a living human brain obtained by magnetic resonance imaging (MRI). The two pictures employ the MRI technique to display slightly different structural features. Courtesy of Dr F. W. Smith and Dr J. A. O. Besson, Departments of Nuclear Medicine and Mental Health, Medical School, Aberdeen.

introduced into the brain via the bloodstream. Positrons emitted by the reporter substance collide with electrons generating γ-rays, the sites of emission of these γ-rays can be determined with suitable detectors. By making measurements around the head and using computer analysis, an image of a 'slice' of brain can be obtained based on the distribution of the reporter substance. This in turn will report some function of the brain depending on the reporter substance chosen. The resolution of the technique is rather poorer (4–8 mm) than CAT or MRI, it is expensive, and it requires a cyclotron on site to generate the positron-emitting isotopes with their short half lives. Nevertheless, PET has generated unique information on brain function.

One application of PET is to obtain images of cerebral blood flow using reporter substances such as $[^{15}O]CO_2$, $[^{15}O]H_2O$ and $[^{11}C]CH_3F$ (Fig. 9.3). These substances distribute in the blood volume and using these kinds of substance, images of the brain in action can be obtained as the blood flow to a particular brain region is thought to increase when that brain region is active. Brain regions that are activated during certain kinds of thinking can be mapped in this way (Roland *et al.* 1987). Information on changes in brain activity in brain disorders can also be obtained by measurements of cerebral blood flow; some results from these studies will be considered later.

Regional cerebral glucose metabolism can be measured by PET if a labelled form of deoxyglucose (usually $[^{18}F]$deoxyglucose) is given to the subject. Neurones take up glucose in proportion to their activity. Deoxyglucose is taken up by neurones and phosphorylated in the same way as glucose but cannot be metabolized. Therefore active

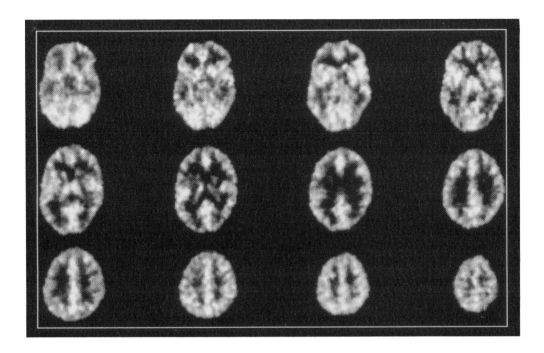

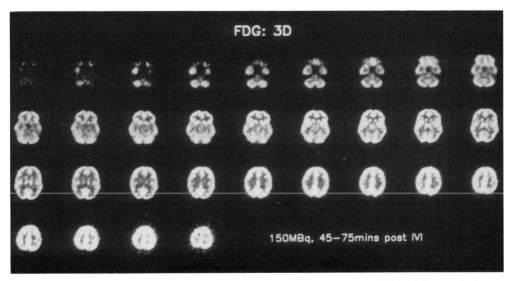

Figure 9.3   Positron emission tomography (PET) used to determine cerebral blood flow and glucose metabolism in human brain. The upper panel shows a series of horizontal sections obtained using the inhaled tracer $[^{15}O]CO_2$ to measure cerebral blood flow. The lower panel shows a series of horizontal sections obtained using the injected tracer $[^{18}F]$ fluoro-deoxyglucose to measure cerebral glucose metabolism. The pictures are by courtesy of Professor R. S. J. Frackowiak, MRC Cyclotron Unit, Hammersmith Hospital, London.

neurones accumulate [^{18}F]deoxyglucose and the PET distribution of this labelled compound provides a picture of active areas of the brain (Fig. 9.3). This has been used to make measurements of brain activity in some neurodegenerative diseases. For example, one of the earliest changes in Huntington's disease may be a reduction of glucose metabolism in the striatum and this may precede the actual losses of neurones that occur (Chapter 11).

Analogous measurements of neuronal activity can be made by measuring oxygen utilization with [^{15}O]O$_2$. These are found to parallel quite closely measurements of cerebral blood flow (Roland *et al.* 1987). This supports the idea that measurements of blood flow reflect tissue activity.

PET is now being applied to the study of neurotransmitter metabolism and receptors. [^{18}F]L-DOPA can be used to label regions of the brain rich in dopamine as it behaves like L-DOPA and is taken up, decarboxylated, and stored with the dopamine. PET studies of the distribution of [^{18}F]L-DOPA have allowed clear illustrations of the striking losses of dopamine in Parkinson's disease to be constructed in living patients; these will be considered in Chapter 10.

Receptors can also be visualized using PET if a suitable ligand labelled with a positron-emitting isotope is available. This has enabled studies to be performed on the drug occupancy of brain D$_2$ dopamine receptors and on numbers of D$_2$ dopamine receptors in the brain in schizophrenic patients (Chapter 13) using the ligands [^{11}C]*N*-methyl spiperone and [^{11}C]raclopride. There are, however, considerable technical difficulties with the studies and the interpretation of the results is not necessarily straightforward (Waddington 1989; Seeman *et al.* 1990).

In Chapter 7 data on the activation of different cerebral cortical regions during the performance of different tasks were presented. These were not obtained using PET but used a somewhat older technique whereby the subject is given a small quantity of the gaseous γ-ray emitting isotope ^{133}Xe. This distributes in the circulation and provides an index of blood flow. The γ-rays detectable outside the head represent only the outer shell of brain which in practice is the cerebral cortex. Therefore if an array of γ-cameras is located on one side of the head, the distribution of the γ-emitter shows the distribution of activated brain areas on one side of the brain; this gives essentially a two-dimensional image of cerebral cortical activity. As discussed in Chapter 7, this technique gives very useful information about the activation of cerebral cortical regions during certain tasks. This technique has now been improved with the introduction of newer reporter molecules e.g. ^{99}Tc^{m}-HMPAO and three-dimensional images of cerebral blood flow are available with the application of tomographic technology. The technique is termed single photon emission computerized tomography (SPECT). It has the advantage over PET that it is cheap and widely available whereas PET is unlikely ever to be widely available. The resolution is comparable to that of PET if the improved technology is used.

Behavioural effects of drugs with defined biochemical properties

Another way to infer information about the function of the human brain is to examine the behavioural effects of drugs whose *in vitro* biochemical actions are well defined. If a specific behavioural change is seen when the drug is administered to a patient, then it can perhaps be inferred that the biochemical system affected by the drug is involved in the behavioural change. For example, if normal volunteers are given selective antagonists of muscarinic acetylcholine receptors such as scopolamine, then they suffer a loss of short term memory. A reasonable inference from this is that cholinergic systems are involved in some way in memory function. This will be elaborated on in Chapter 12 on Alzheimer's disease.

There are several problems with this kind of approach. Very few drugs are absolutely specific and frequently specificity has been established using non-human animal models. If there are species differences these could confound the measurements. Also, the effects of the administered drug on one neuronal system could be to disturb a second neuronal system that is actually responsible for the behavioural change. The problems of specificity can be overcome by using a range of substances and comparing the doses required to change behaviour *in vivo* with their potencies in the *in vitro* test system. If a correlation is obtained between potencies in the *in vivo* and *in vitro* systems for a range of compounds of different potencies and different chemical structures, then this is reasonable evidence that the *in vitro* activity is important for the *in vivo* behaviour. In Chapter 13 I shall describe how such a correlation was obtained for a range of compounds (antipsychotic drugs) between their abilities to alleviate the positive symptoms of schizophrenia and their binding to the D_2 subclass of dopamine receptors. Most of the compounds tested have activities at other receptors, but the correlation with *in vivo* activity is only found for their activity at the D_2 dopamine receptor, supporting the role of this receptor in the anti-schizophrenic action of these drugs and suggesting a role for dopamine neuronal systems in the control of behaviour and emotion.

The approach of using drugs with defined biochemical properties has been taken a stage further by some workers. Some of the drugs whose biochemical properties are well defined and which produce specific behavioural changes are also effective at treating particular brain disorders. One example mentioned above is of the antipsychotic drugs whose ability to block D_2 dopamine receptors seems to account for the antipsychotic action (Chapter 13). Another example is provided by certain drugs used to treat depression (Chapter 14), where the ability of these drugs to inhibit the neuronal reuptake of the monoamine neurotransmitters noradrenaline and 5-hydroxytryptamine (Chapter 5) seems to be important for the antidepressant effect. Thus alterations in monoamine neuronal activity can alleviate depression.

In both cases, satisfactory theories of drug action can be proposed based on specific biochemical changes. In both cases, however, the theories of drug action have been extended, in reverse, to provide neurochemical theories of the disorder. In the case of the antipsychotic drugs it has been suggested that schizophrenia is due to overactivities of brain dopamine systems, whereas in the case of the antidepressant drugs it has been suggested that depression is due to alterations in monoamine neurotransmitter activities. Although these extrapolations are tempting, in the absence of firm information on changes in the particular neurochemical system in the disease, they are unwarranted. It is important to separate theories of drug action from theories of disease and the two examples cited here will be considered in more detail in later chapters.

Neuropsychological testing

Neuropsychological tests provide another approach to determining the nature of brain damage or dysfunction in patients suspected to have such damage or dysfunction. Since overt behaviour depends on brain activity, behaviour should appear abnormal when there is either brain damage or altered function. Numerous cases have been described where circumscribed damage to parts of the brain gives rise to specific changes in behaviour. Such examples have helped in the assignment of functions to regions of the brain, especially in the cerebral cortex. For example in Chapter 2 the example was noted of patients with the speech defect, Broca's aphasia, which results from specific damage to the cerebral cortex of the left hemisphere. There are many other examples, some of which will be mentioned in the following chapters on brain disorders.

Given this background of knowledge on the relationship between changes in behaviour and damage to different regions of the brain, a wide range of tests has been devised to probe this relationship. These are neuropsychological tests which aim to make inference about changes in brain function by defining, as precisely as possible, changes in behaviour. Patients with suspected localized brain damage or dysfunction would then be given a battery of neuropsychological tests and the results of these tests would be interpreted in terms of possible brain changes. The kinds of brain function that can be tested for include intellectual function, memory, language, visual function, and motor function.

I do not intend to describe in detail the tests that are used, rather a few important examples will be given. One test which provides a baseline measure of cognitive function is the Wechsler adult intelligence scale. This test provides separate scores for verbal and performance tests. Verbal tests consist of a series of verbal questions, while the performance tests are more dependent on the manipulation of symbols and pictures. In general, a low score on the verbal test is associated with well defined lesions of the left hemisphere, whereas a low score on the performance test can be found in patients with lesions to the right hemisphere. Memory can be tested for using the Wechsler memory scale. This consists of a series of sub-tests which probe different aspects of memory.

Frontal lobe function can be tested for in a variety of ways. One test is based on the observation that patients with lesions of the frontal lobes have difficulty in switching behaviour patterns when this is required, that is they are said to perseverate. A test has been developed for this called the Wisconsin card-sorting test. This requires that the subject sort a set of cards according to a particular criterion (for example the colour or shape on the card). The subject is told only whether the sorting is correct or incorrect and eventually learns the solution. Once the problem has been solved, the solution is changed and the subject must find the new solution. Shifting away from the earlier solution has been shown to be particularly difficult for patients with frontal lobe lesions, so the Wisconsin card-sorting test can be used to highlight frontal lobe problems. This therefore is a neuropsychological test for changes in human brain function. The interpretation of results is, however, not straightforward: the problems detected could be secondary manifestations of changes in other neuronal systems that affect frontal lobe functions. For example, patients with chronic schizophrenia perform poorly in the test (Goldberg *et al.* 1987) and this has been taken as some evidence for deficits in prefrontal cortex function in these patients. There is some minor evidence for actual changes in prefrontal cortical structure and more evidence for deficits in prefrontal cortical function using cerebral blood flow measurement when these patients are compared with normal controls. The functional deficits shown by cerebral blood flow are also more apparent when the patients are subjected to the card sorting test. However, the prefrontal cortical functional deficits are most likely to reflect actual structural changes elsewhere in the brain—in schizophrenia this is probably due to changes in the structure of the temporal lobes which in turn affects prefrontal cortex function via their interconnections (Chapter 13). Also in both Parkinson's disease (Chapter 10) and Huntington's disease (Chapter 11), apparent deficits in frontal lobe functions have been described using the card-sorting test, probably reflecting the connections between the frontal lobes and the striatum where there is either a lesion (Huntington's disease) or disturbed function (Parkinson's disease).

Epidemiological and genetic approaches

Epidemiological studies of the incidence of a disease can shed light on possible causes, which can be broadly divided into genetic or environmental. Genetic influences might be suspected if there were a strong familial aggregation of the disease, whereas environmental causes might be suspected in the absence of a genetic explanation and in the presence of evidence for a role for an environmental factor. Epidemiological studies can be confusing so a brief description of the terms used will be given here.

Epidemiological studies

A variety of ways are used to express the occurrence of diseases. The *prevalence rate* of a disease is the frequency of occurrence in the general population expressed as a rate. The prevalence can be estimated on a given day (point prevalence) or within a given time interval (period prevalence) and the results will depend on whether the whole population is considered or only a part. The *incidence (or inception)* rate is the frequency of appearance of new cases in the general population. The period prevalence rate therefore is a function of the incidence rate and the duration of the illness. A third mode of expressing the occurrence of a disease is the *expectancy* (*lifetime risk* or *morbid risk*). This is the probability (usually expressed as a percentage) that any individual will develop the disease given exposure during the risk period and sufficient survival.

Measures of the occurrence of a disease are important and can help give information on the underlying causes of the disease. For example, if the prevalence shows a geographical bias which can also be linked to an environmental factor, then this may help understand the causation. Genetic factors can also be important and have been examined by determining the expectancy of diseases in first degree relatives of patients suffering from the particular disease. If the expectancy in the first degree relatives is higher than in the population as a whole, this provides some support for a familial tendency.

This could, however, reflect either inherited genetic factors or shared environmental factors. A dissociation of these two broad groups of factors has been attempted by examining the incidence of the diseases in twin pairs, specifically comparing incidence in monozygotic and dizygotic twin pairs. Monozygotic twins have identical genes whereas dizygotic twins have genes that are no more identical than typical siblings, whereas the environmental influences should be similar within either kind of twin pair. Therefore if there is a greater tendency (concordance) for both twins to suffer from the disease for the monozygotic twin pair compared with the dizygotic twin pair, this is good support for a genetic component to the incidence of the disease. Such twin studies have been criticized and championed on a number of levels; some of these criticisms will be considered when the individual diseases are discussed. Different patterns of occurrence of disorder in twin pairs will be observed if the genetic factor is encoded on the mitochondrial genome rather than the nuclear genome. (Harding 1991; Chapter 10).

Another way to approach the effects of genetics and environment on the incidence of a disease is to examine the incidence of the disease in children adopted away from their natural family. If genetic effects are important, a child whose natural parents have the disorder should still show an increased risk of developing the disorder. An increased risk in such a study will also tend to rule out environmental influences as being important.

Genetic linkage analysis

If epidemiological studies provide good evidence for genetic influences on the occurrence of a disease, the techniques of molecular biology can then be applied in order to attempt to identify the genetic change involved. The most favourable situation for this kind of study will be a disease that shows an autosomal dominant pattern of inheritance. In this case if one parent in a family carries the gene for the disease, then 50 per cent of the children of this parent will carry the disease gene. This is the case for Huntington's disease (Chapter 11) and some cases of Parkinson's disease (Chapter 10) and Alzheimer's disease (Chapter 12), but for the other brain disorders no such clear inheritance patterns are seen.

The approach that is taken in genetic linkage analysis is to identify genetic markers specific for particular parts of the human genome that are inherited in the same way within a family pedigree as the disease. It is then argued that the genetic marker must be close to the disease locus. Once a marker close to the disease locus has been identified it should be possible, through further extensive genetic studies, to identify the gene responsible for the disease. The actual techniques used for this will be considered in detail in Chapter 11 in relation to their use in Huntington's disease. It cannot be over-emphasized that genetic linkage analysis is fraught with problems when there is clear inheritance of the disease; where the inheritance patterns are good only for certain families or where there is an environmental factor important for disease occurrence, the possibility of error is much greater.

A further complication for both epidemiological and genetic linkage studies is inherent in the nature of some of the brain disorders considered in the subsequent chapters. In several of the disorders, frank symptoms of the disorder show only when a threshold of influences or brain changes has been exceeded dependent usually on several interacting factors, both genetic and environmental. This complicates all analyses but a particular problem arises from the likely existence in the population of individuals who have similar brain changes to the symptomatically affected individuals but at a level below the threshold for the occurrence of symptoms. These individuals will not show the clear symptoms of the disorder, although there may be preclinical signs. If the brain changes in these asymptomatic individuals are the same as those seen in patients showing the full disorder, then the occurrence of these subthreshold brain changes in these individuals is important. If, however, inheritance patterns are established only on the basis of the presentation of symptoms, these subthreshold individuals will be discarded as negatives. This will weaken inheritance patterns which would be clearer if the subthreshold changes in the brain in the asymptomatic individuals were also taken into account.

Recommended reading

Abouh-Saleh, M. T. (1990). Brain imaging in psychiatry. *British Journal of Psychiatry*, **157** (suppl. 9), 5–101.

Bouchard, T. J., Lykken, D. T., McGue, M., Segal, N. L., and Tellegen, A. (1990). Sources of human psychological differences; The Minnesota study of twins reared apart. *Science*, **250**, 223–8.

Dodd, P. R., Hambley, J. W., Cowburn, R. F., and Hardy, J. A. (1988). A comparison of methodologies for the study of functional transmitter neurochemistry in human brain. *Journal of Neurochemistry*, **50**, 1333–45.

Fowler, C. J. (1986). The pros and cons of using human brain autopsy samples for radioligand binding experiments. *Trends in Pharmacological Sciences*, 7, 9–10.

Gusella, J. F. (1986). DNA polymorphism and human disease. *Annual Review of Biochemistry*, 55, 831–54.

Hardy, J. A. and Dodd, P. R. (1983). Metabolic and functional studies on post mortem human brain. *Neurochemistry International*, 5, 253–66.

Kolb, B. and Wishaw, I. Q. (1990). *Fundamentals of human neuropsychology* (3rd edn). Freeman, New York.

Sturt, E. and McGuffin, P. (1985). Can linkage and marker association resolve the genetic aetiology of psychiatric disorders? Review and argument. *Psychological Medicine*, **15**, 455–62.

Volkow, N. D. and Tancredi, L. R. (1991). Biological correlates of mental activity studied with P.E.T. *American Journal of Psychiatry*, **148**, 439–43.

Wing, J. K. (ed.) (1978). *Schizophrenia, towards a new synthesis*. Academic Press, London.

10   *Parkinson's disease*

Parkinson's disease is a well defined neurological disorder with a clear loss of brain cells. It was first described in detail by James Parkinson in 1817 in his *Essay on the shaking palsy* and following his description the disease came to be called after him. It is not clear how prevalent the disease was in the nineteenth century and before; indeed, some have speculated that Parkinson's disease may have only arisen in the late eighteenth century, but a disease similar to Parkinson's disease is described in the ancient Indian medical system Ayurveda (Manyam 1990). Parkinson's disease refers to a specific constellation of symptoms in patients, as described below. To this day the underlying cause is unknown and so is termed idiopathic, but there is an innate assumption that true Parkinson's disease does have a clearly defined cause. Similar symptoms can be seen in part in other conditions where the aetiology is much clearer and these are referred to as parkinsonism or parkinsonian syndromes. The distinction between Parkinson's disease and parkinsonism is important but we may learn about the aetiology of Parkinson's disease by studying parkinsonism.

Clinical description

Parkinson's disease is a disease of later life with a mean age of onset of about 60 years of age. It affects about 0.15 per cent of the total population but the prevalence increases to 0.5 per cent of those over 50. Parkinson's disease is a progressive disease with a gradual exacerbation of symptoms. There is no evidence for dietary or infectious influences in Parkinson's disease itself and until recently it was considered that Parkinson's disease was not an inherited disorder. Recently, however, families where the disease does seem to be inherited have been identified and these will be considered below. Epidemiological studies suggest that the incidence of Parkinson's disease is rather uniform, although increased incidence has been linked variously with rural environments, drinking well water, industrialization, and pesticide usage, whereas decreased incidence has been demonstrated for cigarette smokers (Tanner 1989; Koller *et al.* 1990).

The classical features of Parkinson's disease are tremor, rigidity, and disturbances of movement (bradykinesia and akinesia). The tremor exhibits as a resting tremor in the limbs and disappears on movement or during sleep. Rigidity refers to a resistance to passive movement and is often of a jerky or 'cogwheel' nature. There is a generalized paucity of movement (akinesia), especially involuntary movement, and this can account for the 'mask-like' face seen in some patients. Also there is difficulty in initiating voluntary movement and slowness once started (bradykinesia). There are a number of other symptoms, e.g. a stooped posture (Fig. 10.1), speech problems, excessive sweating, and micrographia (Fig. 10.2).

The classical descriptions of Parkinson's disease do not include cognitive changes in the patients but it now seems that there may be specific alterations in some cognitive abilities early in the disease (see later). In the later changes there is also an increased risk of dementia (10–15 per cent increased risk) (Quinn *et al.* 1986).

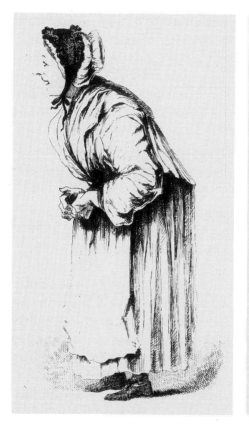 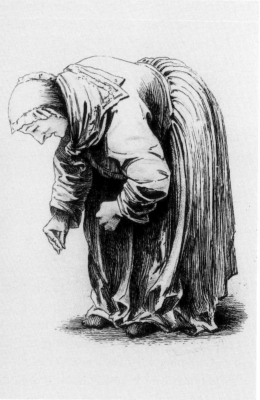

Figure 10.1   The stooped posture of Parkinson's disease. The drawings are of a patient Marie Gavr in 1874 (left) and 1879 (right) and were drawn by Richer, a student of Charcot who in the late nineteenth century in the Salpêtrière Hospital in Paris was responsible for much of the early clinical definition of Parkinson's disease. Note also the hands in the earlier drawing which are held in a particular way. The drawings are taken from *Oeuvres Completes* (Vol. 1) of Charcot (1886) and were kindly supplied by Madame V. Leroux Hugon of the Bibliotheque J. M. Charcot, Salpêtrière Hospital, Paris.

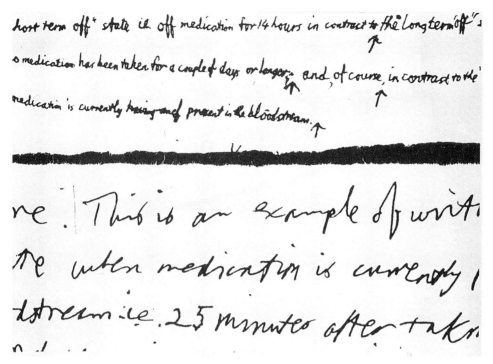

Figure 10.2 Micrographia (very small handwriting) typical of Parkinson's disease. The upper panel shows micrographia clearly, the arrows show the places where the patient paused due to tremor. The lower panel shows the handwriting after taking L-DOPA. Taken from Ferry (1987) with permission.

Neuropathological observations

Post-mortem examination of the brains of Parkinson's disease patients shows a specific degeneration of the substantia nigra (pars compacta) (Fig. 10.3). In addition, round eosinophilic intraneuronal inclusions containing filamentous material called Lewy bodies are frequently seen in the substantia nigra and the locus coeruleus. The presence of Lewy bodies in these brain regions may be diagnostic for Parkinson's disease (Gibb 1989). Lewy bodies are not, however, confined to these catecholamine-containing tissues and are also found in Parkinson's disease in several other brain regions and widely in the autonomic nervous system. Lewy bodies are also found in patients who do not have Parkinson's disease, but to a lesser degree; this may be indicative of low levels of the same degeneration in these patients as is seen in Parkinson's disease (Gibb and Lees 1988).

In 1960 Ehringer and Hornykiewicz measured dopamine levels in human brain and showed there to be a profound (>50 per cent) depletion of dopamine and of its metabolite homovanillic acid in the caudate nucleus, putamen, substantia nigra, and to a

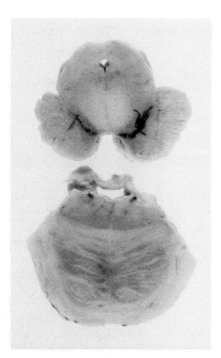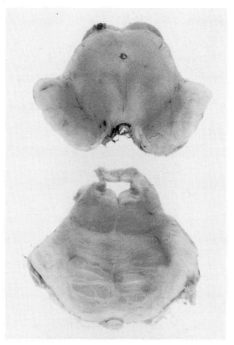

Figure 10.3 The substantia nigra and locus coeruleus of normal (lefthand panel) and Parkinson's disease (righthand panel) patients. The upper photograph in each panel shows a section through the mid brain and the loss of pigmented cells in the substantia nigra can be clearly seen in the parkinsonian case. The lower photograph in each panel shows a section through the pons, illustrating the loss of the locus coeruleus. Courtesy of Dr. S. E. Daniel, Parkinson's Disease Society Brain Bank, London.

lesser extent in the globus pallidus of Parkinson's disease patients (Hornykiewicz 1973). These findings, taken together with the nigral degeneration described above, suggested that in Parkinson's disease there was a specific loss of the mesostriatal dopamine pathway (see Chapters 5 and 7) which runs from the substantia nigra to the neostriatum (caudate nucleus and putamen) and globus pallidus. The loss of this pathway can account for many of the symptoms of the disease owing to the involvement of the neostriatum (caudate nucleus and putamen) in the control of movement (see below). Analysis of dopamine in different regions of the caudate nucleus and putamen has shown that the dopamine loss is much greater in the putamen than in the caudate nucleus; in some regions of the putamen it is greater than 90 per cent, whereas in some regions of the caudate nucleus it is no more than 60 per cent (Kish *et al.* 1988). This suggests some selectivity in the degenerative process. The loss of dopamine in the striatum can now be observed on living patients using positron emission tomography (Chapter 9) (Fig. 10.4). (See Fig. 10.7 also.)

Examination of dopamine neurochemistry in more detail has shown that com-

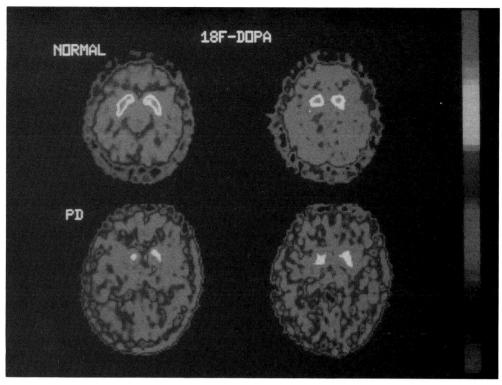

Figure 10.4 Positron Emission Tomography (PET) scan of brain dopamine levels. The patients were given [^{18}F]L-DOPA which accumulates as [^{18}F]dopamine in the striatum and can be visualized from the positron emission of ^{18}F. The upper panel shows normal scans whereas the lower panel shows scans from a patient with Parkinson's disease. The loss of dopamine storage subsequent to loss of mesostriatal dopamine neurones is clear in the patient with Parkinson's disease. The loss is greater in the putamen than in the caudate nucleus. The pictures show horizontal sections through the striata and were kindly supplied by Dr D. Brooks, Hammersmith Hospital.

pensatory changes in dopamine metabolism occur in the residual mesostriatal neurones. The remaining neurones increase their activity, increasing dopamine turnover and release. Thus the ratio of dopamine metabolites to dopamine increases and the activity of tyrosine hydroxylase increases. These presynaptic compensations allow a loss of mesostriatal neurones to occur without significant clinical manifestations until the striatal dopamine levels have declined by at least 80 per cent. This figure of 80 per cent represents something of a threshold which, if exceeded, leads to clinical symptoms of Parkinson's disease.

It might also be expected that a postsynaptic supersensitivity would develop as an additional compensation. The levels of postsynaptic D_1 or D_2 dopamine receptors have been measured in striatum in post-mortem samples of brain from Parkinson's disease patients (Seeman and Niznik, 1990) and there is a general tendency for receptor levels to be increased for patients who had not taken L-DOPA recently before death. Where the patient had taken L-DOPA just prior to death, receptor levels are normal. There is, however, some scatter in the data, emphasizing the problems with post-mortem studies on human tissues which may be seriously affected by the state of the patient at death (Chapter 9). It may also be that the postsynaptic receptor status will vary from patient to patient according to the extent of presynaptic compensation and any postsynaptic degeneration.

Other dopamine pathways are affected, although less severely. There is loss of about 50 per cent of the dopamine cells in the ventral tegmental area, the origin of some of the mesocortical pathway, so that this pathway is partly depleted. Effects on other dopamine pathways are poorly characterized.

Other parts of the brain are also affected in Parkinson's disease; for example, cell loss is seen in the locus coeruleus (origin of noradrenergic neurones) (Fig. 10.3) and the nucleus basalis of Meynert (this is particularly affected in patients who show dementia who may show the same loss of cholinergic neurones seen in patients with Alzheimer's disease (see Quinn *et al.* 1986 and Chapter 12)). There are many reports of changes in other neurotransmitter systems, e.g. GABA, 5-hydroxytryptamine, and certain peptides. Some of these changes may be due to specific alterations in nerve cells outside the mesostriatal axis whereas some may be occurring subsequent to the mesostriatal dopamine cell loss. Certain specific symptoms of Parkinson's disease may be related to these alterations in other systems.

In summary, the major effect in Parkinson's disease is loss of the mesostriatal dopamine pathway with less major alterations in the mesocortical dopamine and locus coeruleus noradrenaline pathways with losses of cholinergic pathways in patients with Alzheimer-type dementia.

Treatments for Parkinson's disease

L-3,4-dihydroxyphenylalanine (L-DOPA)

Prior to the early 1960s, there were few useful medications for Parkinson's disease although anticholinergic drugs such as atropine could be used to achieve some control. The discovery of the depletion of striatal dopamine, however, offered a new approach—replacement of the lost dopamine. Dopamine administered orally is not useful as it does not penetrate the blood–brain barrier, but the precursor of dopamine, L-DOPA, will penetrate the blood–brain barrier and is converted to dopamine in the brain. Carlsson and colleagues had shown in animal experiments in 1957 that administration of L-DOPA would reverse a brain dopamine deficiency (Carlsson *et al.* 1957) and from 1961, tests with L-DOPA began in patients with Parkinson's disease. Early reports using low doses were encouraging but it was not until 1967, when Cotzias and colleagues used much larger doses (4–16 g a day), that significant alleviation of the main symptoms was seen in many patients (Cotzias *et al.* 1967). The high dose of L-DOPA led to certain complications, many of which were due to peripheral decarboxylation of L-DOPA to dopamine before it reached the brain. Thus inhibitors of the decarboxylase enzyme were made that did not pass the blood–brain barrier, e.g. benserazide and carbidopa. These, if administered with L-DOPA, prevented decarboxylation peripherally, whereas L-DOPA in the brain was still converted to dopamine. The dose of L-DOPA required could thus be lowered considerably.

Therapy of patients suffering from Parkinson's disease with L-DOPA (1 g day^{-1}) and a peripheral decarboxylase inhibitor (e.g. carbidopa, 100 mg day^{-1}) is very successful in reducing many symptoms significantly (Fig. 10.2) although there are some side effects such as dyskinesias, psychiatric disturbances, and a reduction in efficacy with time. The majority of patients who have Parkinson's disease with Lewy bodies in the substantia nigra show a modest to very good response to L-DOPA. These figures must be considered in the light of the near total inability to treat the symptoms prior to the advent of L-DOPA.

Mode of action of L-DOPA

The success of the treatment with L-DOPA belies some ignorance over its precise mode of action. Levels of dopamine are certainly raised in the brain after L-DOPA administration, but it is not clear where the decarboxylation is occurring. It may be in the residual mesostriatal neurones, but other striatal neurones have been suggested as sites of the decarboxylation. In addition, it is not clear how the exogenous dopamine acts. Presumably some is stored in the remaining mesostriatal neurones and released as if normal. Indeed, as mentioned before, there is a substantial increase in dopamine release and synthesis in striatum from Parkinson's disease patients. This may account for the lack of clinical symptoms until more than 80 per cent of the mesostriatal neurones are lost and the increased synthetic activity may help in the use of dopamine derived from L-DOPA.

However, if all the dopamine that reaches postsynaptic sites in the striatum does so after release from the remaining mesostriatal cells (even during L-DOPA therapy), then as such a massive cell loss has occurred, this implies the following: either there is a very high redundancy in the mesostriatal innervation of the striatum with the loss of some mesostriatal neurones possibly being compensated for by increased activity in those remaining or dopamine is being released and acting at sites away from the release site. Given that dopamine agonists other than dopamine can elicit some improvement in symptoms (see below), it seems reasonable to suggest that L-DOPA supplies dopamine, some of which is released from residual mesostriatal cells to act over short and longer distances, and some of which is formed in other cells and effectively bathes the striatum.

Occupancy of postsynaptic receptor sites is achieved by both routes, suggesting that control of striatal function is more dependent on the concentration of dopamine present at postsynaptic receptors than on the temporal pattern of impulse flow in the meso-striatal cells. These points will be discussed again at the end of this chapter when the normal function of the striatum is considered.

Problems with L-DOPA therapy

It is important to mention the side effects of L-DOPA therapy and to attempt to account for them as they can be a barrier to the continuation of the therapy. A variety of dys-kinesias occur in response to L-DOPA and seem to be due in part to excessive stimulation of striatal dopamine receptors (see later). Similarly, a variety of psychiatric complications can occur. It has been suggested that these may be related to stimulation of dopamine receptors in the mesocortical dopamine projections. This would be consistent with the involvement of this pathway in some aspects of behaviour and its implication in aspects of schizophrenia (Chapter 13).

In addition to these side effects, after chronic treatment with L-DOPA the clinical improvement in symptoms is markedly reduced in many patients. Patients also exhibit motor oscillations. These can be seen either as the effect of a single dose of L-DOPA lasting for a shorter time ('wearing off') or as unpredictable fluctuations in clinical state (the so called 'on–off phenomenon' where an abrupt change occurs from the mobile to immobile state).

These altered responses to L-DOPA are likely to be due in part to the continuing loss of mesostriatal dopamine neurones. This loss reduces the storage capacity for dopamine as well as reducing the ability to decarboxylate L-DOPA and so the effect of a single dose of L-DOPA lasts a shorter time. Therefore the dopamine levels achieved in the brain become much more dependent on plasma L-DOPA, leading to the fluctuation in clinical response. A further complication can be competition between L-DOPA and dietary neutral amino acids for uptake across the blood–brain barrier, so dietary protein intake should be carefully regulated (Nutt *et al*. 1984). Fluctuations in clinical response have been reduced using continuous intravenous infusion of L-DOPA but, although this emphasizes the importance of plasma L-DOPA levels for clinical response, it is rather impracticable for general use. Slow release formulations of L-DOPA have been developed and may be of some use in reducing the number of daily doses of L-DOPA required (Duvoisin 1989). Subcutaneous or transdermally delivered dopamine agonists may also be of use (see below).

The general loss of efficacy of L-DOPA with time may reflect a need for some normal mesostriatal impulse transmission even when L-DOPA is given and this pathway is being progressively lost. Transplants of fetal nigral cells (see below) may be important here if they can integrate into the circuitry of the brain. It must not be forgotten, however, that Parkinson's disease is a progressive disease, and as other brain cells are lost the therapies described here may become ineffective. It has been suggested that a toxic metabolite of L-DOPA may lead to more rapid degeneration of mesostriatal cells during L-DOPA therapy. The latter idea has led to some concern over when to start L-DOPA therapy, some clinicians favouring delaying the start of treatment as late as possible on the grounds that L-DOPA administration leads to further degeneration. Other clinicians favour starting L-DOPA as soon as possible on the grounds that deterioration in response occurs independently of therapy. I shall return to this point later but a recent study provided no evidence for deleterious effects of L-DOPA (Blin *et al.* 1988).

Dopamine agonist therapy

Dopamine agonists such as apomorphine, bromocriptine, lisuride, pergolide, PHNO, and terguride can be used to control symptoms of Parkinson's disease. They are often not as effective as L-DOPA but provide a lower incidence of some side effects, e.g. dyskinesias, although there may be a slightly higher incidence of others, e.g. psychiatric complications (this may be related to the interaction of these substances with meso-cortical dopamine systems or, for some of the substances, interaction with 5-hydroxy-tryptamine systems). A useful combination, however, seems to be low dose L-DOPA (0.3–0.6 g, plus a decarboxylase inhibitor) together with low dose bromocriptine (16–25 mg). This achieves as good or better control of symptoms than either drug given separately with fewer side effects and less 'wearing off' (Rinne 1985). An alternative therapy which may lead to more stable levels of drug is provided by subcutaneous delivery (apomorphine) or transdermal delivery (PHNO). Subcutaneous apomorphine provides good therapy for some patients helping to reduce periods of immobility (Frankel *et al.* 1990) and this agonist has also been used successfully via intranasal, sublingual, and rectal administration (Kapoor *et al.* 1990; Hughes *et al.* 1991).

The ability of a dopamine agonist to ameliorate the symptoms of Parkinson's disease shows that simple occupancy of striatal dopamine receptors is sufficient to establish normal striatal function independently of mesostriatal neuronal activity. Thus normal mesostriatal neuronal function may be similar, releasing a carefully controlled tonic level of dopamine. Nevertheless, the effectiveness of dopamine agonist therapy tends to diminish with time in the same way as L-DOPA therapy. This can be explained in one of two ways. Firstly, in addition to the exogenously supplied dopamine agonist, there may be a requirement for some kind of regulated dopamine release in the mesostriatal neurones in order to establish proper striatal function. This may reflect the normal small increases in mesostriatal activity in preparation for a movement (see below). As the mesostriatal neurones gradually disappear, this component is lost and the dopamine agonist alone cannot control striatal function adequately.

Secondly, as described in Chapter 5, some of the dopamine agonists used, e.g. bromo-criptine and lisuride, are D_2 dopamine receptor agonists and D_1 dopamine receptor antagonists. It is becoming clear from animal experiments that motor function controlled by mesostriatal dopamine cells is dependent on dopamine having agonist activities at D_1 and D_2 receptors in the striatum (Waddington 1986). Thus early in treatment with a dopamine agonist, the D_2 receptors will be occupied by the exogenous agonist and D_1 receptors may be occupied by the endogenous dopamine. As the mesostriatal cells are lost the situation will alter and, particularly if the drugs have D_1 antagonist activity, control may be lost. This may explain why combined L-DOPA and bromocriptine lose their effect less quickly than the individual drugs. It will be of interest in the future to see the effect of a combination of a potent D_1 receptor agonist and D_2 receptor agonist in controlling the disease for long duration, although spread of the degeneration to other brain pathways may ultimately limit the success of this approach. Apomorphine, with D_1 and D_2 receptor agonist activity, may go some way towards providing these functions.

Selegiline (Deprenyl)

This drug, which is a specific inhibitor of monoamine oxidase B, has been proposed for therapy in Parkinson's disease on the basis that it should reduce the breakdown of dopamine and thus prolong its action (either endogenous dopamine or that supplied exogenously by L-DOPA therapy). Results are variable: the drug on its own does not seem to have a major acute effect although it does seem to potentiate the action of L-DOPA and reduce fluctuations in response.

Some workers, however, believe that the progressive nature of Parkinson's disease is due to the formation of toxic metabolites of dopamine or the activation of exogenous toxins. If monoamine oxidase B played a part in such activation then selegiline therapy might prevent the progression of the disease. A preliminary study which will be considered later supports this.

Amantadine

This antiviral drug can be of some use in treating early Parkinson's disease. It is more useful than the anticholinergics but less effective than L-DOPA. Its mechanism of action is unclear but it has been suggested that it increases dopamine release. It is also a potent antagonist at the NMDA subclass of glutamate receptor (Turski *et al.* 1991).

Neural transplants

There has been much interest recently in the possibility of replacing the lost dopamine in Parkinson's disease by transplanting tissue containing dopamine-releasing cells into the brains of patients with the disease. Two sources of tissue have been considered. The adrenal medulla produces some dopamine and, in experimental animals, adrenal grafts into the striatum corrected motor deficits due to loss of dopamine. The first adrenal transplants in Parkinsonian patients were carried out in Sweden and no long term benefits were reported. In 1987, however, reports from Mexico suggested major clinical improvements in parkinsonian patients with adrenal grafts (Moore 1987). A number of other similar operations have subsequently been performed in the United States and the clinical improvement has been much less and there have been significant complications. In addition, the adrenal graft does not seem to survive so this does not seem a very promising avenue for treatment.

An alternative tissue source would be substantia nigra and fetal tissue would be required in order for the grafted cells to survive. In animal models fetal substantia nigra grafts form synaptic connections and successfully correct motor deficits due to depletion of dopamine. Transplants of fetal nigral cells into Parkinson's disease patients have been performed in a number of centres with mixed results. Some striking improvements have been reported whereas in other cases little or no improvement results (Lindvall 1989). Recent results from carefully controlled clinical studies of fetal nigral implants do show some improvement in the patients (Freed *et al.* 1990; Lindvall *et al.* 1990). The nigral grafts survive for up to a year and the presence of the graft seems to be associated with the clinical improvement. The technique is still, however, experimental, it is not clear why a unilateral graft provides bilateral improvement in motor function in some patients and the ethical issues need careful discussion (Calne and McGeer 1989; Freed 1990). Also at present the improvement from a fetal nigral graft is less than can be achieved with some of the newer drug treatments such as subcutaneous apomorphine (Quinn 1990).

Theories of the aetiology of Parkinson's disease

What needs to be explained here is why a group of nerve cells, the mesostriatal dopamine neurones, undergo a relatively selective degeneration in Parkinson's disease. I shall consider some theories for this.

If we could understand the cause of the degeneration in Parkinson's disease it would enable rational means to be proposed to prevent the disease. It might also help in understanding other degenerative diseases such as Alzheimer's disease (Chapter 12). An auto-immune aetiology has been proposed (Abramsky and Litvin 1978) but Parkinson's disease does not show the hallmarks of an autoimmune disease such as major fluctuations in clinical symptoms. Other explanations must, therefore, be sought and I shall consider broadly two kinds of evidence before attempting to summarize in terms of a theory. Firstly there are families where Parkinson's disease shows some heritability. Secondly there are the different parkinsonian syndromes which show some of the symptoms of Parkinson's disease and have relatively well defined aetiologies related to exposure to environmental agents.

Heritability of Parkinson's disease

The recent discovery of a large kindred showing inherited Parkinson's disease (Golbe *et al*. 1990) has led to a reappraisal of ideas about genetic influences in this disease. The kindred show the apparent inheritance of an early onset form of Parkinson's disease in an autosomally dominant manner with high penetrance. Typically, however, Parkinson's disease does not show a high heritability of this kind and recent studies comparing monozygotic and dizygotic twins concluded that there was no inherited component to Parkinson's disease (Johnson *et al*. 1990). These twin studies may, however, be methodologically flawed: if mitochondrial proteins encoded by genes on the mito-chondrial genome were involved, then the concordance rates in monozygotic and di-zygotic twins would be similar (Harding 1991) unlike a disorder dependent on nuclear genes (Chapter 9). Also, as noted earlier, overt symptoms of Parkinson's disease appear only when a threshold of neuronal loss has been crossed, but there may also be asymptomatic individuals who have a subthreshold neuronal loss due to the same process. Inherited factors might be underestimated if this subclinical damage is not con-sidered in assessing concordance rates although it is difficult to do this. Therefore the possibility must be entertained that in some cases an inherited single gene defect can lead to Parkinson's disease and that in other cases inherited factors may play a role.

Parkinsonian syndromes related to environmental agents

Encephalitis lethargica

Between 1915 and 1926 in central Europe, a viral disease, encephalitis lethargica, affected many individuals. It was more prevalent in adolescents and young adults although it afflicted all ages. The disorder began with influenza-like symptoms and this was followed by behavioural changes including somnolence (this came to be called 'sleeping sickness'). Mortality was high (40 per cent) and at least half of the survivors developed parkinsonism within five years. It has sometimes been suggested that this syndrome is connected with the influenza pandemic of 1918–19 but this seems not to be the case.

   Neuropathological examination showed that the substantia nigra was severely affected and that striatal and nigral dopamine levels were reduced (Hornykiewicz 1973). Despite this apparent similarity at the neuropathological level with Parkinson's disease, the incidence of Lewy bodies is no greater than in the normal population, but neuro-fibrillary tangles (Chapter 12) are seen. The syndrome is separate from Parkinson's disease, being more of a disease of youth, and has a different clinical profile. Some of the confusion surrounding the syndrome is due to the fact that as these patients aged it became increasingly difficult to distinguish them from Parkinson's disease patients.

   The existence of the syndrome shows that a viral infection can induce mesostriatal degeneration and a parkinsonian syndrome. Thus viral aetiologies have been considered for Parkinson's disease, but there is currently no evidence in support of this.

Manganese or carbon disulphide exposure

Industrial exposure to either of these substances induces a syndrome with some of the symptoms of Parkinson's disease, but in neither case is the syndrome identical to Parkinson's disease. Neuropathological examination shows that manganese exposure leads to striatal degeneration whereas carbon disulphide exposure leads, in animals, to degeneration of striatal output pathways. Thus neither syndrome resembles Parkinson's disease at the neuropathological level although structures related to the mesostriatal pathway are affected. The existence of the two syndromes does, however, show that environmental toxins can cause degeneration of specific nerve cells and lead to parkinsonian symptoms.

Antipsychotic drug treatment

An early side effect of treatment of schizophrenia with antipsychotic drugs can be parkinsonian symptoms (extrapyramidal side effects) (see Chapter 13). The symptoms disappear upon withdrawal of the drugs or reduction of dosage and presumably relate to blockade of striatal dopamine receptors of the D_2 subclass. This then is a neurochemical equivalent of loss of mesostriatal control on the striatum and supports the idea that loss of dopamine neurones is responsible for the motor deficits of Parkinson's disease.

Amyotrophic lateral sclerosis: parkinsonian syndrome–dementia complex on Guam

A very high incidence of three degenerative nervous disorders (amyotrophic lateral sclerosis, parkinsonian syndrome, and senile dementia) has been reported on the island of Guam. The occurrence has been linked to water supplies low in Mg^{2+} and Ca^{2+} but high in aluminium or to the consumption of the cycad seed (Garruto and Yase 1986). Preliminary evidence was presented suggesting that the amyotrophic lateral sclerosis could be due to the presence of β-N-methylamino alanine in the cycad seed which acted as an exogenous neurotoxin (Spencer *et al.* 1987). There is much debate on this and it now seems that this substance would have been largely removed before consumption of the flour derived from the cycad seeds (Duncan *et al.* 1990). Therefore either abnormal minerals (Garruto *et al.* 1988) or another substance in the cycad seeds (Spencer *et al.* 1990) are the best candidates for producing the neurodegeneration. These observations provide further circumstantial evidence for environmental effects leading to degeneration of specific neuronal pathways.

1-Methyl-4-phenyl-1,2,3,6-tetrahydro pyridine (MPTP)

This substance was sold in error to heroin addicts in Northern California as a narcotic substitute in 1982 (Langston 1985; Singer *et al.* 1987). These individuals rapidly developed a severe parkinsonian syndrome that very closely resembled Parkinson's disease in terms of symptoms. The resemblance at the neuropathological level was also close, with a profound degeneration of the mesostriatal dopamine pathway. MPTP can also induce a parkinsonian syndrome when administered to primates, but in young animals the brain changes caused by MPTP are more restricted than those seen in Parkinson's disease in humans. In young animals MPTP causes selective damage to the substantia nigra, with other brain areas remaining intact. In elderly primates, however, more extensive pathology is seen with damage to the locus coeruleus and the appearance of inclusion bodies resembling Lewy bodies. The parkinsonian syndrome induced by MPTP treatment of humans and experimental animals therefore provides a rather useful model for Parkinson's disease. It offers a new research tool as well as prompting speculation on the aetiology of the disease.

It seems that MPTP is not the toxic substance, rather MPP$^+$ (Fig. 10.5) is generated by the action of monoamine oxidase B (glial and neuronal). The MPP$^+$ is then taken up by dopamine cells via the normal dopamine reuptake carrier, thus gaining access to the dopamine cells where it is taken into mitochondria in which it inhibits oxidative phosphorylation by inhibiting complex I of the mitochondrial electron transport chain. Thus the cells are depleted of ATP and die. The selectivity of MPTP for aminergic cells is

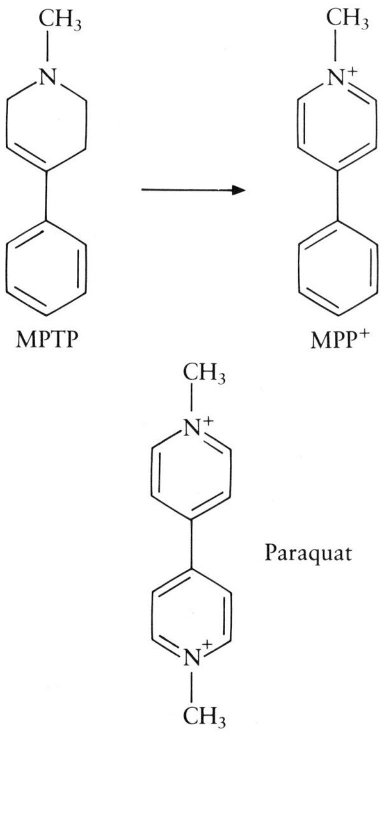

Figure 10.5   The structure of MPTP and its activation to MPP$^+$. The structure of paraquat is shown for comparison.

explained by the presence on these cells (dopaminergic and noradrenergic) of a mono-amine reuptake mechanism for monoamines that will also carry MPP$^+$. The particular vulnerability of the mesostriatal cells may be due to neuromelanin in the cells that acts as a depot for MPP$^+$ (D'Amato *et al.* 1986; Hirsch *et al.* 1988).

The existence of MPTP-induced parkinsonism has led to speculation that Parkinson's disease itself could be caused by an environmental factor. Substances related to MPTP are present in many foods, for example isoquinolines (Singer and Ramsay 1990), and in certain pesticides, for example paraquat, which resembles MPP$^+$ structurally although it is unlikely to share the same mechanism of action (Fig. 10.5). Evidence has also been presented for an increased incidence of Parkinson's disease in agricultural regions of Canada where pesticide usage would be higher. Increased incidence has also been suggested linked variously to industrialization, living in a rural environment, or to the drinking of well water (Tanner 1989; Koller *et al.* 1990). Another class of compound related to MPP$^+$ is the β-carbolines which are metabolites of the naturally occurring indoleamines (Singer and Ramsay 1990). It may therefore be that our environment contains several possible factors that could lead to selective mesostriatal degeneration; this would complicate epidemiological studies which have frequently indicated a general incidence of the disease unrelated to specific environmental factors.

These examples of environmentally determined parkinsonian syndromes and especially the effects of MPTP have highlighted interest in the possibility of an environmental cause for Parkinson's disease as suggested earlier, and the examples of familial Parkinson's disease have led to a resurgence of interest in genetic factors in the occurrence of the disease. Let us consider how a theory might be constructed to account for Parkinson's disease that takes these factors into consideration.

Central to the theory is the inability of brain neurones to divide. The brain cannot, therefore, replace damaged or dead neurones, rendering it very vulnerable to patholog-ical cell loss. Now, there is a normal age-dependent loss of neurones in the mesostriatal dopamine pathway. This is not well documented but appears to be rather slow in the early to middle years with a marked acceleration during the later years ($>$60 years) (Mann 1984; Calne 1989). The cause of the cell loss is unknown but could reflect a gradual oxidative cell damage owing to toxic metabolites of dopamine released by metabolic oxidation by monoamine oxidase, for example hydrogen peroxide. We can-not, however, exclude cell damage due to environmental factors and it could also be that individuals differ in their rates of cell loss owing to genetic differences (see below). The later acceleration of cell loss might reflect increased oxidative damage due to increased turnover of dopamine subsequent to increased cell activity compensating for partial loss of dopamine cells.

Parkinson's disease shows a similar pattern of a relatively low incidence in the middle years with an increased incidence in the later years. This is consistent with a model for

Parkinson's disease of an abnormal loss of mesostriatal neurones superimposed on the normal age-dependent loss of neurones. The abnormal cell loss could be either a single major loss of cells or a gradual loss of cells at a rate above the normal cell loss (Fig. 10.6). In either case the normal rapid acceleration of cell loss in the later years may then reduce the striatal dopamine level to below the threshold of 20% when the clinical symptoms will be seen (Calne and Langston 1983; Calne *et al*. 1986).

The challenge then is to understand the cause of the abnormal cell loss in Parkinson's disease and we must consider here the effects of environmental factors and possible genetic factors. As environmental factors we can consider a possible neurotoxin, perhaps similar to MPTP, and as outlined above there are substances in the environment that might act in this way. A single large exposure or a chronic low level exposure to the toxin would provide for the cell loss. The normal age-dependent loss of cells could also be ascribed to low level exposure to environmental toxins.

There is also evidence that metabolism of iron is disturbed in Parkinson's disease (Dexter *et al*. 1989*b*) and this might add to free radical damage in cells already undergoing oxidative stress through excessive metabolism of dopamine. There is also evidence for increased lipid peroxidation in brains from Parkinson's disease patients (Dexter *et al* 1986, 1989*a*) which would be consistent with ongoing oxidative damage. Related to these observations are the recent descriptions in post-mortem brains from Parkinson's disease patients of deficiencies in complex I of the mitochondrial electron transport

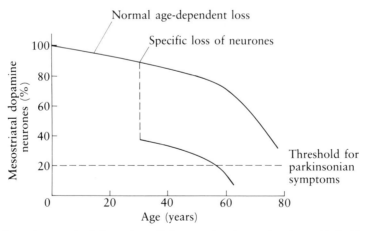

Figure 10.6 Loss of mesostriatal dopamine cells in normal patient and patient with Parkinson's disease. The graph is based on Calne and Langston (1983) and Calne (1989) and shows the normal loss of mesostriatal cells and in Parkinson's disease patients, a large specific loss of cells related to a particular environmental insult superimposed on this gradual loss. This combined with the normal loss due to ageing takes the mesostriatal cell number below 20% and Parkinson's disease results. As discussed in the text, parkinsonian symptoms could also result from a gradual loss of mesostriatal cells at a rate greater than the normal rate of loss and there may be different numbers of mesostriatal cells present at the outset in different patients.

chain (Mizuno *et al*. 1989; Schapira *et al*. 1990*a,b*). As noted above, MPP$^+$ inhibits energy generation in neurones by inhibiting complex I of the mitochondrial electron transport chain so one explanation for the loss of complex I in Parkinson's disease could be that it has been damaged by an MPP-like toxin. An alternative possibility is afforded by recent observations on the mitochondrial genome in Parkinson's disease. In normal ageing and to a much greater extent in Parkinson's disease, deletions of mitochondrial DNA are observed including regions that code for subunits of complex I of the electron transport chain (Ikebe *et al*. 1990; Ozawa *et al*. 1991). This could provide a rationalization for the death of mesostriatal neurones in normal ageing and the greater loss in Parkinson's disease. Cell death would be caused by interference with ATP generation by loss of components of the mitochondrial electron transport chain. The damage to the mitochondrial genome could reflect the effects of free radicals generated during the metabolism of dopamine.

As for inherited genetic factors I can only speculate. One possibility is that individuals have genetically determined differences in the number of mesostriatal neurones. A low number of mesostriatal neurones in an individual would predispose to later Parkinson's disease with the normal age-dependent loss of these neurones, whereas those with high starting numbers of mesostriatal neurones would not get the disease unless other damage also occurred. Other possibilities are that the genetic factor specified is related to detoxification or oxidative stress generally altering the rate of mesostriatal cell loss. It must be emphasized, however, that these putative genetic factors would have a dominant effect only in families where the disease appears to be clearly inherited. In other patients the expression of the genetic factor would play a role alongside environmental factors, otherwise inheritance patterns would be clearer.

A common strand in the discussion above has been that mesostriatal cell loss may be related to oxidative damage perhaps via free radicals, in turn derived from dopamine metabolism or via an MPTP-like toxin. Free radicals derived from dopamine metabolism and MPTP activation depend on activity of the enzyme monoamine oxidase. These considerations have focused interest on monoamine oxidase B as the major subtype of the enzyme in human brain (see Chapter 5). This would be the major generator of free radicals or MPP$^+$-like toxins and so it has been suggested that inhibition of monoamine oxidase B might slow the progression of Parkinson's disease in newly diagnosed patients. A major trial is at present in progress to test this hypothesis where patients are being treated with selegiline (deprenyl), the selective inhibitor of monoamine oxidase B, and tocopherol in order to suppress more general free radical formation (Lewin 1985). Preliminary results (Tetrud and Langston 1989; Shoulson *et al*. 1989) from this and similar trials have shown that selegiline delays the need for L-DOPA therapy in early Parkinson's disease. It is currently not clear whether this is due to the slowing of the disease process or whether selegiline simply prolongs the action of dopamine in the brain but this is obviously a key area of current research.

In summary, therefore, the theory proposed here (Fig. 10.6) is that Parkinson's disease is due to an abnormal loss of mesostriatal cells (acute or chronic) superimposed on the normal age-dependent loss of these cells. When the threshold for neuronal loss is exceeded, Parkinson's disease results. Such a theory can also include the encephalitis lethargica patients. In these patients the virus could have caused a very large degeneration of the mesostriatal cells so that within a few years even young patients developed parkinsonism. Therefore, MPTP-induced parkinsonism, encephalitis lethargica related parkinsonism, and Parkinson's disease itself may be reflections of the same overall pattern, an abnormal mesostriatal cell loss superimposed on the normal age-dependent loss of these cells. A related theory is now being applied to another degenerative disease of brain, Alzheimer's disease (Chapter 12).

This theory for Parkinson's disease predicts that there will be a number of individuals who have subclinical damage to the mesostriatal pathway. These patients will have lost a large proportion of their mesostriatal cells but not enough to produce the clinical symptoms of Parkinson's disease; the presence of Lewy bodies in non-parkinsonian patients is in agreement with this. Some further evidence in favour of this contention comes from parkinsonian-like side effects induced by antipsychotic drugs (see Chapter 13). These drugs are used to treat schizophrenia and a major mechanism of action of these drugs is to block dopamine transmission. Only a proportion of patients taking these drugs show the parkinsonian-like side effects and the incidence of the side effects shows a similar age profile to the incidence of Parkinson's disease. A plausible explanation is that only in those patients who have already lost a substantial proportion of their mesostriatal cells will interference with dopamine transmission lead to parkinsonian-like side effects.

Further evidence in general agreement with the theory comes from patients who have taken MPTP but not developed parkinsonism. These patients show a reduced ability to store striatal dopamine and presumably have lost a proportion of their mesostriatal neurones (Fig. 10.7). Some of these patients have subsequently developed parkinsonian symptoms.

Implications for normal brain function

In Parkinson's disease there is a relatively selective loss of the mesostriatal dopamine pathway which normally runs from the substantia nigra (pars compacta) to innervate the neostriatum (caudate nucleus and putamen) and globus pallidus. The relatively discrete set of clinical symptoms may be treated by replacement of dopamine function either directly with dopamine agonists or indirectly with L-DOPA. These observations have implications for our understanding of the function of the mesostriatal dopamine pathway in the overall expression of motor function by the brain.

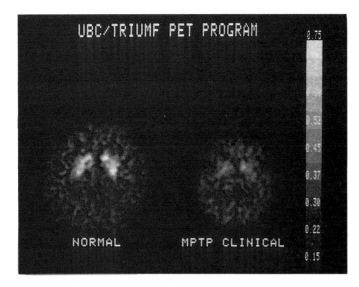

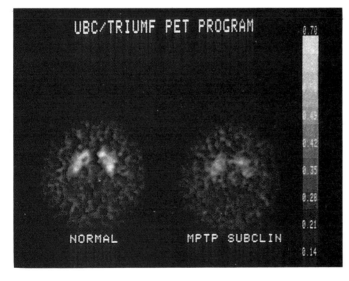

Figure 10.7 Positron emission tomography (PET) study of [^{18}F]L-DOPA accumulation as in Fig. 10.4 in human brain. The upper panel shows a normal scan (left) and a scan from a patient with parkinsonism (right) caused by MPTP. The lower panel shows a normal scan (left) and a scan from a patient who had taken MPTP but was free of parkinsonian symptoms (right). [^{18}F]L-DOPA accumulation in the latter patient is intermediate between that in the normal and the patient exhibiting parkinsonism. The pictures were kindly supplied by Professor D. B. Calne, University of British Columbia.

Normal function of the mesostriatal pathway

I shall now attempt a description of the function of the mesostriatal dopamine pathway based on a synthesis of information in this and in previous chapters (5 and 7). The synaptic target of the mesostriatal dopamine neurones is the striatal medium spiny cell. In Chapter 7 it was suggested that the effects of dopamine might be on the one hand to reduce the basal firing rate of the medium spiny cells, making them more responsive to cortical inputs, and on the other hand to modulate (inhibit) more specifically the cortical inputs to the medium spiny cells. In fact, as will be described in the next section, the functional effects of dopamine are to facilitate transmission in some medium spiny cells and inhibit it in others.

The results of dopamine agonist therapy in Parkinson's disease cited earlier suggest that the mesostriatal cells largely function tonically (acting in a sustained manner over time rather than in a variable or phasic manner) by releasing a controlled level of dopamine, achieving a particular dopamine concentration and this dopamine concentration occupies the postsynaptic receptors to a particular degree. The concentration of dopamine achieved at the target sites is regulated by presynaptic autoreceptors (Chapter 5). Although it was suggested above that following mesostriatal neurone degeneration some dopamine is released and reaches sites distant from the release sites, it is unlikely that dopamine normally reaches sites distant from the release sites. Conventional synapses are formed by mesostriatal neurones and the topographical organization of the mesostriatal innervation of the striatum argues against widespread normal diffusion. The postsynaptic receptors for dopamine (D_1 and D_2) are slow acting receptors (see Chapters 5 and 6). Thus the effects of dopamine in the striatum are slow; this is consistent with tonic release of dopamine.

The role of the medium spiny striatal cell is to convey information about movement (see below) but although the activity of the mesostriatal cells increases slightly in preparation for and during a movement, their activity does not correlate with specific movements unlike that of the striatal cells themselves (Schultz *et al.* 1983). We can suggest therefore that the mesostriatal dopamine cells are acting in a 'gain setting' manner. In preparation for a movement their activity increases slightly, increasing dopamine release to a new higher steady level; this reduces the basal firing rate of some of the medium spiny cells making them more responsive to the impending input of motor information as well as inhibiting some inputs on to dendritic spines. There is also a shift in the balance between striatal output pathways as described in the next section. It is indeed because of its rather slow function and the ability of dopamine to act diffusely that therapy with L-DOPA or exogenous agonist is possible. The implications of these ideas are that permanent therapy with agonists should be possible but reasons have been outlined earlier why this may not be the case. In the long term perhaps the most important is that the disease is progressive and with time other pathway losses occur. Long term research should be aimed therefore at preventing the degeneration.

The mesostriatal dopamine pathway and motor control

Can we learn anything about the normal function of the mesostriatal pathway in motor control from observations of Parkinson's disease patients? In these patients the pathway degenerates and the result is profound motor deficit as well as more subtle cognitive deficits (see below). This would suggest that the pathway is involved in some aspects of motor control and cognition. This can be appreciated better by considering the overall brain pathways in which the striatum participates.

The neostriatum (caudate nucleus and putamen) receives inputs from almost the entire cerebral cortex as well as the thalamus (Fig. 10.8). It sends outputs to the thalamus via the two output nuclei of the basal ganglia, the globus pallidus and the substantia nigra (pars reticulata). From the thalamus, pathways return to specific parts of the cortex and the overall function of the looped circuit is to facilitate activity in the cerebral cortex. This is achieved by striatally driven disinhibition of the thalamocortical projection. The signal from the thalamus to the cortex then enables or facilitates cortically generated motor function. There seem to be some clear subdivisions in these systems (Alexander *et al*. 1986). There is a 'motor circuit' in which information from sensory and motor cortices as well as the supplementary motor area (an area of cerebral cortex thought to be involved in programming, initiating, and excuting movement) is fed

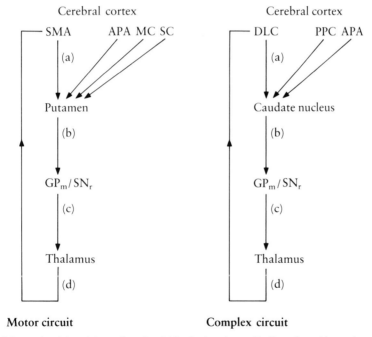

Fig. 10.8 'Motor circuit' and 'complex circuit' in the basal ganglia (based on Alexander *et al*. 1986). In the 'motor circuit', SMA is the supplementary motor area, APA is the arcuate premotor area, MC is the motor cortex and SC the somatosensory cortex. One example of a 'complex circuit' is shown, termed the dorsolateral prefrontal circuit: DLC is the dorsolateral prefrontal cortex, PPC the posterior parietal cortex and APA the arcuate premotor area. The neurotransmitters involved are glutamate ((a) and (d)) and GABA ((b) and (c)) so that input to striatal regions (putamen/caudate nucleus) from several cerebral cortical regions leads to disinhibition of thalamic projections to specific cortical regions, facilitating their activity. The diagram omits certain details which are included in Fig. 10.9. GP_m is the medial segment of the globus pallidus and SN_r is the pars reticulata of the substantia nigra.

into the putamen. Information then proceeds to the globus pallidus and substantia nigra, the thalamus, and then back specifically to the supplementary motor area. Separate distinct 'complex circuits' funnel information from several cortical regions including association regions through the caudate nucleus, the globus pallidus and substantia nigra, the thalamus, and then back to specific frontal cortical areas. Thus the two major regions of the striatum that are severely affected in Parkinson's disease, i.e. the putamen and the caudate nucleus, participate in functionally different circuits, the former being involved in the more purely motor functions while the latter are involved in more cognitive functions. There is some segregation of connections here in that the caudate nucleus connects more to the substantia nigra and the putamen more to the medial segment of the globus pallidus, but the segregation is only partial and varies in different parts of the two subdivisions of the neostriatum.

There is further complexity in the striatal output pathways that needs to be considered. Striatal medium spiny output neurones project to the substantia nigra (pars reticulata) and globus pallidus as outlined above but there are separate populations of neurones projecting to the lateral and medial segments of the globus pallidus (Fig. 10.9). Whereas the medial segment of the globus pallidus can be aligned with the substantia nigra in that both project to the thalamus, the lateral segment of the globus pallidus projects to the subthalamic nucleus which itself projects on to the two output nuclei of the basal ganglia, the substantia nigra and the medial globus pallidus. Therefore there is a direct pathway linking the striatum to the medial globus pallidus/substantia nigra (inhibitory) and an 'indirect' pathway via the subthalamic nucleus (excitatory overall); the balance of activity in the two will determine the output of the system. If the balance is in favour of the 'direct' pathway, as is likely normally, then this will lead to inhibition of the medial globus pallidus/substantia nigra and in turn disinhibition of thalamic neurones that facilitate cortical activity.

Dopamine controls the different pathways differentially. Whereas dopamine elicits a functional facilitation of activity in the 'direct' striatal–medial globus pallidus/substantia nigra pathways it induces a functional inhibition of the 'indirect' striatal–lateral globus pallidus–subthalamic nucleus pathway. Thus dopamine helps set the balance between the 'direct' and 'indirect' pathways in favour of the former. These interactions together with some of the neurotransmitters involved are shown in Fig. 10.9 and will be considered again later in this chapter and also in subsequent chapters (11 and 13). The small increase in dopamine that occurs in preparation for a movement as discussed in the previous section will further alter the balance of activity in the 'direct' and 'indirect' pathways linking the striatum to the medial globus pallidus/substantia nigra in favour of the 'direct' pathway. This will lead to disinhibition of the thalamus and facilitation of cortical activity and hence movement.

The putamen and caudate nucleus together then receive information from sensory and motor cortices as well as prefrontal association regions. Thus the striatum (putamen and

Normal

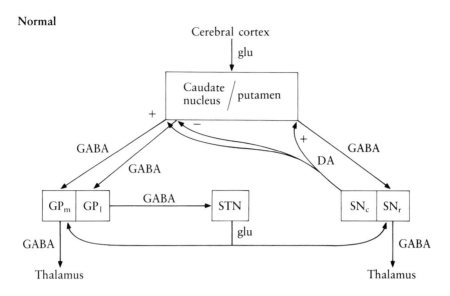

Parkinson's disease

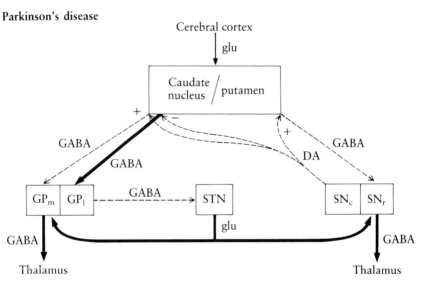

Figure 10.9 Striatal–pallidal–nigral interactions. The upper diagram shows the normal pathways through the neostriatum (caudate nucleus-putamen) and globus pallidus and substantia nigra. Dopamine control is lost in Parkinson's disease, leading to the functional changes depicted in the lower diagram. In the upper diagram the 'direct' pathway from the striatum to the medial globus pallidus (GP$_m$) and the pars reticulata of the substantia nigra (SN$_r$) is shown. In this pathway cortical drive leads to disinhibition of thalamic activity (see Fig. 10.8). The 'indirect' pathway is via the lateral globus pallidus (GP$_l$) and subthalamic nucleus (STN) and this will tend to oppose the activity in the 'direct' pathway so that a balance must be established between the two. Dopamine neurones from the pars compacta of the substantia nigra (SN$_c$) control the 'direct' and 'indirect' pathways differently so that in Parkinson's disease, when the dopamine neurones are lost there is an overall increased inhibition of the thalamus and this ultimately reduces thalamic drive to the cerebral cortex (Fig. 10.8). The net result is a reduction in impulse flow in the cortical–thalamic–cortical circuit and a reduced facilitation of cortically generated motor function (see also Fig. 11.4 and 11.6).

caudate) is at the interface between thought and action: it has been suggested that the striatum and the pathways through it are involved in motor planning, specifically in selecting and assembling the motor programmes that comprise the motor plan. This is likely to be achieved via striatally driven disinhibition of the projection from the thalamus to the cortex which enables or facilitates cortically generated movement. These motor programmes would not be stored in the striatum, rather they would originate from the cerebral cortex. Because of the existence of segregated 'motor' and 'complex' circuits based on the putamen and caudate respectively, it can be seen that the putamen is involved in the more purely motor aspects whereas the caudate nucleus is responsible for more cognitive aspects.

It has been shown earlier that in Parkinson's disease, although there is a generalized deficit of dopamine in the striatum, this is much more severe in the putamen than in the caudate nucleus, at least in the early stages of the disease when motor problems are paramount. It has been suggested that the dopamine deficits in the caudate nucleus may not be great enough to cause a major disruption of dopamine function given the compensatory changes in the remaining mesostriatal cells (Kish *et al*. 1988). Thus the motor deficits can largely be accounted for by disruption of putamen function by the loss of dopamine. Impulse passage in the 'motor circuit' outlined above will be impaired resulting in slowness in initiating movement and slowness in movement. In terms of the complex interactions shown in Fig. 10.9, we can rationalize this as loss of dopamine control over medium spiny putamen cells leading to functional inhibition of the 'direct' putamen—medial globus pallidus/substantia nigra pathway and functional facilitation of the 'indirect' putamen—lateral globus pallidus pathway. The balance between the 'direct' and 'indirect' pathways shifts in favour of the 'indirect' pathway. This will lead to a facilitation of subthalamic nucleus activity and hence facilitation of the subthalamic nucleus control over the substantia nigra and medial globus pallidus. The net result is a reduction in impulse flow in the 'motor circuit' linking the cerebral cortex, striatum, thalamus, and cerebral cortex and a net reduction in cortical drive from the thalamus which is exhibited as a reduction of motor function (Fig. 10.9).

Although this discussion has become very complex it is important in understanding Parkinson's disease but can also help us understand why dyskinesias may result from L-DOPA therapy. Dyskinesias are unwanted movements that appear when high doses of L-DOPA are encountered during long-term L-DOPA therapy. Crossman (1990) has suggested that the origin of the dyskinesias is disturbed control by dopamine of the striatum leading to preferential action of dopamine on the putamen—lateral globus pallidus neurones leading to their inhibition and subsequent inhibition of the subthalamic nucleus. This disturbs the balance of striatal output pathways in favour of the 'direct' pathway so that there is excessive drive to the cerebral cortex, and dyskinesias can result. In later chapters I shall return to these ideas in accounting for different forms of unwanted movement in Huntington's disease (Chapter 11) and schizophrenia (Chapter 13).

Whereas the motor deficits in Parkinson's disease are clear and can be explained in terms of the impaired normal striatal function, this is not the case with cognitive deficits. The very existence of cognitive deficits (other than dementia, which is a late symptom in some patients) has been debated but it does seem that there are clear but subtle cognitive deficits e.g. impaired ability to use spatial information for motor function, inability to shift 'mental set' (perseveration), memory problems, or mood alterations.

Recent studies have stressed deficits in tasks related to self-directed behavioural planning and have suggested that this is related to deficits in the activities of prefrontal cortical regions (Taylor *et al*. 1986*a,b*; Gotham *et al*. 1988; Morris *et al*. 1988; Brown and Marsden 1990). It is as though there is a decreased ability to control the attention of the internal processes of the brain and this causes problems in planning action and thought. This has also been interpreted as a reduction in central processing capacity. Problems with frontal cortical function may be explained in two ways, both of which may contribute to the cognitive deficits of Parkinson's disease. Firstly there is extensive linkage of the frontal cortical association regions with the caudate nucleus in the complex (cognitive) loop referred to earlier. The mesostriatal innervation of the caudate nucleus declines in Parkinson's disease and although the decline is not as great as for the putamen, there is likely to be disruption of function in the caudate nucleus and hence in the cognitive loop (Figs 10.8 and 10.9). That the cognitive changes are rather subtle is consistent with the relative sparing of the caudate nucleus. Similar cognitive changes are seen in Huntington's disease (Chapter 12) where caudate nucleus efferent pathways are damaged and in progressive supranuclear palsy where a severe mesostriatal dopamine loss in the caudate nucleus is seen (Kish *et al*. 1985).

Secondly there is a loss of mesocortical dopamine pathways in Parkinson's disease. These innervate frontal cortical regions and so disruption of function may occur. Thus there is ample scope for minor diffuse changes in cognitive, frontal cortical type functions in Parkinson's disease.

Recommended reading

Agid, Y., Cerrera, P., Hirsch, E., Javoy-Agid, F., Lehericy, S., Rousman, R., and Ruberg, M. (1989). Biochemistry of Parkinson's Disease 28 Years Later: a critical review. *Movement Disorders*, **4**, supplement 1, S126–44.

Albin, R. L., Young, A. B., and Penney, R. B. (1989). The functional anatomy of basal ganglia disorders. *Trends in Neurosciences*, **12**, 366–75.

Crossman, A. R. (1990). A hypothesis on the pathophysiological mechanisms that underlie levodopa or dopamine agonist induced dyskinesias in Parkinson's Disease: implications for future strategies and treatments. *Movement Disorders*, **5**, 100–8.

Duvoisin, R. (1987). History of parkinsonism. *Pharmacology and Therapeutics*, **32**, 1–17.

Lang, A. E. (1987). Manipulating the dopaminergic system in Parkinson's Disease. *Pharmacology and Therapeutics*, **32**, 51–76.

Langston, J. W., Irwin, I., and Ricaurte, G. A. (1987). Neurotoxins, parkinsonism and Parkinson's Disease. *Pharmacology and Therapeutics*, **32**, 19–49.

Lindvall, O. (1989). Transplantation into the human brain: present status and future possibilities. *Journal of Neurology, Neurosurgery and Psychiatry*, supplement, 39–54.

Martin, W. R. W. (1987). The contribution of PET scanning to understanding metabolism and drug actions in the basal ganglia. *Pharmacology and Therapeutics*, **32**, 77–87.

Marsden, C. D. (1982). The mysterious motor functions of the basal ganglia. *Neurology*, **32**, 514–39.

Marsden, C. D. (1990). Parkinson's Disease. *Lancet*, **335**, 948–52.

Marsden, C. D. and Parkes, J. D. (1977). Success and problems of long term levodopa therapy in Parkinson's Disease. *Lancet*, **i**, 345–9.

11   *Huntington's disease*

Huntington's disease (chorea) is a well defined neurological disorder which first gained recognition from the work of George Huntington. The disease came to be named after Huntington, who studied the incidence of chorea in families in East Hampton, Long Island, New York in the late 1800s. The disease is an inherited one and families of Huntington's disease sufferers in different parts of the world may be traced back to emigrés from Europe in the 1600s. For example, many of the New England group of sufferers may be traced back to brothers who left Bures St Mary, Suffolk, UK for Salem, Massachusetts in 1630 (Critchley 1984) (Fig. 11.1). Indeed it has been suggested that some of the 'witches of Salem' may have suffered from the disease.

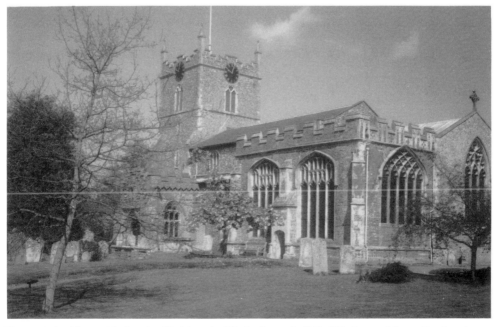

Figure 11.1   The parish church of St Mary the Virgin, Bures, Suffolk, UK. Some of the earliest immigrants to the United States came from Bures and it is thought that the genetic defect of Huntington's disease was carried by three brothers from Bures who settled in Salem, Massachusetts (Critchley 1984). Photograph by the author.

Clinical description

Huntington's disease is a rare inherited disease affecting 0.01 per cent of the population. It has a mean age of onset between 35 and 42 years and is progressive, death occurring on average 17 years after the onset of the full disease.

The principal symptoms of the full disease are involuntary, choreiform (dance like) movements and dementia. The movements are characteristically out of control, continuous, and jerky with many parts of the body affected. Eventually speech and the ability to stand and walk may become impaired. In addition to the chorea, there is a slowness of voluntary movement (bradykinesia) not unlike that seen in Parkinson's disease (Thompson *et al*. 1988). The dementia is different from the dementia of Alzheimer's disease (Chapter 12). Whereas there are thinking and learning difficulties, apraxia, aphasia, and agnosia are absent in Huntington's disease (Smith and Mindham 1987).

The disease has an insidious onset and may first manifest as changes in personality or rather minor signs of movement problems such as unsteadiness or clumsiness. The personality changes may include emotional disturbances such as depression and cognitive impairment and may be apparent up to ten years before the full disease presents. Owing to the inherited nature of the disease, given a positive family history, diagnosis is not difficult and there is an inexorable progression to death frequently by choking or pneumonia. Suicide is also more common than in the general population.

A minor proportion of cases show juvenile onset (<15 years) with bradykinesia, epilepsy, dementia, and ataxia and a very rapid course. On the other hand, late onset cases (>60 years) show a slower progression and less severe symptoms.

The disease is an autosomal dominant one whereby the child of an affected parent has a 50 per cent chance of inheriting the gene. Penetrance is 100 per cent in that given the presence of the inherited gene, the disease will be expressed. Heterozygous and homozygous patients are clinically indistinguishable (Wexler *et al*. 1987); the significance of this will be considered below. Studies of the inheritance of the age of onset indicate that the expression of the Huntington's disease gene may be modified by a small number of other genes.

Individuals at risk will frequently have had children by the time the disease becomes apparent and, on average, 50 per cent of their children will then get the disease. The decision by children of an affected parent not to have children themselves would prevent further occurrence of the disease. This would, however, be unnecessary in half of the cases and, in the absence of a foolproof test for the Huntington's disease gene, such advice has serious ethical ramifications. Fortunately, molecular genetic analysis of Huntington's disease families (see below) has provided gene probes related to markers on chromosome 4 which can be used to predict with a high degree of accuracy whether an individual will develop the disease, given good familial inheritance data. Limited predictions are also possible when less extensive familial data are available. The accuracy of the test will increase when the actual gene has been identified.

The testing of potential carriers of the gene will, however, pose further ethical problems. Application of the test will free half the individuals from the burden of the worry of developing the disease whereas for the other half the test result will be equivalent to a death sentence given the absence of any effective treatment. When an accurate test is available, prenatal diagnosis and selective abortion should lead to a major reduction in incidence but this has further ethical problems.

Neuropathological observations

Post-mortem examination of the brain from Huntington's disease patients shows a generalized shrinkage which may be as much as 20 per cent in advanced cases. There are losses of neurones from a number of structures including the neostriatum (caudate nucleus, and putamen), globus pallidus, cerebellum, and cerebral cortex. The changes seen depend very much on the extent of progression of the disease. Glial cell numbers may appear to be increased but this may reflect preservation of glia relative to neurones.

The earliest changes in the brain of a Huntington's disease patient seem to occur in the striatum where a number of cell types are lost. The striatum also shows the greatest loss of neurones in advanced cases where up to 95 per cent of the striatal neurones are lost, although then changes in other regions are apparent. The atrophy of the striatum may be clearly seen in post-mortem sections (Fig. 11.2) and some tissue loss can be detected using magnetic resonance imaging (Fig. 11.3). Within the striatum, specific parts of the

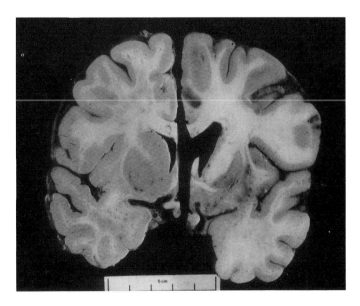

Figure 11.2 Sections of post-mortem human brain from normal (left) and Huntington's disease (right) patients showing the degeneration of the striatum. Courtesy of Dr G. P. Reynolds, Sheffield University.

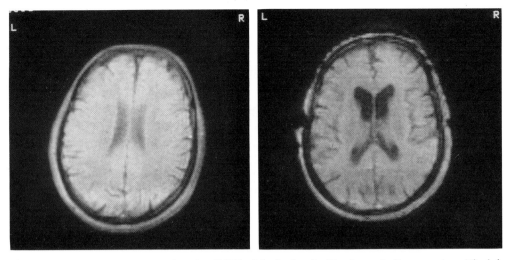

Figure 11.3 Magnetic resonance imaging (MRI) of the brain of a Huntington's disease patient. The left picture shows a horizontal MRI scan of the brain of a normal patient whereas the right picture shows a similar scan from a patient with Huntington's disease where the ventricles show some enlargement owing to loss of brain tissue. Courtesy of Dr F. W. Smith and Dr J. A. D. Besson, Departments of Nuclear Medicine and Mental Health, Medical School, Aberdeen.

caudate nucleus and putamen seem to be affected more as determined by microscopic examination in early stages of the disease but in later stages large areas of both structures are affected.

Imaging techniques using positron emission tomography in living patients are now being applied and have highlighted an early reduction in glucose metabolism in the striatum, especially in the caudate nucleus. This may indicate that the earliest pathological changes in Huntington's disease represent some alteration to cell metabolism which leads to cell death in the caudate nucleus and putamen. There are also some indications of changes in metabolic enzymes responsible for energy production in neurones in brain tissue from Huntington's disease patients (Carter *et al*. 1989).

Extensive post-mortem neurochemical analyses have been performed on Huntington's disease brain. These are best understood by reference to the known cell types and their neurochemistry in the striatum (Fig. 11.4). Early studies indicated substantial loss of the neurotransmitter GABA from the substantia nigra and globus pallidus as well as loss of the associated biosynthetic enzyme glutamic acid decarboxylase in the striatum and substantia nigra. Choline acetyl transferase levels were also decreased in the striatum so that it seemed that a generalized degeneration of striatal cells was occurring in agreement with the neuropathological observations.

There is considerable variability in many of the post-mortem neurochemical observations and this reflects the problems in working with such tissue, e.g. state of the

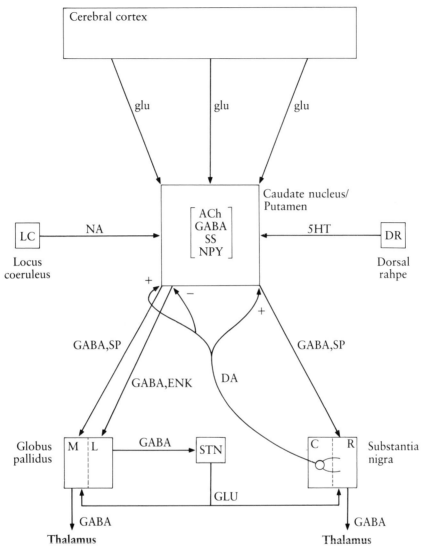

Figure 11.4 The principal connections of the neostriatum (caudate nucleus/putamen) (after Martin 1984; Alexander *et al.* 1986; McGeer *et al.* 1987*b*; Albin *et al.* 1989). The diagram is not exhaustive and further details are contained in the references. M and L refer to the medial and lateral segments of the globus pallidus, C and R to the pars compacta and reticulata of the substantia nigra, and STN to the subthalamic nucleus. In the pars compacta, dendrites of dopamine cells are shown extending into the pars reticulata (Moore and Bloom 1978). The major outputs from the globus pallidus and substantia nigra are to the thalamus (see also Fig. 10.9). Neurotransmitters are shown as follows: glu, glutamate; NA, noradrenaline; 5HT, 5-hydroxytryptamine; SP, substance P; ENK, enkephalin; DA, dopamine. Neurotransmitters in brackets in the caudate/putamen are in interneurones (Ach, acetylcholine; SS, somatostatin; NPY, neuropeptide Y).

patient at death, post-mortem delays, pre-mortem drug treatments, and extent of progression of the disease (Chapter 9). Also, it may be difficult to ascribe a meaning to a neurochemical measurement when such major neuronal losses are occurring in some cell types. More recently, attempts have been made to grade patients according to the severity of their disease and with the examination of more homogeneous samples of tissue a more consistent picture seems to be emerging, with a loss of a particular group of cells in the striatum with preservation of other cell types. The cells that are lost are of the medium spiny type from their appearance and contain the neurotransmitter GABA which coexists with either substance P or met-enkephalin. These cells project to the globus pallidus and substantia nigra where substantial decreases in these substances are seen. Some of the earliest neurochemical changes may be in cells projecting from the striatum to the lateral segment of the globus pallidus (GABA/enkephalin) and cells projecting from the striatum to the pars reticulata of the substantia nigra (GABA/ substance P cells). It is interesting to see how, with more careful neurochemical examination of more defined samples from patients in earlier stages of the disease, the original picture of a rather diffuse atrophy of the striatum can now be seen to be the final result of rather specific early changes in defined neuronal populations. Choline acetyl transferase is also reported to be reduced in the striatum in some studies but not in others; it has been suggested that this may reflect cellular damage rather than loss.

Neurones that project to the striatum do not seem to be as severely affected and although there is some cell loss this is not as great as in the medium spiny cell populations. Thus levels of dopamine, noradrenaline, and 5-hydroxytryptamine are either normal or slightly increased. Levels of glutamate are either normal or slightly decreased in advanced cases (see also Perry and Hansen 1990).

The relative preservation of dopamine neurones may contribute to the chorea as suppression of dopamine activity with antagonists can control the chorea whereas L-DOPA tends to exacerbate these symptoms. This may reflect the selective losses of certain striatal cell types as described above and the differential sensitivity of striatal neurones to dopamine. Mechanisms for this effect will be considered below. The dopamine cells may also be overactive as they lose the normal inhibition they receive from striatal GABA cells.

Some cells within the striatum seem to be unaffected in Huntington's disease; these contain the peptides somatostatin and neuropeptide Y along with an enzyme activity termed NADPH diaphorase. Because of the relative preservation of these cells, levels of these peptides are substantially increased in the striatum of Huntington's disease patients. Striatal somatostatin receptor levels are, however, reduced (Palacios *et al.* 1990).

In summary, the changes in Huntington's disease are complex, but early effects are seen in the striatum and specifically in neurones projecting from the striatum to the globus pallidus and substantia nigra.

Treatment of Huntington's disease

There are few effective ways to treat Huntington's disease and no means to halt the progression. Attempts at treatment have been made based on alleviating the GABA and cholinergic deficits, modelled on the success of dopamine replacement in Parkinson's disease. Neither has been successful. In the case of GABA, this may be because the GABA system is a fast system and simple replacement of GABA does not mimic normal function. In addition, GABA replacement may affect pathways downstream from those degenerating. In the case of the reported cholinergic deficit, the targets for the acetylcholine neurones (GABA cells) are lost. Alternatively baclofen, the $GABA_B$ receptor agonist, has been reported to be of some benefit in Huntington's disease and it may elicit its action by inhibiting the release of glutamate. These findings are preliminary and need confirmation.

The only treatment currently available is to use dopamine antagonists. These give some relief of the choreic symptoms. The effect of these drugs presumably reflects an interference with the action of dopamine from the mesostriatal cells on residual striatal cells; this will be considered in more detail later. As further striatal cell loss occurs, this relief becomes less effective. Even when the choreic symptoms are suppressed the bradykinesia remains and patients are still functionally impaired (Thompson *et al.* 1988).

There is some hope that treatments may become available based on understanding the pathogenesis of the cell loss. If, as described below, this occurs subsequent to release of an excitoxin (a substance that excites (depolarizes) the neurones to such an extent that toxic or degenerative effects result), then inhibition of its effects might halt the progression. Another possibility is the use of neural transplants, but this would need to be applied early in the disease before widespread neuronal loss had occurred. Also, the degenerative process that produces Huntington's disease might affect the transplant, rendering this approach ineffective.

Theories of the aetiology of Huntington's disease

The cause of the brain degeneration in Huntington's disease is unknown and, as in the case of Parkinson's disease (Chapter 10), there is a relatively selective loss of a population of cells together with a more diffuse loss. The major distinction between the two diseases is the clearly inherited nature of Huntington's disease. This facet, together with the application of molecular genetics as outlined below, should lead to the discovery of the underlying genetic defect. This should enable the cause of the degeneration to be understood and it seems likely that the knowledge gained will also be useful in understanding other degenerative diseases of the brain. From this understanding of Huntington's disease it may be possible to propose rational therapies, but in the longer term this may be unnecessary as a genetic test for the disease will allow affected fetuses to be identified. As noted earlier, patients that are heterozygous or homozygous for Huntington's disease are clinically indistinguishable (Wexler *et al.* 1987). This shows that Huntington's disease is not due to elimination of an essential gene, otherwise homozygosity would be lethal. As heterozygosity and homozygosity seem equally deleterious, the disease could reflect the loss or reduction of an enzyme activity that must exceed a strict threshold, or it could reflect the conferment of a novel property on a structural or regulatory protein.

There has been speculation on the aetiology of the disease, centering on the possibility of the production of an endogenous toxin which leads to the degeneration. There is no reason why an exogenous toxin could not also be considered as exogenous toxins have been shown to be able to produce brain degeneration, for example, parkinsonism can be induced by MPTP (Chapter 10). In terms of the comments above, if the toxin were endogenous then the genetic change in Huntington's disease would be associated with its over-production or poor detoxification. For exogenous toxins some defect in detoxification might be anticipated.

Kainic acid and quinolinic acid have been considered as potential toxins acting via excitatory amino acid receptors. Also, the endogenous neurotransmitter glutamic acid has been considered in the same context (Perry and Hansen 1990). These would lead to over-stimulation of the target cell and cell death. Kainic acid injection into the striatum of rats replicates many of the neurochemical alterations seen in Huntington's disease. It does not, however, produce the selective changes outlined above and quinolinic acid has been considered instead. In experimental animals after striatal injection this substance produces neurochemical changes similar but not identical to those seen in Huntington's disease (Ellison *et al.* 1987; Beal *et al.* 1988; Davies and Roberts 1988*a,b*).

Quinolinic acid is indeed made in human brain and a genetic over-production within striatal cells or reduced detoxification would need to be postulated to account for Huntington's disease. Quinolinic acid is thought to exert its action via glutamate receptors of the NMDA subclass. There are preliminary observations supporting and refuting this role for quinolinic acid and the suggestion needs further evaluation (Marx 1987; Reynolds *et al.* 1988; Schwarz *et al.* 1988). There is also some evidence that excessive glutamic acid could give rise to degeneration in the brain (Olney and Gubareff 1978) and in this case it would be necessary to argue that some defect in glutamate metabolism gave rise to the disorder. It is of interest that in post-mortem brain samples taken from Huntington's disease patients, NMDA receptors are selectively lost (Young *et al.* 1988). This would at least be consistent with the presence of NMDA receptors on the degenerating cells. If excessive agonist action at NMDA receptors is responsible for the disease, then blockade of NMDA receptors might prevent the toxic action and act as a therapy for those identified as at risk for the disease. Specific NMDA receptor inhibitors are being developed, e.g. MK801 (Marx 1987).

Molecular genetics in the analysis of Huntington's disease

Huntington's disease is clearly inherited in an autosomal dominant manner and in many affected families the inheritance can be traced back through several generations. This makes the disease ideal for analysis by molecular genetics in order to identify the gene product responsible for the disorder (genetic linkage analysis, Chapter 9). This approach has been successfully used in Duchenne muscular dystrophy to identify the defective gene product, dystrophin (Rowland 1988; Zubrzycka-Gaarn *et al.* 1988; Mandel 1989), and substantial progress has been made in a similar analysis of Huntington's disease (Watt and Edwards 1984; Gusella 1989; also Martin and Gusella (1986) in the recommended reading list).

The analysis of an inherited disease in this way consists of a series of defined stages. I shall consider these for Huntington's disease but they act as a prototype for the analysis of other inherited diseases of the brain, e.g. familial Alzheimer's disease (Chapter 12) and bipolar depressive illness (Chapter 14). Further information on this approach is given in the review by Baron and Rainer (1988). The stages are as follows:

1. Families are identified where the inheritance of the disease is clear and well defined clinically. Blood samples are obtained from all members of the family. In the case of Huntington's disease, early work used one family in Venezuela and another in Iowa, USA.
2. DNA obtained from the blood samples is cut into defined fragments using enzymes (restriction endonucleases). The fragments are analysed by electrophoresis, generating a pattern of fragments that is a 'fingerprint' for the individual. Differences in the DNA between individuals will cause the enzymes to cut at different points, so generating different fragment patterns or polymorphisms (restriction fragment length polymorphisms or RFLPs). Only a part of the DNA fragment pattern is analysed at one time by applying a radioactive probe which is a fragment of DNA which will hybridize to part of the DNA and enable a pattern to be visualized by autoradiography (Fig. 11.5).
3. Analysis of the separated DNA fragments by successive application of different probes will enable a variety of RFLPs to be uncovered. The inheritance of these RFLPs can then be compared with the inheritance of the Huntington's disease gene. Co-inheritance indicates that the gene for the disease is in the vicinity of the enzyme cutting site.
4. Once a RFLP has been identified that is frequently inherited with the disease gene, its chromosomal location can be determined. In the case of Huntington's disease, RFLP analysis showed the gene to be on the short arm of chromosome 4 although at the time of writing the precise gene responsible for the disease has not been identified. Further genetic analysis will enable this to be achieved.

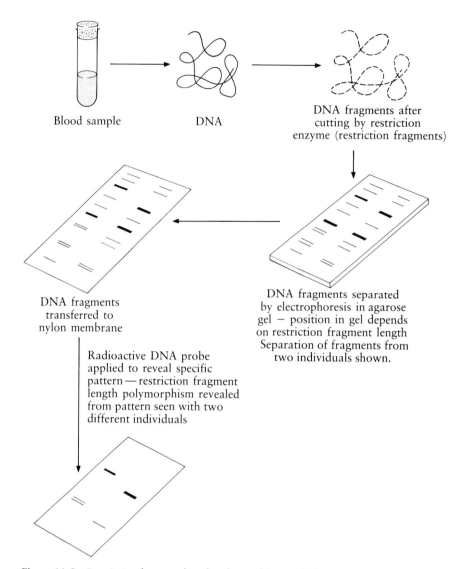

Figure 11.5   Restriction fragment length polymorphism analysis.

5. Once the gene has been identified, the nucleotide sequence can be determined and hence the amino acid sequence of the gene product predicted. Comparison with computer databases of known proteins will show whether this is a known protein. If it is not then it will be necessary to determine the nature of the protein involved. This is not a trivial exercise but it may be approached immunologically using antibodies against defined peptide sequences to locate the protein as in the case of dystrophin

(Zubrzycka-Gaarn *et al*. 1988; Mandel 1989) or it may require the generation of transgenic mice (Gusella 1989).

6. Identification of the gene for the disease will allow a genetic test to be developed. The advantages and ethical problems of this test have been considered earlier. Identification of the gene should also aid considerably in devising treatments for the disease.

Disordered brain function in Huntington's disease

It seems that, at least in the early phases of Huntington's disease, there is a relatively selective loss of particular striatal cell types, specifically those associated with striatal output pathways to the globus pallidus and substantia nigra. The behavioural effects are the involuntary choreiform movements, slowness of voluntary movement, and a form of dementia.

In Chapter 10 the role of the neostriatum (caudate nucleus and putamen) in planning motor function was analysed. The striatum may be involved in selecting and assembling the individual motor programmes that comprise the motor plan. The striatum receives extensive connections from the prefrontal association and sensorimotor regions of the cerebral cortex and after passage through the striatum, information contained in these pathways is passed on to the substantia nigra and globus pallidus, then to the thalamus and back to the cerebral cortex. The thalamocortical projection is important for facilitating cortical activity associated with movement. Separate complex (cognitive) and motor strands exist in these pathways based on the caudate nucleus and putamen respectively (Alexander *et al*. 1986).

Many attempts have been made to provide theories of disrupted brain function in Huntington's disease based on the loss of striatal output pathways, but there are some problems in accounting for the choreic symptoms which can be likened to an uncontrolled readout of individual motor programmes. More recently the example of another motor disease has been noted, namely that of ballism where the patient exhibits an exaggerated form of chorea with uncontrolled movements of the limbs. This disease seems to be caused by the loss of the subthalamic nucleus which might therefore be important for suppressing unwanted motor programmes or controlling which ones are finally read out (Crossman *et al*. 1988).

Indeed in Chapter 10 in the discussion of motor function in Parkinson's disease, it was shown how two pathways link the striatum to the basal ganglia output nuclei, the medial globus pallidus/substantia nigra. These were the 'direct' pathway, forming a direct neuronal link, and the 'indirect' pathway via the lateral segment of the globus pallidus and the subthalamic nucleus. Activity in the 'direct' pathway leads overall to facilitation of cortically generated motor activity and motor function whereas the 'indirect' pathway opposes this. Normally a balance between the two exists but in favour of the 'direct' pathway (Fig. 11.6). It can be seen that in ballism, loss of the subthalamic nucleus will

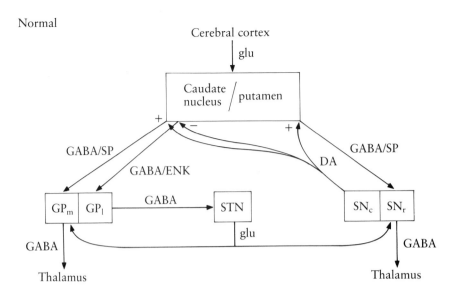

Normal

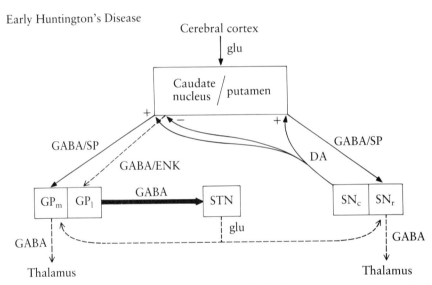

Early Huntington's Disease

Figure 11.6 The diagram, which should be compared with Fig. 10.9 shows the striatal-pallidal-nigral interactions in brains from normal patients and patients with early Huntington's Disease. In the upper diagram the 'direct' and 'indirect' pathways from the neostriatum (caudate nucleus/putamen) to the medial globus pallidus (GP_m) and pars reticulata of the substantia nigra (SN_r) are shown. Normally a balance is set between these two pathways in favour of the 'direct' pathway so that cortically driven striatal activity leads to disinhibition of thalamic activity and thalamo cortical activity occurs facilitating movement.

In early Huntington's Disease (lower diagram) there is a loss of neurones containing GABA and enkephalin (ENK), linking the striatum to the lateral globus pallidus (GP_l) and disrupting the activity of the 'indirect' pathway. The net result is a shift in the balance between the 'direct' and 'indirect' pathways in favour of the former. This leads to reduced pallidal/nigral inhibition of the thalamus and increased thalamo-cortical activity. Since the thalamocortical projections facilitate cortically generated movement patterns this may lead to excessive and unwanted movements (chorea).

In later Huntington's Disease there will be a loss of all striato-pallidal/nigral pathways and this will lead to increased pallidal/nigral inhibition of the thalamus and decreased thalamocortical facilitation of cortically generated movement patterns (bradykinesia).

(GP_m and GP_l are the medial and lateral segments of the globus pallidus. SN_c and SN_r are the pars compacta and pars reticulata of the substantia nigra. STN is the subthalamic nucleus. DA, dopamine, glu, glutamate, SP, substance P, ENK, enkephalin).

alter the balance in favour of the 'direct' pathway. The enabling or facilitating signal from the thalamus to the cerebral cortex will be increased leading to uncontrolled motor activity.

In early Huntington's disease there is a loss of the inhibitory pathway projecting from the striatum to the lateral segment of the globus pallidus. This is part of the 'indirect' pathway from the striatum to the basal ganglia output nuclei, the medial globus pallidus/substantia nigra. Thus the early changes in Huntington's disease would lead to a change in the balance between the 'direct' and 'indirect' pathways in favour of the former, leading to uncontrolled motor activity which is exhibited as chorea (Fig. 11.6). As the striatal degeneration spreads there will be a more general loss of striatal outputs to the globus pallidus (both segments) and substantia nigra, leading to a disruption of information flow in the motor and complex loops through the striatum. The enabling or facilitating signal from the thalamus to the cortex is lost. This will give rise to bradykinesia and an impairment of movement leading to rigidity. I should at this point make the comparison with Parkinson's disease where bradykinesia is also seen. I argued in Chapter 10 that in Parkinson's disease, the loss of the mesostriatal dopamine influence on the striatonigral output cells disrupts information flow in the basal ganglia motor circuit linking the cerebral cortex to the thalamus. Here I have argued for disruption of information flow in late Huntington's disease in the same motor circuit but by actual cell death rather than altered activity. The consequence is, however, the same, i.e. impaired information flow and bradykinesia.

Can we also account for the ability of dopamine antagonists to suppress the choreic symptoms early in the disease? As indicated above, it is now thought that early in the disease there is a selective loss of medium spiny striatal cells projecting to the lateral globus pallidus. These neurones form the first part of the 'indirect' pathway linking the striatum and substantia nigra/medial globus pallidus and the loss of this 'indirect' pathway leads to an imbalance in the striatal output pathways in favour of the 'direct' link. In Chapter 10 it was shown that whereas dopamine performs a 'gain setting' function on striatal neurones, it has overall a facilitatory effect on the 'direct' pathway and an inhibitory effect on the 'indirect' pathway. If, early in the disease, there is an imbalance in favour of the 'direct' pathway, which itself is facilitated by dopamine, then blockade of dopamine receptors may go some way to resetting the balance of striatal outputs and suppressing the chorea. This will be by reducing the facilitation of dopamine on the 'direct' pathway and reducing the inhibition of dopamine on the residual 'indirect' pathway.

A further aspect of this is that the dopamine mesostriatal cells are thought to be inhibited by activity in the striatonigral output cells via the dendrites of the mesostriatal cells in the substantia nigra which extend from the pars compacta to the pars reticulata (Fig. 11.4). This inhibition will be partly lost as the striatal output neurones are lost. The mesostriatal dopamine cells may therefore be overactive; this will further affect the imbalance in the striatal output pathways. Blockade of dopamine receptors may counteract this.

The early dementia of Huntington's disease may also be associated with disruption of striatal function (Brandt and Butters 1986; Smith and Mindham 1987). Patients exhibit problems in planning, organizing, and scheduling activities, slowed thinking, deficits in learning information, and psychopathological problems. Such alterations in behaviour are also seen in part in 'frontal lobe syndrome' where the frontal cortex is damaged. Given the extensive connections, via the complex (cognitive) loop, of the frontal association cortex with the caudate nucleus, where degeneration occurs early in Huntington's disease, such similarities are not surprising (Starkstein *et al.* 1988). Indeed, some patients present first only with neuropsychological problems which can be attributed to an early deficit in caudate nucleus function even without frank cell loss (Reid *et al.* 1988). It suggests, however, that the caudate nucleus has a role far beyond control of motor function: similar symptoms have been noted in Parkinson's disease. Huntington's disease patients also show problems in the acquisition of skills, indicating a role for the striatum in such memory processes. A more severe global dementia may result as brain degeneration spreads to other regions.

Recommended reading

Albin, R. L., Young, A. B., and Penney, J. B. (1989). The functional anatomy of basal ganglia disorders. *Trends in Neurosciences*, **12**, 366–75.

Bird, E. D. (1980). Chemical pathology of Huntington's disease. *Annual Review of Pharmacology and Toxicology*, **20**, 533–51.

Brooks, D. J. and Frackowiak, R. S. J. (1989). PET and movement disorders. *Journal of Neurology, Neurosurgery and Psychiatry*, Special supplement, 68–71.

Crossman, A. R. (1987). Primate models of dyskinesia: the experimental approach to the study of basal ganglia related involuntary movement disorders. *Neuroscience*, **21**, 1–40.

Harper, P. S. (1986). The prevention of Huntington's chorea. *Journal of the Royal College of Physicians London*, **20**, 7–14.

Kowall, N. W., Ferrante, R. J., and Martin, J. B. (1987). Patterns of cell loss in Huntington's disease. *Trends in Neurosciences*, **10**, 24–9.

Martin, J. B. (1984). Huntington's disease. *Neurology*, **34**, 1059–72.

Martin, J. B. and Gusella, J. F. (1986). Huntington's disease, pathogenesis and management. *New England Journal of Medicine*, **315**, 1267–76.

Vonsattel, J. P., Myers, R. H., Stevens, T. J., Ferrante, R. J., Bird, E. D., and Richardson, E. P. (1985). Neuropathological classification of Huntington's disease. *Journal of Neuropathology and Experimental Neurology*, **44**, 559–77.

12 *Alzheimer's disease*

By the end of the nineteenth century the concept of senile dementia was well defined whereby elderly patients showed severe disturbances of memory and thought. Dementia is, however, a rather broad descriptive term (see Fig. 12.1) and can be the result of a variety of conditions, e.g. cerebrovascular problems (multi-infarct dementia), Pick's disease, Huntington's disease, or Parkinson's disease. The most common condition resulting in dementia is, however, Alzheimer's disease.

Alzheimer's disease is named after Alois Alzheimer (Fig. 12.2) who, working in Germany, published in 1907 the results of post-mortem neuropathological observations

Definition of dementia from the Royal College of Physicians (1981)
Dementia is the global impairment of higher cortical functions including memory, the capacity to solve the problems of day-to-day living, the performance of learned perceptuo-motor skills, the correct use of social skills and control of emotional reactions, in the absence of gross clouding of consciousness. The condition is often irreversible and progressive.

Diagnostic criteria for dementia (DSM III-R)
A. Demonstrable impairment in short and long term memory
B. At least one of the following:
   (1) impairment in abstract thinking
   (2) impaired judgement
   (3) other disturbances of higher cortical function, e.g. aphasia, apraxia, agnosia, 'constructional difficulty'
   (4) personality change
C. The disturbance in A and B significantly interferes with work or usual social activities or relationships with others
D. Not occurring exclusively during the course of delirium
E. Either 1 or 2
   1. There is evidence for a specific organic factor judged to be aetiologically related to the disturbance.
   2. In the absence of such evidence an aetiologic organic factor can be presumed if the disturbance cannot be accounted for by any non-organic mental disorder accounting for cognitive impairment.

Figure 12.1 Definitions of dementia. The definition given by the Royal College of Physicians is taken from Black *et al*. (1981) whereas the criteria laid down by the American Psychiatric Association for diagnosis of dementia are abridged from the Diagnostic and Statistical Manual of Mental Disorders (DSM III-R) (American Psychiatric Association 1987). The criteria are satisfied in the case of Alzheimer's disease but can also be seen in other neurological diseases discussed in this book e.g. Huntington's disease and Parkinson's disease.

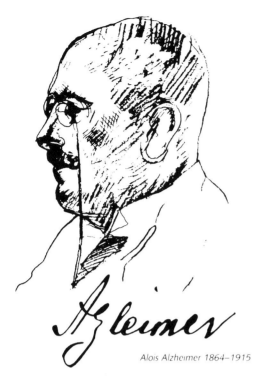

Alois Alzheimer 1864–1915

Figure 12.2   Alois Alzheimer. Taken from Thomas and Isaac (1987) with permission.

on a 56-year-old demented patient who showed the now classical hallmarks of the disease, plaques and tangles in the brain. This presenile form of dementia with the accompanying neuropathological observations came to be called after Alzheimer. It became increasingly clear, however, that the neuropathological changes seen in presenile dementia (<65 years) were also seen in senile dementia (>65 years). Therefore the term Alzheimer's disease has latterly come to be used for both disorders. There is still some suggestion that the early and late onset forms of the disease may be different; this will be discussed further below. It is also not clear to what extent genetic and environmental influences are generally important.

Alzheimer's disease is of great importance in developed countries where, with an increasingly ageing population, large numbers of people will suffer from this devastating disease. Not only is the population ageing at present, but the number of people over 75 years old is increasing disproportionately. This is the group with the highest risk of Alzheimer's disease.

The cost of caring for patients with dementia is enormous both financially and socially. One reflection of this is the tremendous increase in interest from drug companies, many of whom have 'Alzheimer projects' and some of whom have set up entire institutes dedicated to the development of drugs to combat the symptoms of dementia. Interest in Alzheimer's disease has therefore increased considerably and it has even been the subject of a 'best selling' novel, *Strong medicine* (Hailey 1985).

Clinical features

Alzheimer's disease is generally a disease of old age and so its prevalence increases with increasing age: its prevalence in that proportion of the population over 80 years old is about four times that in the population over 65 years old. In contrast, the prevalence in those under 65 years is low and less well defined. About 5 per cent of the population over 65 years of age suffer from dementia and of these between one- and two-fifths can be firmly diagnosed clinically as having Alzheimer's disease. The actual occurrence may be somewhat higher due to problems in differential diagnosis. A definite diagnosis can only, at present, be obtained through histopathological examination of brain tissue either at biopsy or autopsy; no definitive biochemical test applicable during life is yet available.

In some families the disease seems to be clearly inherited as an autosomal dominant disease (familial Alzheimer's disease), but in many cases of Alzheimer's disease such a mode of inheritance is not apparent; these have been labelled as sporadic. For the sporadic cases there does, however, seem to be an increased risk of suffering from the disease if a person has a first degree relative with the disease and the risk seems to increase further the earlier the onset of the disease in that relative. Familial clustering could be due to genetic effects or shared environmental factors. Limited and rather uncertain data are available on the occurrence of Alzheimer's disease in monozygotic and dizygotic twin pairs and these do not support an important genetic influence. In family studies, however, the apparent penetrance of any candidate gene may be reduced in families where the disease is inherited but there is a late age of onset of the disease, owing to death by other causes before the disease has a chance to present. Therefore genetic factors may be being underestimated—recent studies have indicated that the risk of developing Alzheimer's disease approaches 50 per cent in first degree relatives of patients who already have the disease if these relatives survive into their 80s and 90s. The comparable figure for control relatives is only 10 to 15 per cent. This could indicate, therefore, that some of the apparently sporadic forms of the disease in fact represent an autosomal dominant genetic disorder with age-dependent expression (Breitner 1990). The importance of inheritance could then be much greater than is generally suspected and may account for a substantial proportion of cases. Therefore the disease may take the form of an autosomal dominant inherited disease with age-dependent expression and there may also be non-genetic, apparently sporadic cases. Environmental factors will be very important for the latter form but may also play a role in expression of the genetic tendency of the former cases.

Patients present initially with a variety of fairly innocuous symptoms not dissimilar to those seen in normal ageing, but the disease is insidious and progressive. The disease can present in a variety of ways considered by some to represent distinct subtypes. In general, in the early stages there is an impairment of memory for recent events, disorientation (spatial), impaired concentration, and sometimes alterations to the personality. Mood and behavioural symptoms (aggression, depression, and wandering) may be of considerable social and economic importance in determining the care patients need. Later, all aspects of memory fail progressively and patients often exhibit aphasia (loss of language), apraxia (impairment of purposeful movements), and agnosia (loss of recognition of objects). Judgement and the capacity for abstract thought also become impaired. Finally there is a gross disturbance of all intellectual function, marked neurological defects sometimes emerge, e.g. disorders of movement, and patients become increasingly incapacitated, showing progressive wasting.

In some studies patients over 65 years old have been found to survive for a shorter time than those patients who are under 65 years old at onset but the relationship between survival time and age at onset is not straightforward (Burns *et al*. 1991). The symptoms in the younger group tend to be more severe but this may be due to the length of time the disease runs in this otherwise healthier group. From clinical observations alone, the diagnosis of Alzheimer's disease cannot always be made with complete certainty; this requires neuropathological analysis.

Neuropathological observations

Post-mortem examination of the whole brain from patients with Alzheimer's disease generally shows shrinkage of the gyri and enlargement of the ventricles. The shrinkage is often more pronounced in the frontal and temporal lobes of the cerebral cortex where it may reach 20–30 per cent. There is also a similar loss of white matter. There may be changes in both the breadth and thickness of the cerebral cortex; these changes may be more apparent in young patients. This brain atrophy is illustrated in post-mortem sections and in CAT and MRI scans (Fig. 12.3). Although brain shrinkage is a common feature of Alzheimer's disease, it is not diagnostic as some shrinking occurs normally with ageing and not all Alzheimer's disease patients, especially late onset cases, show obvious shrinkage. Cerebral atrophy is also seen in other neurodegenerative disorders, e.g. Huntington's disease (Chapter 11).

Microscopically, there is some evidence for cell (neurone) loss in certain brain regions. Clear losses of neurones have been demonstrated from subcortical nuclei, e.g. locus coeruleus, raphe, and nucleus basalis of Meynert and in the amygdala and hippocampus. It has not been as easy to demonstrate convincingly that there is cell loss from the cerebral cortex, but it does seem likely that there is a substantial loss of the large pyramidal neurones, particularly in frontal, parietal, and temporal regions, and there this cell loss correlates with the degree of dementia. Extensive dystrophic changes in neurites (dendrites and axon terminals) have also been reported. There is also some evidence for

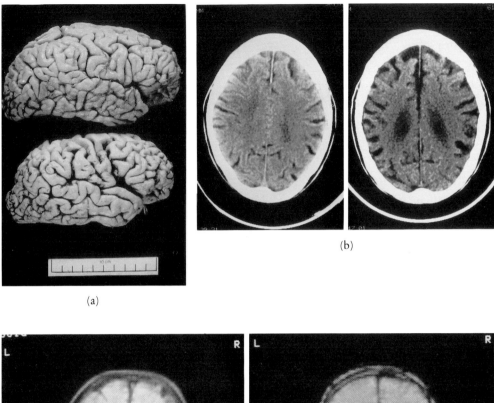

(a)

(b)

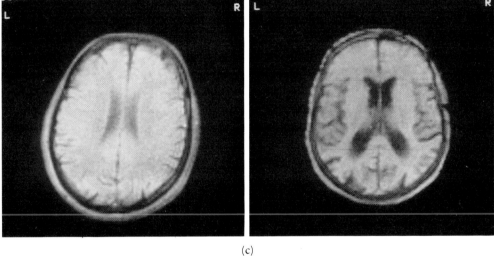

(c)

Figure 12.3 Brain degeneration in Alzheimer's disease. In (a) exterior views of a normal brain (upper) and a brain from a patient with Alzheimer's disease (lower) are shown. The shrinkage in the lower brain is clear (courtesy of Dr G. P. Reynolds, Sheffield). In (b) CAT scans of brain from normal (left) and Alzheimer's disease patients (right) are shown illustrating the shrinkage. The pictures show a horizontal section and are courtesy of Dr A. Burns, Institute of Psychiatry, London. In (c) MRI scans of brain from normal (left) and Alzheimer's disease patients (right) are shown illustrating the ventricular enlargement. The pictures show a horizontal section and are courtesy of Dr F. W. Smith and Dr J. A. O. Besson, Departments of Nuclear Medicine and Mental Health, Medical School, Aberdeen.

glial cell proliferation. It has been suggested that the reduction in cortical breadth is due to the loss of cortical columns of cells (see Chapter 7) which may result from the neuronal loss. It must be emphasized that there is cell loss from these particular brain regions in normal ageing, but the losses described above are in excess of those seen in normal ageing (Coleman and Flood 1987). The reduction in neuronal density combined with reduced cortical breadth results in a considerable reduction in functional capacity of the cerebral cortex in Alzheimer's disease.

Whereas studies on gross brain atrophy conducted *post mortem* have generally shown the most extensive neuropathology to be within the frontal and temporal lobes, more recently the use of imaging techniques for measuring cerebral blood flow and glucose metabolism applied to living patients have highlighted the parietal lobe as a major site of dysfunction (Friedland *et al.* 1985; Tamminga *et al.* 1987; Burns *et al.* 1989). More recent neuropathological studies have found extensive degeneration in the parietal lobe as well as in the temporal and frontal lobes (Fig. 12.4) (Najlerahim and Bowen 1988*a*,*b*, 1989; Bowen *et al.* 1989; Esiri *et al.* 1990). It has been suggested that the parietal lobe may be more affected in the early onset form of the disease with the temporal lobe more affected in the late onset form (Wilcock *et al.* 1988). Subcortical dysfunction is present in both cases. I shall return to this point later.

Some of the clearest neuropathological features of Alzheimer's disease are seen histologically. Senile or neuritic plaques (Fig. 12.5) accumulate in the cerebral cortex in normal ageing and to a much greater extent in Alzheimer's disease. Plaques are seemingly round or spherical structures 15–20 μm in diameter consisting of a peripheral rim of abnormal neuronal processes (neurites) and the processes of glial cells (astrocytes) surrounding a core of amyloid protein composed of 6–10 nm diameter fibrils. Plaque formation may precede and eventually lead to neuronal loss (Duyckaerts *et al.* 1988). Deposition of aluminium and silica in the form of aluminosilicates has been demonstrated in plaques by some workers (Brown 1990) and recently the plaque core protein (β-protein) has been isolated as a peptide of about 40 amino acids in length derived from

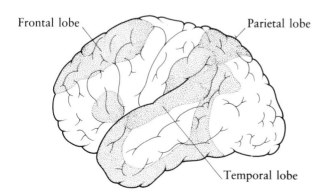

Figure 12.4   The regions of the cerebral cortex most affected in Alzheimer's disease. Degeneration in brain regions indicated is seen in terms of pyramidal neurone loss, reduced cerebral glucose metabolism, and loss of certain neurochemical markers.

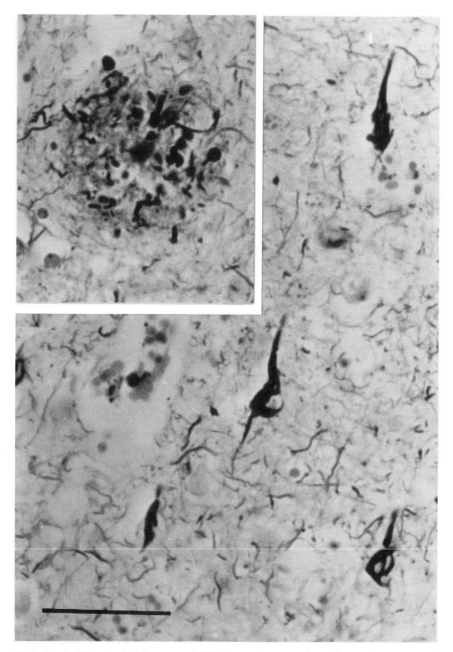

Figure 12.5 Typical histological features of Alzheimer's disease. Three 'flame shaped' neurofibrillary tangles are shown towards the right of the figure and a single neuritic plaque in the inset. Note the central core surrounded by abnormal neurites in the latter. Many of the coarser black processes in the background are neuropil threads which are also composed of paired helical filaments. Bar = 50 μm. Courtesy of Dr P. Luthert, Institute of Psychiatry, London.

a much larger precursor (Fig. 12.6). The relevance of differential processing of this precursor in Alzheimer's disease will be discussed later. There is also extensive deposition of a similar amyloid protein in the walls of cerebral blood vessels.

The neurofibrillary tangle (Fig. 12.5) is another important histological feature of Alzheimer's disease. This consists of paired helical filaments in a double helix, total diameter 20 nm, found in the cytoplasm particularly of the pyramidal cells of the cerebral cortex and hippocampus. The areas of cerebral cortex most affected by tangle formation are the temporal, parietal, and frontal lobes. Neurofibrillary tangles are found in specific patterns in the different layers of the cerebral cortex; this will be described later. Tangles are not generally found in the cerebral cortex of normal aged patients but their occurrence in Alzheimer's disease is not completely specific as they are also observed in other syndromes exhibiting dementia, for example dementia pugilistica, progressive supranuclear palsy, amyotrophic lateral sclerosis–parkinsonism–dementia complex of Guam (Chapter 10). Thus tangle formation may be a rather non-specific marker of neuronal insult. Also, some patients with Alzheimer's disease show abundant plaques but no tangles, suggesting that plaques are the more specific markers of the disease. The structure of the tangle is beginning to be understood: it contains a core protein of M_r about 100 000; the microtubule-associated tau protein is also an important structural component (Wischik *et al*. 1988). The cellular degradation marker protein ubiquitin has also been localized to tangles (Gallo and Anderton 1989) and studies have inferred that tangles may also contain neurofilament proteins and the amyloid β-protein. It has been suggested that neurofibrillary tangles are in fact composed of the same β-protein that is the building block of the plaque cores, but this is controversial (Anderton 1987; Guiroy *et al*. 1987). Tangles are also seen in the subcortical nuclei where neuronal loss has been reported.

Two other discrete microscopic abnormalities are often reported in Alzheimer's disease brain, particularly in the hippocampus. These are granuolar vacuolar degeneration and Hirano bodies. The former refers to clear, round cytoplasmic zones 4–5 μm across with a centrally stained core. The latter are extracellular, rod shaped eosinophilic inclusion bodies found predominantly in the hippocampal pyramidal cell layer. The significance of these changes remains unknown.

Neurochemical observations

There are alterations in the levels of many neurotransmitters during normal ageing, but a specific pattern of neurochemical changes is emerging in Alzheimer's disease. The first and most striking observation was reported in 1976, this being a loss of up to 70 per cent from the temporal and parietal lobes of the cerebral cortex and hippocampus of Alzheimer's disease patients of the cholinergic marker enzyme responsible for acetylcholine synthesis, choline acetyltransferase (CAT). Smaller losses of CAT were seen in other areas. The impairment of acetylcholine synthesis correlates with the severity of the dementia and extensive neuropathological investigations have shown that there is a loss of cholinergic pathways linking the nucleus basalis of Meynert to the cerebral cortex and the septum to the hippocampus. The loss of these pathways accounts for the neuronal loss in the nucleus basalis (see above). The early discovery of these changes and the relative ease of demonstration meant that 'cholinergic hypotheses' of Alzheimer's disease until recently dominated ideas concerning the nature of the disorder; many of these ideas now seem less tenable.

More recently, specific reductions in markers for 5-hydroxytryptamine and noradrenaline neurones have been observed in the cerebral cortex in Alzheimer's disease. These are due to selective loss of projections to the cortex from the dorsal raphe and locus coeruleus respectively. The degree of cell loss in the three subcortical nuclei (nucleus basalis/septum (cholinergic), raphe (5-hydroxytryptamine), and locus coeruleus (noradrenergic)) is similar in post-mortem brain samples (Wilcock *et al*. 1988) although the noradrenergic system is less affected in biopsy samples (Bowen 1990). The equivalent losses of neurones from two or more subcortical nuclei suggests that the degeneration of these cell groups projecting to the cerebral cortex occurs subsequent to some other change, for example cortical degeneration (Fig. 12.7). These observations also underline the broad inappropriateness of 'cholinergic hypotheses' of Alzheimer's disease.

These changes relate to neurones projecting to the cerebral cortex, but there is also a major loss of neurones from the cerebral cortex itself (see above). Thus it would be expected that significant neurochemical changes would be found there. The only consistent change demonstrated early on was in the neuropeptide somatostatin whose levels are reduced. It has been very difficult to demonstrate changes in other cortical neurotransmitters, e.g. glutamate, aspartate, or GABA (Jones and Hendry 1986), and this may be partly because of the widespread involvement of these substances in other more generalized metabolic processes in neurones. Also, if cell loss occurs and the breadth of the cortex is reduced to maintain a normal cellular packing density, then the levels of neurotransmitters when expressed per unit volume may not alter appreciably even though the actual number of functioning cortical neurones will have dropped significantly. Recent neurochemical studies taking this effect of atrophy into account do indicate significant losses of markers for the neurotransmitter glutamate in the frontal and temporal cortex and significant losses of cells in the parietal and temporal lobes (Neary *et al*. 1986; Procter *et al*. 1988*a*,*b*, 1990; Cowburn *et al*. 1990). Since glutamate is the neurotransmitter of the cortical pyramidal neurones, its loss would be consistent with depletion of this cell type in Alzheimer's disease (Bowen 1990).

Another index of cellular activity that has been investigated is glucose metabolism. Biopsy studies from Alzheimer's disease patients have shown hypermetabolism which may reflect mitochondrial uncoupling or a compensatory increase in metabolism of surviving nerve terminals in response to loss of other neurones (Procter *et al*. 1988*a,b*). In contrast, studies of regional cerebral glucose metabolism in living patients using positron emission tomography have shown asymmetrical reductions in glucose metabolism in frontal, parietal, and temporal cortices; these changes in glucose metabolism occur quite early in the disease (Haxby *et al*. 1990). These changes might reflect early signs of neuronal degeneration and there is a good correspondence between areas of the brain where neuronal degeneration is observed and where reduced glucose metabolism is seen (Najlerahim and Bowen 1988*a,b*). Intriguing circumstantial evidence for altered mitochondrial function in Alzheimer's disease has come from studies on the mitochondrial electron transport chain in platelets from such patients (Parker *et al*. 1990). A deficiency in cytochrome oxidase (complex IV) activity was seen and this may indicate a defect in oxidative phosphorylation and energy production. If this is also found in the brain it could be associated with defective tissue metabolism. It is of interest that in another neurological disease considered in this book, Parkinson's disease (Chapter 10), there are also indications of mitochondrial dysfunction.

Thus in Alzheimer's disease there is a loss of pyramidal neurones from the cerebral cortex and a loss of neurones from the cholinergic, 5-hydroxytryptamine and noradrenergic pathways innervating the cortex. There is also a loss of neurones from the amygdala and hippocampus. As speculated above, it is felt that the primary neurone loss is cortical but I shall discuss this in more detail later.

Theories of the aetiology of Alzheimer's disease

As outlined earlier in this chapter, there are specific cellular and neurochemical alterations in the brain in Alzheimer's disease. The underlying cause of these changes is, however, not understood. A number of factors have been suggested that could contribute to the changes in the brain and these are considered below. At the end of this section an attempt will be made to put these ideas together into a unifying hypothesis. The importance of these considerations lies firstly in that an understanding of the aetiology of Alzheimer's disease may lead to effective therapies or preventative measures and secondly, understanding the degeneration in Alzheimer's disease may help us understand brain degeneration in a variety of other diseases.

Genetic factors

There has been much discussion of the importance of genetic factors in Alzheimer's disease (see for example Wright and Walley (1984) and Kay (1989)) and I have alluded to this earlier. In some families, Alzheimer's disease seems to be inherited as an autosomal dominant disorder, but in many cases such a clear pattern of inheritance is not seen. However, it has been suggested that many more cases of Alzheimer's disease than previously suspected are familial but that the inheritance patterns are obscured by death from other causes (Breitner and Folstein, 1984).. This may account for the apparent increased heritability of Alzheimer's disease for early onset patients. Recent observations that the risk of Alzheimer's disease in first degree relatives of patients with the disease approaches 50 per cent if the relatives live into their 80s and 90s supports the idea (Breitner 1990). These observations point to the importance of genetic factors in Alzheimer's disease, but the situation is far from clear. In particular it is not clear whether the disease is genetically homogeneous.

The importance of specific genes for Alzheimer's disease is further emphasized by the example of Down's syndrome (Oliver and Holland 1986). Down's syndrome is a genetic disease (trisomy 21, i.e. presence of an additional copy of chromosome 21 or part of this chromosome) and all patients who survive for more than 40 years show the neuropathological hallmarks of Alzheimer's disease, that is plaques and tangles in their brains. In addition, about a third of the patients develop a dementia similar to that seen in Alzheimer's disease. The link between Down's syndrome and Alzheimer's disease is strengthened by the observation of an increased occurrence of Down's syndrome in relatives of Alzheimer's disease patients.

In the light of these findings, attempts have been made to identify a gene responsible for Alzheimer's disease by applying genetic linkage analysis to families where clear inheritance has already been seen (see Chapter 11 for a discussion of the molecular biology techniques used here). There was much excitement when the genetic linkage studies identified chromosome 21 as the site of the familial Alzheimer's disease gene (although the actual gene itself had not been identified) and this intensified when the gene for the amyloid plaque core protein (β-protein) was also located on chromosome 21 (Hardy 1988). The excitement was quelled when further analysis showed that the familial Alzheimer's disease gene and the β-protein gene were not identical. Several studies, but not all, have shown, however, that the β-protein gene is located very close to the region of chromosome 21 required to produce Down's syndrome (Tanzi *et al*. 1989). There may be an extra copy of the β-protein gene and plaque formation in Down's syndrome may therefore result from overproduction of the β-protein. Disturbances in β-protein metabolism could also be important for Alzheimer's disease itself.

The linkage of familial Alzheimer's disease to a marker on chromosome 21 appears, however, only to hold for families where the disease shows an early onset. For families where the disease shows late onset, there is no linkage to chromosome 21 markers (Marx 1988). There may be linkage to markers on chromosome 19 in the late onset familial patients (Martin *et al*. 1990) but environmental agents may also be important for the occurrence of the late onset familial disease (Farrer *et al*. 1990). This genetic heterogeneity will complicate the search for the genes involved. This search is already complex and tortuous because of the limited number of families with clear and defined inheritance patterns (Tanzi *et al*. 1989).

The long term aim of these studies is to identify a genetic defect in Alzheimer's disease and this is likely also to lead to genetic tests for susceptibility to Alzheimer's disease. The ethical problems of such tests will be severe given the lack of any suitable therapy and the likely large number of people concerned.

Environmental factors

Alzheimer's disease could be caused by an environmental toxin. This possibility is strengthened following the finding that parkinsonism can be induced by MPTP (Chapter 10). Epidemiological studies on Alzheimer's disease itself do not, however, give much support for the role of such environmental agents (although see below). There is some evidence that Alzheimer's disease is more common in western countries than in Japan and the developing countries. Whether this reflects genetic or environmental factors is not clear.

One substance that has received much attention in this context is aluminium. Administration of aluminium salts to experimental animals induces the formation in their brains of filamentous structures resembling, but not identical to, the paired helical filaments of Alzheimer's disease tangles. Aluminium has been detected in cells containing tangles and in plaques in Alzheimer's disease brains; in these plaques it is thought to be in the form of aluminosilicates, although there is some debate over this (Brown 1990). There is some recent epidemiological evidence linking the level of aluminium in drinking water to the prevalence of Alzheimer's disease (Martyn *et al.* 1989).

It is not clear at present whether aluminium is a causative or permissive agent in Alzheimer's disease or whether aluminium accumulation is a late event in the disease process. Some information can be obtained by considering the amyotrophic lateral sclerosis–parkinsonism–dementia complex seen on the island of Guam (see also Chapter 10). These patients have among their symptoms a severe dementia and post-mortem examination of the brain shows neurofibrillary tangles (but no neuritic plaques). Thus there is some resemblance to Alzheimer's disease. It has been suggested that the disease is associated with low Ca^{2+}/Mg^{2+} and high aluminium in drinking water (Garruto and Yase 1986) and more recently a role for a potential neurotoxin from cycad nuts consumed by the patients has been suggested (Spencer *et al.* 1987, 1990). It is possible that the combination of these factors (low Ca^{2+}/Mg^{2+}, high Al^{3+}, and a neurotoxin) can cause brain degeneration leading to dementia.

The tendency to accumulate aluminium in the brain seems to vary between brain regions with the hippocampus, septum, amygdala, and cerebral cortex showing a higher tendency than other brain regions (Pullen *et al.* 1990). Since these are the brain regions where there is extensive pathology in Alzheimer's disease, this differential accumulation of aluminium could provide a mechanism whereby increased environmental levels of this substance, for example in drinking water, could produce regionally specific brain changes. Mechanisms for aluminium toxicity have been proposed (Blair *et al*. 1990).

Although not strictly an environmental factor, head injury, for example in a car accident, in earlier life has been cited as a predisposing factor for later Alzheimer's disease. The significance of this is unclear but it may indicate that minor brain damage can lead eventually to degenerative changes. This idea is supported by the observation of a form of dementia (dementia pugilistica) in boxers. In this syndrome there are motor impairments, and problems with speech and memory, and neuropathologically, neurofibrillary tangles are seen along with a loss of the cholinergic marker enzyme CAT. Whereas earlier studies reported an absence of senile plaques, more recently deposits showing immunoreactivity to the amyloid β-protein have been described in the brains of patients with this syndrome (Roberts *et al*. 1990). These β-immunoreactive deposits may be immature forerunners of the neuritic plaques of Alzheimer's disease.

Transmissible agents

Speculation that a transmissible agent may be important in Alzheimer's disease has centred around the human diseases Creuzfeldt–Jakob disease, Gerstmann–Straussler syndrome, and kuru, and the animal diseases scrapie (affecting sheep and goats), transmissible mink encephalopathy and bovine spongiform encephalopathy (Pain 1988; Holt and Phillips 1988). In these diseases, which seem to be related, there is vacuolation of the nerve cells, leading to spongiform brain tissue, occasional plaques and tangles, and in the human diseases, progressive and severe dementia. Fibrillar structures (scrapie associated fibrils) have also been identified in scrapie brain but these are different from the amyloid fibrils and paired helical filaments of Alzheimer's disease (Somerville 1985).

Gerstmann–Straussler syndrome is a familial disease following an autosomal dominant pattern of inheritance with complete dominance (Collinge *et al*. 1990). The other spongiform encephalopathies are not usually familial and transmission of these diseases is quite difficult and most easily accomplished by deliberate or accidental contact between infected brain material and a second brain (Holt and Phillips 1988). Within a species and in some cases between species, however, transmission seems to be possible by oral consumption of infected tissue. Even so, the disease takes time to develop and the responsible agents have been termed 'unconventional' or 'slow' viruses. Prusiner (1982) has isolated an 'infectious' agent from scrapie infected animals which seems to be largely protein in nature and may be related to the fibrils mentioned earlier, although the presence of some nucleic acid cannot be ruled out. He has termed this a prion (proteinaceous infectious particle) and it would constitute a novel form of infectious agent. The major protein constituent of this, PrP, has been characterized and shown to be a normal gene product. Understanding how this normal gene product leads to the disease is a major challenge (Westaway *et al*. 1989; Gabizon and Prusiner 1990;

Weissman 1991). In Gerstmann–Straussler syndrome it has been shown that there is a mutation in the gene coding for PrP (Collinge *et al.* 1990).

Despite the similarities between these diseases and Alzheimer's disease, there are considerable differences; there is no evidence for the transmission of Alzheimer's disease via an exogenous agent and the similarities must remain a tantalizing speculation (although see Manuelidis *et al.* 1988).

Processing of the plaque core precursor protein

Cloning of the gene for the amyloid β-protein that forms the plaque core has shown that it is derived from a much larger precursor. Four mRNA species have been found corresponding to the precursor molecule each derived by alternative splicing. These code for proteins of 695, 714, 751, and 770 amino acids in length. The precursor molecule is expressed widely in neural and non-neural tissues from normal and Alzheimer's disease patients, suggesting that it has some fairly general important function. Hydropathicity analysis of the amino acid sequence suggests that it consists of a large extracellular domain and short intracellular domain linked by a short transmembrane domain (Fig. 12.6). This would be typical of a molecule with important activities at the cell surface such as a receptor or cell adhesion molecule—there is some evidence for the latter role. Indeed, membrane bound forms of the precursor (M_r 12 000) have been described. This then raises the question of why the metabolism of this normal protein is altered in Alzheimer's disease, giving rise to the senile plaques. I shall return to this later.

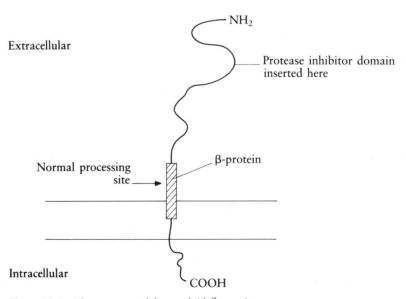

Figure 12.6   The structure of the amyloid β-protein precursor.

One clue to this comes from the recognition that one of the domains present in the 751 and 770 amino acid forms of the precursor is a 56 amino acid species encoded by a separate exon and showing a high degree of homology with a serine protease inhibitor. In fact, a large part of the amino-terminal part of the precursor that is secreted by various cultured cells is identical to the protease inhibitor nexin II. Further evidence for the importance of proteases in plaque formation comes from the identification of the protease inhibitor α_1-antichymotrypsin in plaques.

The different forms of the precursor protein show differential expression in different tissues with the 695 amino acid form predominating in brain. This form lacks the protease inhibitor domain and it will be of great interest to define in detail the regulation of expression of the different forms in normal and Alzheimer's disease brain (Ishiura 1991). The β-protein itself has recently been shown to be present in a wide range of tissues in Alzheimer's disease patients including skin (Joachim *et al.* 1989). This shows that the deposition of β-protein is not solely due to neural damage and the presence of the protein in skin may allow a simple test for the disease to be developed.

The amyloid β-protein constitutes a rather small part of the precursor molecule but other parts of the precursor molecule have been found in senile plaques, suggesting that some processing of the precursor molecule occurs locally in the vicinity of the plaque itself. Soluble forms of the precursor containing parts of the amyloid β-protein have also been found (Palmert *et al.* 1989). This raises the possibility that deposition of amyloid (in blood vessels) and plaques may be from circulating forms of the precursor. This is unlikely, however, as the circulating forms do not contain the full β-protein sequence.

It seems that cleavage of the precursor molecule to release the β-protein is not its normal metabolic fate. The normal cleavage point is within the β-protein sequence yielding the soluble protein forms (Fig. 12.6). This normal cleavage must be due to a specific protease and when amyloid is deposited as in Alzheimer's disease there must be a change in the processing pathway.

The challenge then is to understand why the metabolism of this normal protein, the β-protein precursor, is so disturbed in Alzheimer's disease. A plausible hypothesis is that there is some alteration in the proteolytic processing or gene expression of the precursor that gives rise to larger than normal amounts. These larger amounts cannot be dealt with adequately by the normal metabolic route for the precursor and the alternative pathway is used, giving rise to the intact β-protein and amyloid and plaque deposition. The example of Down's syndrome is instructive here where there may be an elevated expression of the β-protein precursor owing to the genetic defect in this disease. This could overload the normal proteolytic pathway leading to β-protein generation, amyloid, and plaques. There is some evidence for over-expression of the precursor in certain regions of Alzheimer's disease brains although this is controversial. Further circumstantial evidence in support of these ideas comes from the demonstration of a mutation in the β-protein precursor in some but by no means all families where Alzheimer's disease is inherited (Goate *et al.* 1991). The mutation may disturb the metabolism of the β-protein precursor. Additional evidence comes from studies on transgenic mice over-expressing one form of the β-protein precursor. These mice develop immature neuritic plaques in their brains (Quon *et al.* 1991).

It is clear from this discussion that proteolytic processing is important for the understanding of amyloid β-protein deposition. The presence of a protease inhibitor domain in the β-protein precursor could be important here and alterations in precursor processing could be related to differential inhibition of the processing enzymes.

The use of more refined analytical techniques based on antibodies specific for the β-protein has shown that there is a much wider distribution of β-protein deposits in brains from Alzheimer's disease patients than was revealed by conventional histology. The deposits appear as immature preamyloid plaques in the absence of neuritic change and suggest that disturbances in β-protein metabolism may represent an early event in the changes of Alzheimer's disease. Therefore the mature plaques taken to be the hallmarks of Alzheimer's disease may take up to 30 years to reach maturity. In terms of the speculation above this could represent a gradual accumulation of material over many years and would not occur to the same extent in normal individuals owing to their possible lower expression of or greater processing capacity for the precursor. Some possible mechanisms that could lead to the cellular damage are considered in the next section. Clearly, understanding the basis of plaque formation will be very important for understanding the basis of the disease.

Growth factors

It seems likely that the maturation and survival of nerve cells in the central nervous system depends on low molecular weight growth factors. Thus a degenerative disease of the brain like Alzheimer's disease could be associated with defective growth factor action. This speculation is given circumstantial support by the structural resemblance between the precursor for the β-protein of the plaque core and the precursor for epidermal growth factor which consists of similar domains. Thus some products of the processing of the β-protein precursor could be related to cellular growth factors and disturbances in their action could result in plaque formation or alter cell division and maturation. Both neurotrophic and neurotoxic effects of the β-protein have been described and these could contribute to the development of the neuropathological changes seen (Yankner *et al.* 1990*a*). There are also reports of beneficial effects of nerve growth factor (NGF) on neuronal survival and a trial of this substance is being considered in Alzheimer's disease patients. NGF has, however, also been shown to promote expression of the β-protein precursor and a substantial potentiation of the neurotoxic effects of the β-protein by NGF has been reported (Yankner *et al.* 1990*b*). Therefore any trial of NGF will need to be carefully supported by animal experiments (Marx 1990; Everall and Kerwin 1990).

Metabolic disturbances

In vivo imaging of glucose uptake using positron emission tomography has shown that there is a reduction in glucose utilization in certain brain areas (frontal, parietal, and temporal cortices). These changes can occur fairly early in Alzheimer's disease when metabolism is disturbed or neuronal degeneration is beginning. Some evidence has been presented for an increase in cell metabolism in biopsy samples of cerebral cortex and this could reflect mitochondrial uncoupling or a compensatory increase in metabolism in the remaining neurones in the tissue that has already lost some cells. Together, these studies are consistent with early metabolic changes in neurones that may lead to cell death.

Nasal infection theory

A study of the anatomical distribution of the degeneration of neurones in different brain regions from Alzheimer's disease patients has shown that severe degeneration occurs in association regions of the frontal, temporal, and parietal lobes of the cerebral cortex, whereas sensorimotor regions are relatively less affected. An exception to this is the olfactory system. The hippocampus and amygdala are also severely affected and frequently more so than the cortical regions (Pearson *et al.* 1985; Lewis *et al.* 1987; Esiri *et al.* 1990). Tangle formation is more severe in layers III and V of the cerebral cortex containing pyramidal cells (Chapter 7). These are the cells giving rise to connections between different cortical regions (layer III) and cells giving rise to output pathways to subcortical regions of brain such as the basal ganglia (layer V) (Fig. 7.4).

Two sets of neuroanatomical observations can be cited to explain the pattern of degeneration. First, neuroanatomical studies of the cerebral cortex have shown that the different association regions are connected by cortico-cortical fibres based on pyramidal cells and the association regions in turn connect to the hippocampus via the entorhinal cortex (Jones and Powell 1970). Secondly, the degree of cortical degeneration in different regions seems to correlate roughly with the extent of connections to the amygdala; regions with heavy connections, such as the association cortex of the temporal lobe (largely limbic cortex), having extensive degeneration while regions with few connections such as sensory cortical regions showing little degeneration. The amygdala also connects to the hippocampus and the three principal subcortical nuclei affected in Alzheimer's disease (nucleus basalis, raphe, and locus coeruleus) (Esiri *et al.* 1990). Figures 12.7 and 12.8 outline some of these interrelationships.

Thus the regions of the brain most affected in Alzheimer's disease are interconnected by nerve fibres that could offer routes for the spread of some toxic or infectious agent.

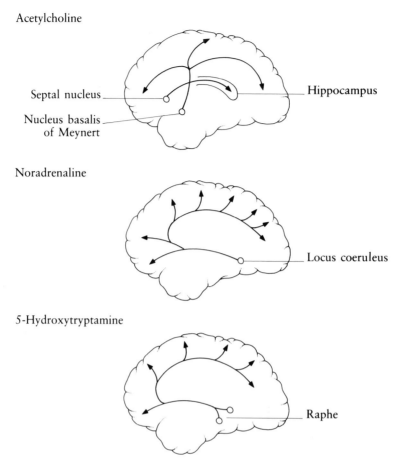

Acetylcholine

Septal nucleus

Nucleus basalis
of Meynert

Hippocampus

Noradrenaline

Locus coeruleus

5-Hydroxytryptamine

Raphe

Figure 12.7 The cerebral cortex and its connections to subcortical nuclei in relation to Alzheimer's disease. The pathways containing the neurotransmitters acetylcholine, noradrenaline, and 5-hydroxytryptamine are shown as these degenerate in Alzheimer's disease. See also Fig. 7.14.

Whereas motor, somatosensory, and primary visual areas of the cerebral cortex are relatively spared in Alzheimer's disease, the olfactory cortex is frequently badly affected and so the olfactory bulb, via the neurones in the olfactory epithelium of the nose, could be the site where a toxic agent gains access to the brain and spreads transneuronally along the interconnections outlined above (Saper *et al.* 1987). Spread along nerve cells would be via axonal transport (Chapter 3).

   The olfactory bulb is connected both to the amygdala, and thence to the association regions of the cerebral cortex, and to the entorhinal cortex and thence sequentially to the association regions of cerebral cortex. Entry of a toxic agent via the olfactory bulb would lead to differential degeneration as described. In support of such a 'nasal infection theory', recent observations on the olfactory epithelium have highlighted abnormal

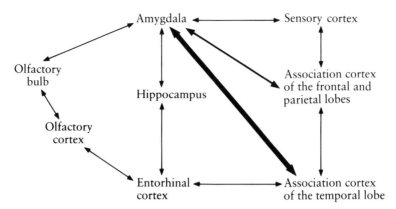

Figure 12.8 Neuronal pathways linking the olfactory bulb to the cerebral cortex and subcortical nuclei. The diagram shows the reciprocal interconnections between the different association regions of the cerebral cortex and the hippocampus, amygdala, and olfactory bulb as single lines. Lines of varying intensity represent connections between the amygdala and the sensory and different association regions of cerebral cortex. These interconnections allow for entry of a toxic agent into the brain via the olfactory bulb followed by sequential spread along the neurones connecting the olfactory cortex, entorhinal cortex, and association regions or spread to the amygdala and then to the different association regions, with different degrees of spread to the association regions and sensory regions according to their degree of interconnectedness with the amygdala. Either of these routes accounts for the high degree of pathology seen in the amygdala and hippocampus and the decreasing pathology seen in the temporal, fronto-parietal, and sensory cortices.

neurites and abnormal antigenicity in the neurones of the olfactory epithelium in Alzheimer's disease (Altman 1989). Alzheimer's disease patients also have olfactory deficits so these pieces of evidence support the idea that there is damage to the olfactory system. Although such a hypothesis would be suitable for the spread of a virus or other toxic agent that gains access to the brain from the exterior via the olfactory system, the nature of the toxin is unknown. Evidence against the proposal that the olfactory system is a primary pathological site comes from studies showing that while olfactory deficits do occur in Alzheimer's disease, they do not occur early in the disease (Serby *et al*. 1991).

The consequences of the interlinked degenerative changes outlined above are that large areas of the cerebral cortex are affected and the hippocampus is isolated from its inputs and outputs (Hyman *et al*. 1984). Degeneration of the cholinergic, noradrenergic, and 5-hydroxytryptamine cells projecting to the cerebral cortex would then be secondary to the degeneration occurring in the amygdala and cerebral cortex and again may reflect transneuronal spread of some pathogen.

Synthesis of theories on the aetiology of Alzheimer's disease

It should be clear from the above discussion that speculation on the aetiology of Alzheimer's disease has ranged widely. This partly reflects the paucity of real knowledge on the topic. In consequence, some of the factors considered may only have a peripheral relevance to Alzheimer's disease, e.g. 'slow viruses' (prions) where the syndromes associated bear only a passing resemblance to Alzheimer's disease.

It is also important in understanding the aetiology of Alzheimer's disease to distinguish early and late changes. For example at present it seems that formation of neuritic plaques represents an early stage in the disease process. Understanding the mechanism of their formation and the regulation of expression of the β-protein precursor gene on chromosome 21 and the effects of environmental factors on this will be of great importance. Similarly, alterations in cellular metabolism may occur fairly early, so understanding these will be important too. The precise timing and sequence of the different neuronal changes is a third area of importance in understanding the pathogenesis of this disease. The status and timing of certain other alterations in Alzheimer's disease is becoming less clear. For example, the tangles seem to be fairly non-specific markers of neuronal damage so although important in relation to the capacity of affected cells to function, they may not tell us about the specific disease process but may reflect a neuronal death that is induced by other changes.

It may be that there is more than one way to achieve the syndrome that we recognize as Alzheimer's disease. This is the case for parkinsonism where several ways are recognized for achieving the same specific brain degeneration and clinical picture. In the case of parkinsonism (Chapter 10) it was suggested that there was a threshold of neuronal loss beyond which symptoms were seen. A similar idea has been proposed for Alzheimer's disease (Roth 1986; Calne *et al.* 1986). In normal ageing there is cell death and formation of plaques and tangles in some brain regions, whereas in Alzheimer's disease there is more extensive cell death and formation of plaques and tangles. Alzheimer's disease symptoms might only appear when a certain threshold of cell death is reached. Below the threshold only the symptoms of normal ageing are seen.

The threshold of cell loss could be reached by some insult to the brain leading to a large loss of cells which, if superimposed on normal ageing, takes the cell loss past the threshold. Alternatively, loss of cells at a rate greater than normal could take the patient past the threshold. An accelerated loss of cells rather than a single major loss now seems more likely as I shall speculate below.

In the familial forms of the disease, the autosomal dominant nature suggests that a single gene defect is responsible for the appearance of symptoms and therefore for the loss of neurones. As discussed before there is also evidence for inherited genetic effects in many of the apparently sporadic cases of Alzheimer's disease. These cases may also be due to an autosomal dominant disorder but with age-dependent expression of the disease. The age of onset in these cases may be dependent on some of the environmental factors outlined above. Therefore Alzheimer's disease may be in large part an autosomal dominant disease with age-dependent expression and only where the age of onset is early will the disease appear clearly familial because when there is a late onset many potential sufferers will have died of other causes before the disease presents. At present it does not seem that the disease is genetically homogeneous but it will be of great interest ultimately to identify the genes involved as this will help generally in understanding the causation of the neuronal loss and the occurrence of the disease.

There may also be other forms of Alzheimer's disease that are less dependent on genetic influences where the threshold of neuronal loss is reached after a combination of influences has exerted effects. This could be due to environmental influences, some of which have been described earlier. Genetic influences could contribute but at a low level. These forms of the disease would then appear sporadic.

At present it seems that a critical factor in the loss of cells (neurones) in the brains of patients with Alzheimer's disease is the formation of neuritic plaques (see before). The formation of immature plaques may commence in early life subsequently leading to neuronal loss at a rate greater than normal. This then leads to the development of mature plaques with the neurotrophic and neurotoxic effects of the β-protein contributing to this. There is now evidence in some familial cases of Alzheimer's disease and for Down's syndrome that altered metabolism of the plaque core β-protein precursor may be associated with the development of the disease. Perhaps the different genetic factors and environmental influences each in some way alter the metabolism of the β-protein precursor and either singly or in combination lead to the classical neuropathological signs of Alzheimer's disease (Fig. 12.9).

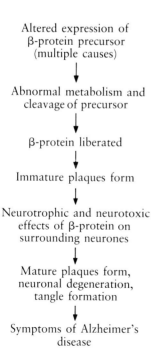

Figure 12.9 Speculative scheme for the aetiology of Alzheimer's disease. The scheme suggests that the generation of amyloid-containing neuritic plaques is central to the disorder. The influences leading to Alzheimer's disease (genetic factors, head injury, nasal infection, and aluminium) are proposed to affect the metabolism of the amyloid β-protein precursor and hence plaque deposition.

In considering the cases of Alzheimer's disease which are not obviously familial, there has been much discussion about whether late onset and early onset (senile and presenile) forms should be considered as separate entities. The early onset form tends to show more severe symptoms with frequent visuospatial dysfunction, more severe changes in the brain, and greater evidence for genetic influences, whereas the late onset form appears more sporadic with less severe symptoms and brain changes (Rossor *et al*. 1984; Bondareff *et al*. 1987). In terms of the symptoms and brain changes, the differences are quantitative rather than qualitative and the greater genetic influence on the early onset cases may simply reflect death by other causes obscuring the inheritance pattern in the late onset cases. The quantitative difference in severity of symptoms may reflect the time the disease has to run from its onset to death. In terms of the theory of Alzheimer's disease outlined earlier, it may be unnecessary to postulate distinct early and late onset forms of the disease. Rather, one should examine the influences (genetic, environmental) leading to the same constellation of symptoms.

There is, however, some evidence emerging with the application of imaging techniques and more detailed histological examinations that the parietal lobes may be more severely affected in early onset cases whereas the temporal lobes are more affected in late onset cases (Wilcock *et al*. 1988; Burns *et al*. 1989). Whether the differences reflect different pathological processes remains to be seen but if the differences are borne out in more extensive studies, it will be important in future work to segregate early and late onset cases when studying the relationship of biochemical or neuropathological parameters to the disease.

Treatments for Alzheimer's disease

Several treatments have been tried for Alzheimer's disease with only marginal success and it is fair to say that at present any drug that would help with the symptoms would be useful (Mayeux 1990): no treatment is available to halt the inexorable progress of the disease. The treatments that have been tried are mostly directed towards the memory disturbances of Alzheimer's disease, but it has been suggested that the aggressive and antisocial behaviour of some patients may be just as distressing if not more so and therefore also should be attempted to be treated.

Several substances have been used which have multiple pharmacological actions altering neurotransmitters, oxygen usage, and blood flow in the brain. Hydergine (a mixture of ergot alkaloids) is a widely used example of this kind of substance but gives only minor improvements in cognitive function in Alzheimer's disease (Thompson *et al*. 1990).

Significant effort has been expended by the pharmaceutical industry on attempts to modulate cholinergic function in order to improve cognitive function in Alzheimer's disease. The discovery of the deficit in the cholinergic pathway linking the nucleus basalis and cerebral cortex in Alzheimer's disease led to parallels being drawn with the markedly successful treatment (using L-DOPA) of the dopamine deficit in Parkinson's disease. Attempts have been made to treat the cholinergic deficit in Alzheimer's disease using precursors of acetylcholine (e.g. choline and lecithin), which might raise acetylcholine levels, anticholinesterases (e.g. phystostigmine and tetrahydroaminoacridine), which should prevent destruction of acetylcholine, and directly acting muscarinic cholinergic agonists (e.g. bethanechol), which should mimic the action of acetylcholine. Some small cognitive improvements have generally been reported with the latter two approaches although a recent study with tetrahydroaminoacridine reported somewhat greater effects (Eagger *et al.* 1991). Some improvement in performance has also been reported after administration of the nicotinic acetylcholine receptor agonist nicotine which seems to improve attention and information processing but not memory (Sahakian *et al.* 1989). Overall, however, the approach of cholinergic therapy seems too optimistic. The cholinergic defect is not the only defect in Alzheimer's disease and indeed the loss of pyramidal cells from the cerebral cortex may be much more significant in terms of thought processes. Also the nature and function of the cholinergic pathway (see next section) do not render it easily amenable to a replacement therapy. If, as outlined earlier, there are fewer changes in the brain of late onset cases of the disease with cholinergic changes being prominent, then these patients might benefit more from cholinergic therapy.

Other treatments are currently being considered based on modulation of 5-hydroxytryptamine and GABA systems, but if an early loss of cortical pyramidal cells occurs in Alzheimer's disease then, unless the resultant decline in cerebral cortical function can be reversed, it is not easy to see how any treatment can have a major effect. If the neurotransmitter involved in the cortex is glutamate, then as this is a fast acting neurotransmitter it will be difficult to perform a replacement therapy that restores a rapid, time-dependent action. One possibility would be to increase the activity of the remaining cortical pyramidal cells. This approach is being pursued based on the manipulation of the glycine modulatory site of the NMDA subclass of glutamate receptor (Chapter 6) (Bowen 1990). Some fanciful suggestions have appeared in the press that neuronal transplants of cholinergic cells may help in Alzheimer's disease. These would be subject to the same constraints outlined above.

Thus the therapeutic outlook is bleak and the main hope in Alzheimer's disease rests in understanding the basis of the brain degeneration which will eventually allow this degeneration to be prevented or its progress, at least, to be restricted or slowed.

Relation of brain changes seen in Alzheimer's disease to normal brain function

In Alzheimer's disease there is a specific clinical picture and a corresponding specificity in the loss of certain cell types from the brain. Thus cortical pyramidal neurones, cholinergic, 5-hydroxytryptamine, and noradrenergic neurones innervating the cerebral cortex, and cholinergic neurones innervating the hippocampus are lost. It should be possible to relate the functional and cellular losses and I shall make some attempt at this here.

It seems likely that much of our thinking and storage of memory takes place in the cerebral cortex and in Alzheimer's disease there are selective losses of cells in the temporal, parietal, and to a lesser extent frontal lobes. Particularly affected are the association areas of the cerebral cortex which are involved in higher order brain function. The association cortex in the parietal and temporal lobes is thought to be involved in the integration of sensory information from several sensory modes and may influence higher sensory function, language, and perception of body space. Thus it is not surprising that in Alzheimer's disease, aphasia, agnosia, and apraxia are prominent symptoms. Some parts of the temporal lobe (limbic association cortex, Chapter 7) are involved in memory and emotion and the frontal lobe also has a role in emotion, so damage in these areas can contribute to the personality changes in Alzheimer's disease. As the cortical neurone loss spreads to these three regions, the Alzheimer patient will have severe problems with cognition and formation of new memories, and later will suffer loss of memory altogether as these association areas critical for higher function are severely compromised.

There has been much speculation about the importance of the loss of cholinergic cells innervating the cerebral cortex and hippocampus to memory and cognitive dysfunction in Alzheimer's disease (Collerton 1986). There are disturbances of short term memory in humans given anti-cholinergic drugs such as scopolamine, although these are not identical to the changes in Alzheimer's disease; also, in experimental animals, lesions of the cholinergic pathways to the cerebral cortex disrupt behaviour in certain aspects of memory tests. The hippocampus, which becomes virtually disconnected from its inputs and outputs in Alzheimer's disease (Hyman *et al*. 1984) is also known to be important in memory function, perhaps in laying down of memory although it also participates in other functions as discussed in Chapters 13–15. Thus there is ample support for a role of cholinergic pathways lost in Alzheimer's disease in some aspects of memory function, perhaps the laying down and retention of new memories. Therefore the loss of the cholinergic pathways may be responsible for some of the loss of short term memory.

As this deficit has been a particular target for pharmaceutical intervention, I shall consider whether it is likely to be reversed by drug therapy. The cholinergic pathways to the cortex are topographically organized, influencing discrete regions of the cortex, and are active in response to certain aspects of behaviour so it can be speculated that parts of the pathways are activated when certain aspects of memory are encoded (Richardson and Delong 1988). Any pharmaceutical intervention would involve generalized activation of cholinergic pathways and it is not at all easy to see how this could ameliorate the memory deficit. Earlier changes in the cerebral cortex place further constraints on this approach as discussed above.

Losses of neurones in the 5-hydroxytryptamine and noradrenergic pathways may contribute to some of the psychiatric problems of Alzheimer's disease, as such pathways have been implicated in affective disorders (Chapter 14); the loss of neurones from the amygdala may also be important in this regard owing to the important role of this brain region in emotional function.

Recommended reading

Bartus, R. T. (1989). Alzheimer's disease: current and emerging topics on age related neurodegeneration. *Neurobiology of Ageing*, **10**, 381–650.

Harrison, P. J. (1986). Pathogenesis of Alzheimer's disease—beyond the cholinergic hypothesis: discussion paper. *Journal of the Royal Society of Medicine*, **79**, 347–52.

Kay, D. W. K. (1989). Genetics, Alzheimer's disease and senile dementia. *British Journal of Psychiatry*, **154**, 311–20.

Mann, D. M. A. (1988). Alzheimer's disease and Down's syndrome. *Histopathology*, **13**, 125–37.

Marchbanks, R. M. (1982). Biochemistry of Alzheimer's disease. *Journal of Neurochemistry*, **39**, 9–15.

Muller-Hill, B. and Beyreuther, K. (1989). Molecular biology of Alzheimer's disease. *Annual Review of Biochemistry*, **58**, 287–307.

Jorm, A. F. (1987). *Understanding senile dementia*. Croom Helm, London and Sydney.

Pitt, B. (ed.) (1987). *Dementia*. Churchill Livingstone, Edinburgh.

Roth, M. and Iversen, L. L. (eds.). (1986). Alzheimer's disease and related disorders. *British Medical Bulletin*, **42**, 1–115.

Schneck, M. K., Reisberg, B., and Ferris, S. H. (1982). An overview of current concepts of Alzheimer's disease. *American Journal of Psychiatry*, **139**, 165–73.

Selkoe, D. J. (1989). Amyloid β-protein precursor and the pathogenesis of Alzheimer's disease. *Cell*, **58**, 611–12.

Selkoe, D. J. (1989). Biochemistry of altered brain proteins in Alzheimer's disease. *Annual Review of Neuroscience*, **12**, 463–90.

Selkoe, D. J. (1990). Deciphering Alzheimer's disease: the amyloid precursor protein yields new clues. *Science*, **248**, 1058–60.

Selkoe, D. J. (1991). The molecular pathology of Alzheimer's disease, *Neuron*, **6**, 487–98.

Wright, A. F. and Whalley, L. J. (1984). Genetics, ageing and dementia. *British Journal of Psychiatry*, **145**, 20–38.

Wurtman, R. J. (1985). Alzheimer's disease. *Scientific American*, **252** (1), 48–56.

13   *Schizophrenia*

. . . poor Ophelia, divided from herself and her fair judgement without the which we are pictures or mere beasts . . .

Shakespeare, *Hamlet*

The term schizophrenia (splitting of psychic functions) was first introduced in 1911 by Eugen Bleuler to denote the breakdown of integration between emotions, thought, and actions. It is a very difficult disease to consider especially in biochemical terms because of problems in diagnosis. The symptoms are rather heterogeneous and even to this day there can still be disagreements about diagnosis despite the introduction of modern operational criteria: definitions may also be influenced by cultural factors.

Nevertheless, the disease is of much interest for several reasons. It has a high incidence in the general population; it is the disease most popularly associated with 'madness'; and certain highly creative and notable individuals may have suffered from it. Diagnosis of schizophrenia also overlaps with political and social concepts of normal behaviour and has provoked strong reactions. The diagnosis has been abused, most notably in totalitarian states where it has been used as a reason for institutionalization and deprivation of freedom.

Clinical features

The annual incidence of schizophrenia is between 0.1 and 0.5 per 1000 depending on the diagnostic criteria used. This represents a lifetime risk of about 1 per cent. Epidemiological studies have shown no great geographical variation in the incidence but there is a slight but definite tendency for the birth time to be skewed towards the winter and spring months. There is some circumstantial evidence that environmental pathogens such as viruses may be involved in causation and there has been much speculation on this point. There is evidence for a role of hereditary influences and for obstetric complications on the incidence of schizophrenia. Psychosocial influences such as significant life events and interactions within the family also appear to be important in precipitating episodes of schizophrenia.

Symptoms

Schizophrenia is an example of a psychosis, that is a severe mental disorder in which there is impaired judgement and loss of contact with reality. The symptoms seen in different cases of schizophrenia are similar in nature but often variable in form and this may contribute to diagnostic problems. Certain groups of symptoms may be defined which may or may not be expressed in a particular patient. These are as follows:

1. *Thought disorder*. The form and stream of thought are manifest in a disconnected way. There may be a loosening of the structure and coherence of thought so that the patient's thoughts are difficult to follow. In addition there may be blocking, slowing, or poverty of thought which may manifest as reduction (poverty) of speech.

2. *Abnormal beliefs or delusions*. These may be delusions that the patient is being persecuted, delusions of reference (events in the world have specific reference to the patient), delusions of control, and delusions about the possession of thought. For example the patient may believe that his thoughts are not under his control, are being inserted by external influences, or are being broadcast to or shared with others.

3. *Abnormal experiences or perceptual disturbances*. These often take the form of hallucinations. The most common are auditory hallucinations, characteristically of the patient's own thoughts spoken out loud or of others commenting on the patient's actions. Other kinds of hallucinations are visual, olfactory, and tactile. Sometimes the abnormal experiences are interpreted in a delusional way.

4. *Mood disorders*. There may be mood alterations in schizophrenia at different times, for example, depression, anxiety, or facile euphoria. Characteristically there is a disconnection between mood and other aspects of functioning so that different moods are expressed inappropriately, e.g. the patient laughs heartily when describing the death of a close relative. This is known as incongruous affect. There may also be a blunting or flattening of affect which is a sustained emotional indifference or diminution of emotional response.

5. *Motor alterations*. This can be increased motor function, such as restlessness or purposeless overactivity, or reduced function with the patient remaining immobile for long periods. The type of schizophrenia demonstrating these alternating motor changes is known as catatonic but is much less common than in the past.

6. *Changes in social function*. This refers to a gradual withdrawal from social interaction which will affect work performance. In the extreme case the patient may withdraw completely from social interaction, showing a lack of drive or initiative or may break social conventions embarrassingly (for others). The underlying personality often shows a permanent change.

Symptoms such as delusions, thought disorder, perceptual disturbances, incongruous mood, and increased motor function are referred to as positive symptoms as they are supranormal, whereas poverty of speech, loss of emotional responsiveness, reduced motor function, and social withdrawal are often referred to as negative symptoms as they represent deficits from normal function.

The age at onset tends to be in late adolescence or early adulthood. Some patients present with an acute schizophrenic episode where the positive symptoms predominate whereas others may show an ultimately chronic long term schizophrenic illness with a predominance of the negative symptoms. There are, however, many variations and combinations of symptoms in different patients and one particular symptom can predominate in a particular patient. For example, some patients may have mainly paranoid delusions whereas others may appear catatonic, showing primarily disorders of motor function (see above).

It has been suggested that there is a core of true negative symptoms that comprise the so-called 'defect' state of chronic schizophrenia (diminished affect/emotional range, and poverty of speech) and that other apparently negative symptoms such as apathy and social withdrawal are complex reactions to the psychosis, in particular the positive symptoms (Crow 1989). The defect state may then persist as a background for periodic phases of positive symptoms. This is an important distinction for the success of drug treatments since it has been suggested that true negative symptoms (defect state) may be less responsive to existing drugs than are the positive symptoms. If a broader definition of negative symptoms is used then some of these may appear to be more amenable to drug treatment; this has led to some controversy in the literature.

The heterogeneity in symptoms makes for considerable problems in diagnosis (see below) and it should be made clear that for a disorder such as schizophrenia we are dealing with a syndrome based on the presence of a cluster of clinical symptoms rather than a precisely defined disease. This is further complicated by the presence of some symptoms of affective disorders (Chapter 14) in some schizophrenics—it has been suggested that schizophrenia and affective disorders may be separate ends of a continuum of psychotic disorders. There have been many attempts to categorize schizophrenics into groups with particular symptoms mainly with the aim of ultimately defining separate disease entities. Most of these categorizations have not proved to be of long term use or validity so that we are left with a heterogeneous group of patients many of whom show various combinations of the symptoms outlined above. It seems likely therefore that there are a number of factors involved in the disease presentation and I shall attempt to tease these out below. One categorization of schizophrenia which has been very influential recently is that of Crow (1980, 1985) into type I (primarily acute) and type II (primarily chronic) groups of patients. This categorization will be considered in more detail later in this chapter in the section on aetiology.

Diagnosis

It is important to consider the way schizophrenia is diagnosed as, when attempts are made to correlate neuropathological or neurochemical changes with the illness, the kinds of correlations seen will be very dependent on the diagnostic criteria used. Over the years there have been major differences in the diagnostic methods used particularly between the United States and Europe. Nowadays diagnostic criteria are much narrower and based on symptoms together with the course of the disorder.

One important past influence has been the so called 'first rank' symptoms defined by Schneider (Table 13.1). These used to form the basis of diagnosis in the UK but do not address the duration of the illness. Therefore other definitions have been developed based on the symptoms and course of disease; the operational criteria of DSM III-R of the American Psychiatric Association (Table 13.2) take account of this. Patients with a poor outcome are identified because a six month duration is required for diagnosis. It is important to determine the diagnostic criteria used when reading any research data for schizophrenic patients.

Table 13.1   Schneider's 'first rank' symptoms of schizophrenia

Hearing thoughts spoken aloud
'Third person' hallucinations
Hallucinations in the form of a commentary
Somatic hallucinations
Thought withdrawal or insertion
Thought broadcasting
Delusional perception
Feelings or actions experienced as made or influenced by others

This table is taken from Gelder *et al.* (1989) and lists the symptoms considered by Schneider to be of 'first rank' importance and which, when present in a patient enabled a diagnosis of schizophrenia to be made. They are now recognized not to be specific for schizophrenia.

Outcome of illness

The acute (positive) symptoms of schizophrenia usually respond, at least partially, to treatment with antipsychotic drugs (see below). Further acute episodes of symptoms may recur and maintenance therapy with antipsychotic drugs can be of use in preventing this relapse. The long term outcome of an acute schizophrenic attack is very variable. Some patients recover completely whereas some never fully recover, showing residual deficits or the more negative symptoms of the chronic state with the deleterious effects on social interaction and employment prospects. In between these two extremes there

Table 13.2   Criteria for diagnosis of schizophrenia as outlined in DSM III-R of the American Psychiatric Association

A. Presence of characteristic psychotic symptoms in the active phase: either (1), (2) or (3) for at least one week (unless the symptoms are successfully treated).
  1. Two of the following:
     (a) delusions
     (b) prominent hallucinations
     (c) incoherence or marked loosening of associations
     (d) catatonic behaviour
     (e) flat or grossly inappropriate affect
  2. Bizarre delusions (i.e. involving a phenomenon that the person's culture would regard as totally implausible, e.g. thought broadcasting or being controlled by a dead person).
  3. Prominent hallucinations (as in 1b).
B. During the course of the disturbance, functioning in such areas as work, social relations, and self-care is below the highest level achieved before the disturbance.
C. Schizoaffective disorder and mood disorder with psychotic features have been ruled out.
D. Continuous signs of the disturbance for at least six months. The six month period must include an active phase (as in A) during which there were psychotic symptoms with or without a prodromal or residual phase as defined below.
  Prodromal phase. A clear deterioration in functioning before the active phase of the disturbance with at least two symptoms defined below.
  Residual phase. Following the active phase of the disturbance, persistence of at least two of the symptoms defined below.
  Prodromal or residual symptoms
  1. Marked social isolation or withdrawal.
  2. Marked impairment in role functioning as wage earner, student or home maker.
  3. Markedly peculiar behaviour.
  4. Marked impairment in personal hygiene and grooming.
  5. Blunted or inappropriate affect.
  6. Digressive, vague, over elaborate or circumstantial speech or poverty of speech or poverty of content of speech.
  7. Odd beliefs or magical thinking, influencing behaviour and inconsistent with cultural norms.
  8. Unusual perceptual experiences.
  9. Marked lack of initiative, interests, or energy.
E. It cannot be established that an organic factor initiated and maintained the disturbance.

are a variety of possibilities with repeated acute episodes and varying degrees of disablement. It has been estimated that about a quarter of patients make a full recovery whereas about a quarter remain severely disturbed, about half of the latter group requiring long term hospitalization. The remaining half of the patients diagnosed as schizophrenic have a more or less severe disorder with fluctuating episodes over many years. Antipsychotic drugs have, however, helped greatly in the management of symptoms.

The basis of the different outcomes is not understood and is likely to be a reflection of the original heterogeneity of the patients. Features have been proposed that are associated with good or poor outcome and these are outlined in Table 13.3. These are

Table 13.3 Factors predicting the outcome of schizophrenia

Good prognosis	Poor prognosis
Sudden onset	Insidious onset
Short episode	Long episode
No previous psychiatric history	Previous psychiatric history
Prominent affective symptoms	Negative symptoms
Older age at onset	Young age at onset
Married	Single, separated, widowed, divorced
Good psychosexual adjustment	Poor psychosexual adjustment
Good previous personality	Abnormal previous personality
Good work record	Poor work record
Good social relationships	Social isolation
Good compliance	Poor compliance

From Gelder *et al.* (1989).

general guidelines and have no absolute predictive value. It seems that the degree of social stimulation received by a patient may be an important factor here. This can refer to the effects of the hospital environment, significant events experienced by the patient, and the interactions with the patient's family. An intermediate level of social stimulation is optimal for the outcome, too much social stimulation (especially critical) leading to exacerbation of the positive symptoms, while too little exacerbates the negative symptoms. Interactions with the patient's family will be considered in more detail later.

Hereditary influences

Although it has been debated at length, there seem to be clear hereditary influences in the occurrence of schizophrenia. Studies within families show that the lifetime expectancy for developing schizophrenia is about 10 per cent in the first degree relatives of schizophrenic patients, compared with the general population rate of 1 per cent. The risk to a sibling of a schizophrenic where there is also one affected parent is 17 per cent and if both parents are affected this rises to 46 per cent. These increased risks could be due to genetic influences but could also represent environmental or familial effects, e.g. dietary habits, child rearing practices, or viruses. These different influences can be dissected by looking at the occurrence of schizophrenia in monozygotic and dizygotic twin pairs and in adopted children of affected versus non-affected parents. Concordance rates for monozygotic twins (who have identical genes) are about 48 per cent when the index twin has schizophrenia whereas they are about 17 per cent for dizygotic twins, who have genes no more similar than typical siblings. Concordance rates for monozygotic twins are similar whether the twins are reared together or apart, suggesting that genetic factors are of importance. Being adopted away from biological relatives with schizophrenia does not reduce the risk, suggesting that the familial tendency is largely due to genetic factors.

These findings have been strongly criticized on a number of levels (Rose *et al*. 1984; Pam 1990). These authors have underlined the difficulties in carrying out studies of adoptions and twins. The age of adoption will vary and will be very important in determining the influence of the biological and adoptive parents. Similarly there is a selective effect in the adoptive placements which may produce a familial tendency even with non-biological adoptive parents. With respect to the twin studies, these authors argue that monozygotic twins are likely to be treated more similarly than dizygotic twins by their parents, which may account for some of the concordance difference. Claridge (1985) has emphasized, however, that on some ratings monozygotic twins may be less similar than expected so that the monozygotic/dizygotic comparison could actually underestimate genetic effects. Despite these caveats, the prevailing view is still that there is an important genetic component in schizophrenia, but the above remarks underline the importance of considering environmental influences.

There are also cases of schizophrenia who show no familial history of the disorder and in these patients environmental factors could be of particular importance. There has been much interest in the possibility that obstetric complications at birth might lead to an alteration in brain development and that this could lead to schizophrenia in some patients. There are some data to support this idea. This will be considered in more detail later when aetiological theories are discussed.

Recently a study has been made of the offspring of monozygotic twin pairs who are themselves discordant for schizophrenia, i.e. only one twin has the disorder (Gottesman and Bertelsen 1989). The offspring of both the affected and unaffected twins have roughly equal risks of suffering from schizophrenia. This suggests that a genetic tendency for schizophrenia can lie dormant but be passed on to offspring. Environmental stressors may then determine whether the genetic tendency is expressed. These findings suggest that the genetic influence on schizophrenia could have been underestimated in the twin studies described above but that environmental factors of various kinds are important in whether this genetic tendency is expressed.

Genetic linkage studies in families where schizophrenia occurs have been performed using the technique of restriction fragment length polymorphism analysis, a technique that was outlined in connection with Huntington's disease (Chapter 11). One such study reported linkage of schizophrenia to a marker on chromosome 5 (Sherrington *et al*. 1988) but several other studies failed to find such a linkage (Owen and Mullan 1990; Watt and Edwards 1991). This could reflect genetic heterogeneity between families or it could represent the complexity of such a study in a disease like schizophrenia where there may be aetiological diversity.

Psychosocial influences

It often seems that significant life events (positive and negative) precede a schizophrenic attack. These are, however, not specific for precipitating schizophrenia and may precede other psychological and non-psychological illness. Also there is evidence (considered in more detail later in this chapter) that critical, overinvolved or hostile family interactions can lead to poor outcomes for schizophrenic patients. These psychosocial influences have their effects on susceptible individuals and susceptibility may be determined by genetic factors and environmental factors as described above.

Neuropathological observations

Over the past hundred years there have been tantalizing suggestions of neuropathological abnormalities in brains of schizophrenics, especially from air encephalographic studies. There have also been many negative observations and until fairly recently the general opinion was that there were no major pathological changes.

This picture has been transformed with the advent of modern techniques which allow evaluation of the brain status of schizophrenics in life. Computerized axial tomography (CAT) scanning (Chapter 9) confirmed earlier work using air encephalography showing lateral ventricular enlargement in schizophrenics. This has subsequently been found in varying degrees in both acute and chronic patients and does not seem to be progressive. Ventricular enlargement is probably, therefore, present in many patients presenting with a schizophrenic illness.

Ventricular enlargement is not associated with antipsychotic drug therapy but it is also not a change specific for schizophrenia as ventricular enlargement is also seen in affective disorders (Chapter 14). Nevertheless, these changes in the brain may be of some importance. There are some indications that the enlargement of ventricles in schizophrenia is associated with environmental insults, for example birth complications.

Careful morphometric studies of post-mortem brains have subsequently shown that there is no generalized atrophy of the brain in schizophrenia but that there are minor reductions in overall brain size together with selective reductions in the size of temporal lobe structures such as the amygdala, hippocampus, and associated parahippocampal gyrus. These changes may be lateralized to the left hemisphere of the brain (Brown *et al.* 1986; Johnstone *et al.* 1989; Crow *et al.* 1989). Studies of the organization of neurones in brains from schizophrenics have shown cell loss and disruption in similar temporal lobe structures. In the hippocampus from patients with schizophrenia there is evidence for pyramidal cell disorientation which may indicate a disorder of neuronal migration during development (Conrad *et al.* 1991) and similar evidence has been presented for neurones in the parahippocampal gyrus (Jakob and Beckmann 1988). Magnetic resonance imaging has also shown reductions in temporal lobe size in schizophrenia

(Suddath *et al*. 1989; Andreasen *et al*. 1990). There is no evidence of gliosis which might have indicated a pathological process occurring in adulthood.

A further study has highlighted alterations in neuronal number in the prefrontal and anterior cingulate cortex in schizophrenia (Benes *et al*. 1986; Benes and Bird 1987). These findings are of interest in the light of studies on regional cerebral blood flow and glucose metabolism in schizophrenics which have provided evidence of reduced frontal lobe function (hypofrontality) in some studies, although these have not always been replicated (Waddington 1990). Clear evidence of frontal lobe abnormalities has been demonstrated when patients are given tests that specifically require frontal lobe function e.g. the Wisconsin card sorting test (Chapter 9). Diminished performance in the test and no increase in frontal cortical cerebral blood flow during the test are seen in schizophrenic patients (Weinberger 1988). Non-schizophrenics perform better in the test and show increased frontal cortical blood flow when performing the test.

Therefore there seems to be clear evidence of structural differences between brains from normal and some schizophrenic patients with the differences mostly being seen in the temporal lobe. There is some evidence, mostly functional, for abnormalities of frontal lobe function. The cause of these differences is unknown but there seems to be little evidence of an ongoing disease process so that a developmental alteration must be considered.

Neurochemical observations

A vast research effort has been expended over recent years with the general aim of uncovering a specific neurochemical defect in schizophrenia. Much of the work has been misguided and the results have been confounded by effects of drug treatments the patients had been receiving. It is of value here to consider the possible approaches that can be taken to uncover a putative neurochemical defect as this can serve as a paradigm for similar studies in other diseases (see also Chapter 9).

Firstly, it is necessary to have a clinically well defined group of patients and appropriate controls. As we have seen earlier, diagnosis of schizophrenia is difficult and different observers have used different definitions of the disease. Although more homogeneous diagnostic criteria are now being applied it can be seen that the results obtained in neurochemical studies may be very dependent on the patients tested and the diagnostic criteria used.

Secondly, a measurement must be made of a neurochemical parameter. This can be made in an accessible body fluid in life, for example, urine, blood, or cerebrospinal fluid, or in post-mortem brain samples. Additionally, *in vivo* imaging techniques are beginning to be applied to the measurement of specific neurochemical parameters as well as more general parameters such as cerebral blood flow.

Many measurements have been made of neurotransmitters or their metabolites in urine, blood, and cerebrospinal fluid on the basis that these may mirror brain levels of the same substances. Although these measurements are relatively easy to perform it seems unlikely that specific changes in neurotransmitter function in the brain will be reflected in changes in body fluids rather distant from the brain. Where an enzyme or receptor is present both on a blood cell, and in the brain, for example monoamine oxidase, then the rationale for measuring blood parameters as a mirror of brain parameters is better. Even then it is necessary to know that the blood cell enzyme is identical and under similar regulation to the brain counterpart. This seems unlikely in most cases. The prospect for meaningful measurements of brain function based on measurements in post-mortem brain are little better. Measurements in brain are at least made in the correct place but the problems of post-mortem delay, post-mortem changes, and the uncertain state of the patient around the time of death, including drug treatments, can confound these measurements. Most promising are the newer imaging techniques for making non-invasive measurements of neurochemical parameters in life. Examples of these have been given in Chapter 9 and some specific examples for schizophrenia will be given below.

Virtually all of the known neurotransmitters have been considered at one time or another as candidates for defective or altered neurotransmitter systems in schizophrenia and which would then be responsible for the observed symptoms. Much of the impetus for considering particular neurotransmitters has been inspired by the ability of certain psychotropic drugs to induce in normal individuals symptoms resembling more or less closely those seen in schizophrenics. Given that the particular drug is known to affect a particular neurotransmitter system, then it has been argued that perhaps that neurotransmitter system is altered in schizophrenia. Measurements of the neurotransmitter or its metabolites have then been carried out in schizophrenics. The neurotransmitters that have been examined in this way are acetylcholine, noradrenaline, dopamine, GABA, glutamate, 5-hydroxytryptamine, and many peptides; only in the case of dopamine and glutamate is there any real indication of an alteration.

The impetus for considering dopamine as an altered neurotransmitter in schizophrenia came from two observations (Fig. 13.1). Firstly, amphetamine can induce in humans a state that closely resembles paranoid schizophrenia. Amphetamine causes release of dopamine from nerve ending stores although at high doses it also releases noradrenaline and 5-hydroxytryptamine. Secondly, the antipsychotic drugs that can be used to treat the symptoms of schizophrenia are thought to act via blockade of dopamine receptors of the D_2 subclass. These two observations prompted the corollary that the symptoms of schizophrenia might be due to overactivity in the functioning of dopamine systems (the 'dopamine hypothesis' of schizophrenia). However, examination of dopamine and its metabolites and the enzymes responsible for dopamine synthesis and degradation in post-mortem brain have given no consistent evidence for changes in dopamine neurotransmission in schizophrenia. One study reported an asymmetric increase in dopamine in the amygdala in schizophrenics (Reynolds 1983, 1989). The

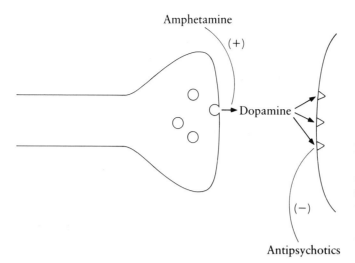

Figure 13.1 Basis of the 'dopamine hypothesis' of schizophrenia. The diagram shows a dopamine synapse and the effects of drugs (amphetamine and antipsychotics) that lead to the proposal of a 'dopamine hypothesis'.

increase was on the left side and is of interest as it is consistent with some lateralized neuropathological changes in temporal lobe structures and other indications of asymmetry which will be discussed later. It is not known, however, to what extent the changes were dependent on the drug treatments as many of the patients tested would have been taking antipsychotic drugs prior to death.

The characteristics of dopamine receptors in the striatal regions of post-mortem brains from schizophrenic patients have been examined energetically and a fairly consistent finding has been an elevated number of dopamine receptors of the D_2 subclass. That there is an increase in D_2 dopamine receptors does not seem to be in dispute; what is disputed is the cause of this elevation. Many of the patients will have been on antipsychotic drug medication in life and the ability of these drugs to block D_2 dopamine receptors may have caused the increase (up-regulation) in receptor numbers (Chapter 6). However, brains taken from patients reliably known not to have taken antipsychotic drugs have also been tested and do show an elevation of D_2 dopamine receptors. It has also been argued that even in patients who have taken neuroleptics in life, there is an increase in the number of D_2 dopamine receptors above that due to the drug (Seeman and Niznik 1990).

Recently, imaging techniques have been used with receptor-specific ligands labelled with positron emitting isotopes e.g. [^{11}C]methylspiperone. Using these methods it should be possible to determine whether there has been an increase of D_2 dopamine receptors in the brains of living schizophrenics. In three studies which examined patients before they received drugs, one study reported an increase in receptor number, two did not. There are significant methodological difficulties with these techniques, so more work needs to be done for a definitive answer (Waddington 1989; Martinot *et al.* 1990).

Glutamate systems have been examined more recently in post-mortem brain as suitable probes have become available. Evidence has been presented for alterations in glutamate function in the frontal and temporal lobes from post-mortem schizophrenic brains (Kerwin *et al.* 1988; Kerwin 1989; Deakin *et al.* 1989; Harrison *et al.* 1991). These changes may relate to the specific neuropathological alterations in these brain regions outlined above.

In summary, then, there is surprisingly little firm information about neurochemical changes in schizophrenia. There is some evidence for changes in dopamine systems mainly at the level of receptors. This 'dopamine hypothesis' of schizophrenia has some problems: centrally active dopamine agonists are only weakly psychotogenic whereas the hypothesis would predict high psychotogenic activity. Also, the antipsychotic effect of the drugs occurs rather slowly and probably later than the blockade of D_2 dopamine receptors. These problems and some resolutions of them will be considered in the next section. There are also indications of changes in glutamate systems in the regions of the brain where neuropathological alterations have been observed.

Treatments for schizophrenia
Antipsychotic drugs

This class of drugs, also called major tranquillizers or neuroleptics, is rather diverse chemically, including several families of compounds (Leysen and Niemegeers 1985). Key members of each family are given in Table 13.4. All of these classes of compound are effective in treating some symptoms of schizophrenia. The different classes of compound do, however, differ in their side effects.

These drugs are most effective at treating the positive symptoms of schizophrenia, such as hallucinations or delusions, and less effective at treating the negative symptoms of chronic schizophrenia, although some studies report beneficial effects on both kinds of symptoms. The responsiveness of the negative symptoms to drug treatment may depend on the definition of negative symptoms. It has been suggested that the 'true' negative symptoms such as diminished affect (mood) and poverty of speech are not drug responsive. However, apparent negative symptoms such as apathy and social withdrawal, which may in fact be secondary reactions to positive symptoms, may be drug responsive (Crow 1989). The atypical drug clozapine may be useful for the treatment of true negative symptoms although it has side effects (Kane *et al.* 1988).

Antipsychotic drugs are also useful in preventing relapse if given after an acute attack has been controlled. Continued oral dosing can be used or a depot form of the drug, e.g. flupenthixol decanoate can be administered at approximately monthly intervals. In this approach the decanoate derivative of the drug is injected intramuscularly in an oily base from which it is slowly released and de-esterified to give the parent compound

Table 13.4 The structures of some antipsychotic drugs and their chemical classes

PHENOTHIAZINES

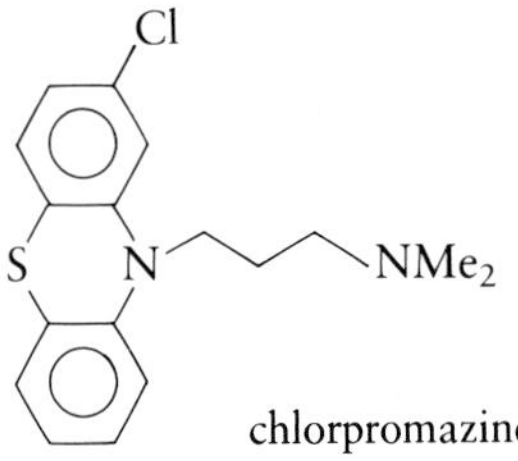

chlorpromazine

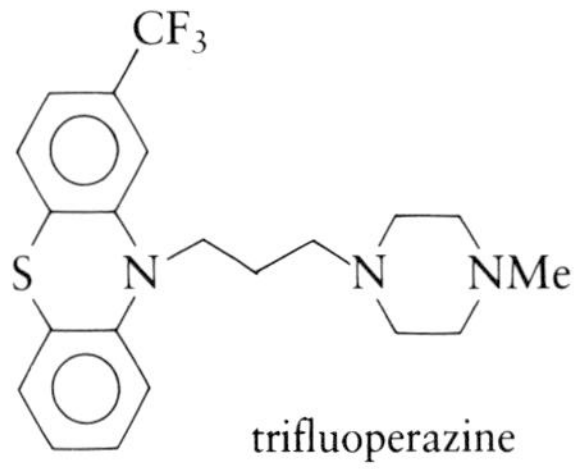

trifluoperazine

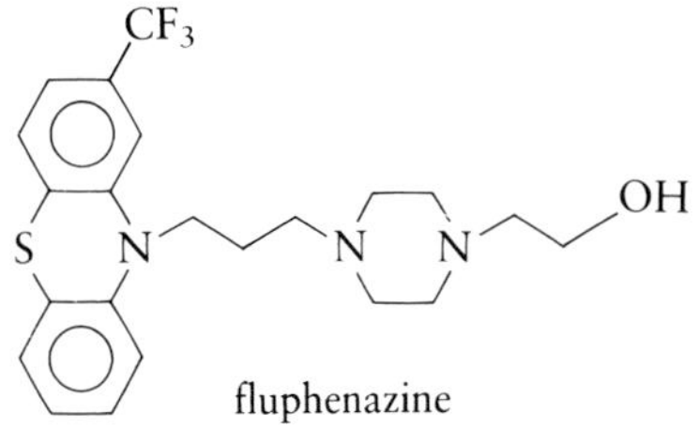

fluphenazine

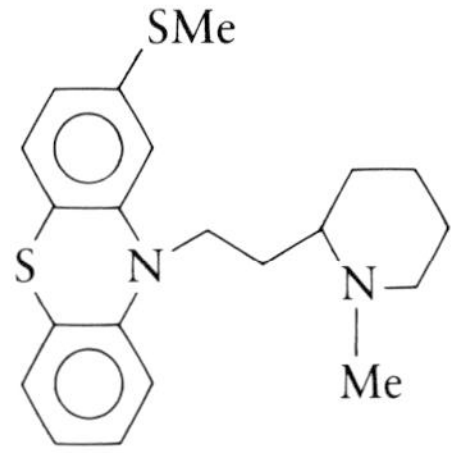

thioridizine

DIPHENYLBUTYLPIPERIDINES   pimozide

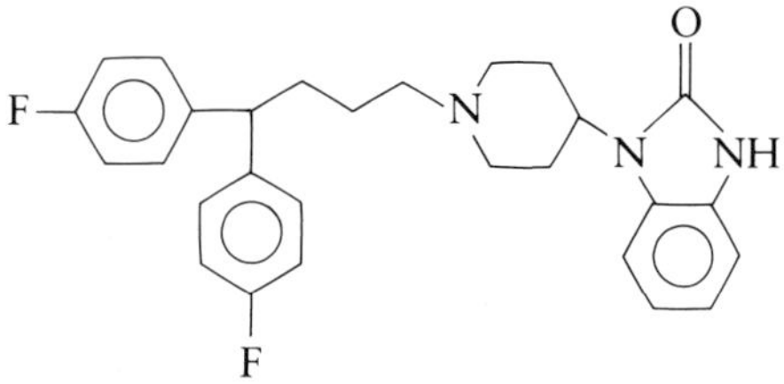

THIOXANTHENES   flupenthixol

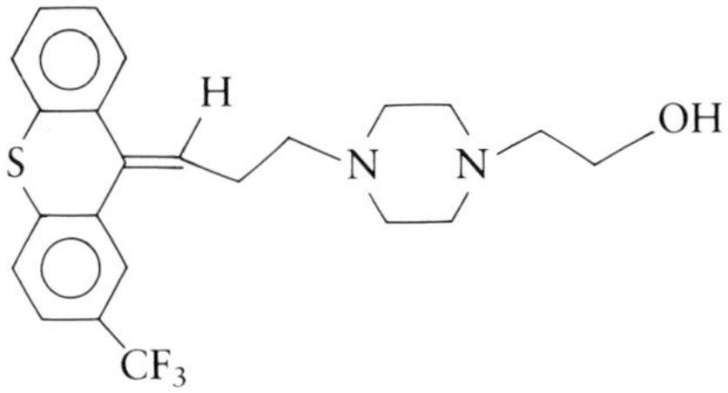

BUTYROPHENONES   haloperidol

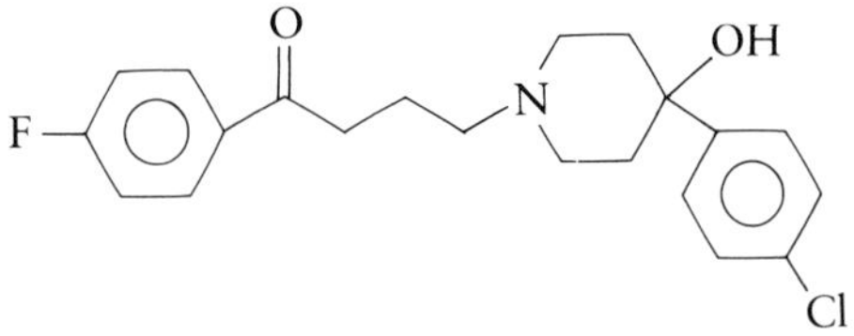

DIBENZODIAZEPINES   clozapine

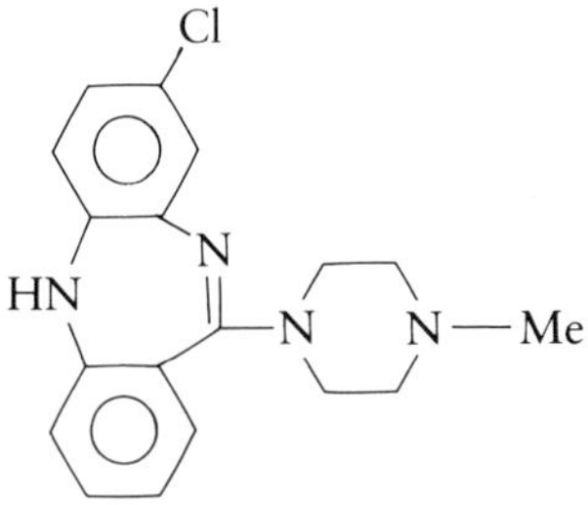

SUBSTITUTED BENZAMIDES   sulpiride

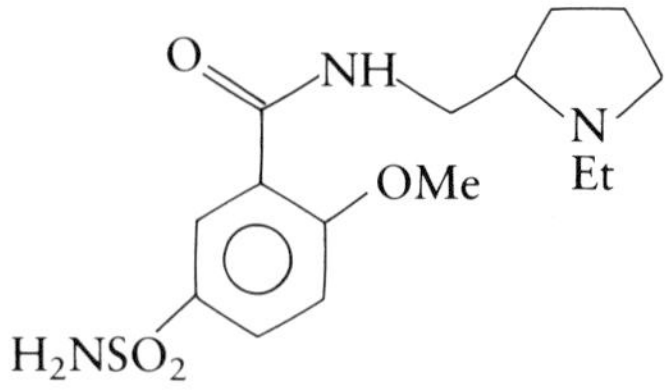

flupenthixol. It has to be remembered that continued use of antipsychotic drugs can lead to dyskinesias which often persist, so maintenance therapy has to be undertaken cautiously.

It is of some interest to understand the mode of action of antipsychotic drugs in treating schizophrenia as this may lead to a greater understanding of the disease process. It is generally accepted now that a key site of action of such drugs is the D_2 dopamine receptor. Support for this comes from correlations of the sort shown in Fig. 13.2 where an excellent correlation is observed between the average daily dose of a drug for treating schizophrenia and its binding to the D_2 dopamine receptor *in vitro*. The correlation is impressive and surprisingly good given the imprecision of the measurements and the factors that must influence the clinical dosage required. Although antipsychotic drugs are also active variously at a number of other receptors, such as D_1 dopamine, 5-HT_2 5-hydroxytryptamine, α_1-adrenergic, H_1 histamine, sigma opiate, and muscarinic acetylcholine receptors, no such correlations are observed for these other systems. Additional D_2-like dopamine receptors have recently been discovered through gene cloning. For example, the D_3 dopamine receptor located in limbic brain regions may be

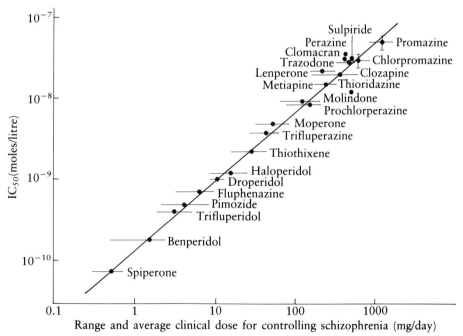

Figure 13.2 Correlation between the average daily dose of antipsychotic drugs for treating schizophrenia and the affinities of the drugs for brain D_2 dopamine receptors. Redrawn from Seeman (1980) with permission. The y-axis gives the concentration of the drug required to inhibit radioligand binding to D_2 dopamine receptors *in vitro* by 50 per cent (IC_{50}). These IC_{50} values are therefore a measure of the ability of the drugs to bind to D_2 dopamine receptors.

important for antipsychotic drug action in addition to D_2 dopamine receptors (Strange 1991*c*). Interactions of some drugs with sigma receptors may also contribute to their antipsychotic activity (Strange 1991*a*).

The idea that blockade of D_2 dopamine receptors is responsible for the antipsychotic effect of these drugs has stimulated interest in the idea that dopamine systems are overactive in schizophrenia as discussed earlier. Although there is some evidence in favour of this latter idea it is also possible that the blockade of D_2 dopamine receptors by antipsychotic drugs could be balancing a disturbance in some other non-dopamine system. It is important, as discussed in Chapter 9, to separate clearly theories of drug action from theories of disease. In the present case it seems that a large part of the therapeutic action of antipsychotic drugs can be ascribed to their activities at D_2 dopamine receptors: that is a theory of drug action. The extension of this to a theory of psychosis based on overactive dopamine neuronal systems (the 'dopamine hypothesis') is not warranted unless there is good evidence for such overactivity. As discussed in the previous section, the evidence is rather meagre.

There are also some difficulties with the idea that the antipsychotic effect is mediated at the D_2 dopamine receptor. It might be predicted that the antipsychotic effect would be exerted once the drugs had reached a steady state plasma or tissue level. Circulating prolactin levels are controlled in an inhibitory manner by dopamine via D_2 dopamine receptors in the anterior pituitary gland (Chapter 5), so a measure of D_2 dopamine receptor blockade may be obtained from the increase in plasma prolactin upon administration of an antipsychotic drug. Prolactin levels rise and reach a steady state level after about a week of drug treatment and remain elevated during chronic drug treatment. Therefore D_2 dopamine receptors are blocked to a steady state level within a week and remain blocked (Crow *et al.* 1977).

In contrast, the antipsychotic effects of the drugs take several weeks to reach a maximum level, so there is a discrepancy between the time course of receptor blockade and clinical effects. Pituitary receptors might be more accessible than those in the brain, thus accounting for the differences in time course. However, new imaging techniques provide a way of examining receptor blockade in the brain of a living patient, and use of positron emission tomography and a suitably labelled antipsychotic drug has shown that D_2 dopamine receptors are blocked to a level of 70 per cent or more, depending on the drug used, and that this level of blockade is achieved within a few hours of treatment (Sedvall *et al.* 1986).

There is therefore a clear discrepancy between the rate of occupancy of brain D_2 dopamine receptors by an antipsychotic drug and the appearance of the antipsychotic effect. This suggests that although the antipsychotic effect depends on occupancy of the D_2 dopamine receptor, other changes in the brain must follow to account for the antipsychotic effect. Further evidence for this comes from experiments where patients taking antipsychotic drugs have the drugs withdrawn. The reappearance of psychosis (positive symptoms) can occur well after the drug is likely to have disappeared from the patient's circulation.

This has prompted a series of trials where experimental animals are treated with antipsychotic drugs for varying periods of time and indices of dopamine function measured. It should be recalled that there are several dopamine neurone systems with different projection fields (Chapter 5) and it seems that these behave differently following antipsychotic drug treatment.

The firing rates of the dopamine neurones themselves are all increased following short term treatment with antipsychotic drugs. This reflects the blockade of the autoreceptors on the neurones that control cell firing. The effects on mesostriatal neurones are greater than for those mesocortical neurones projecting to the prefrontal and cingulate cortices as the latter neurones lack impulse and synthesis regulating autoreceptors (Chapter 5) and fire more quickly. They do, however, possess release-modulating autoreceptors and so occupancy of these by the antipsychotic drug accounts for the increased firing in those cells.

Upon more long term antipsychotic treatments, the mesostriatal neurones (including those projecting to motor regions, such as the caudate/putamen, and limbic regions, such as the nucleus accumbens) adapt to the presence of the drug so that their activity gradually returns towards the basal level and eventually they enter a state of inactivity termed depolarization block. In contrast, the meso-prefrontal–cortical and meso-cingulate–cortical neurones do not adapt in the same way and their firing rate remains elevated during prolonged antipsychotic drug treatment. As the latter neurones lack certain kinds of autoreceptor, it must be the presence of these on the mesostriatal neurones that allows them to adapt.

Postsynaptic dopamine receptor function has also been assessed and, as expected, after a short treatment with antipsychotic drugs, indices of postsynaptic receptor function are inhibited. Upon long term treatment there are compensatory increases in D_1 and D_2 dopamine receptor number (up-regulation, Chapter 6) but as the receptors are blocked to a level of about 70 per cent at an early stage in the antipsychotic therapy, this may not be of great significance to the overall function of the dopamine system. There may therefore be small compensatory increases in postsynaptic sensitivity in response to drug blockade but there is no evidence to suppose that the changes do not occur in all the terminal fields of the different dopamine neurones.

The net result of long term antipsychotic treatment will therefore be to inhibit generally the activities of dopamine systems (the receptors are blocked to a level of about 70 per cent) but also to alter the balance of functional activities in the different dopamine neuronal populations in favour of relatively increased activity in the meso-prefrontal–cortical and meso-cingulate–cortical neurones (Fig. 13.3). This increased presynaptic activity may partly overcome the postsynaptic blockade of receptors. The balance will not be altered until the adaptive processes have occurred in the other neurones and, as

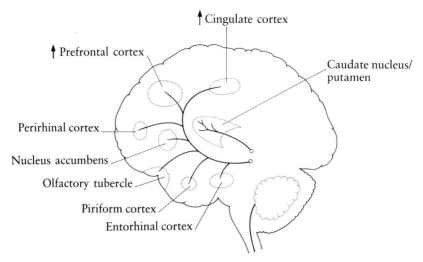

Figure 13.3 Mechanisms of action of antipsychotic drugs. The diagram shows the different dopamine neuronal systems and the relative activities of these upon chronic antipsychotic medication. Antipsychotic drugs inhibit postsynaptic dopamine receptor actions generally, but neurones innervating the prefrontal and cingulate cortices maintain an increased firing rate during chronic therapy whereas the other dopamine neuronal populations show reduced firing rates.

these are relatively slow, this provides a possible explanation for the prolonged time course of antipsychotic therapy in humans. Therefore the antipsychotic effect can be ascribed to the antipsychotic drugs having two effects on dopamine neuronal systems. On the one hand, the antipsychotic drugs will inhibit functional activity in all the dopamine systems by postsynaptic blockade and presynaptic changes (reduction in firing) in some neurones. On the other hand, the antipsychotic drugs will shift the balance among the different neuronal populations in favour of relatively greater activity in those mesocortical neurones innervating the prefrontal and cingulate cortices. These regions of the brain are important for the control and organization of behaviour, mood, emotion, and evaluation of outcomes. The positive symptoms of schizophrenia (treated by the antipsychotic drugs) can be viewed as disturbances of these functions so that specific effects of antipsychotic drugs on these brain regions could provide a rationalization of the antipsychotic effect. As will be suggested below, the effects of the antipsychotic drugs on these brain regions may be to counteract altered functions elsewhere in the brain.

Blockade of D_2 dopamine receptors in the motor regions of the striatum will also occur. It is thought that blockade of striatal dopamine receptors leads to some of the side effects associated with antipsychotic medication which will be considered in the next section.

How do these ideas relate to brain function? It is of interest that both the prefrontal and cingulate cortices participate in analogous but separate cortico-striato-thalamo-cortical circuits. Examples of these basal ganglia circuits have already been discussed in relation to Parkinson's disease and Huntington's disease (Chapters 10 and 11) and Fig. 13.4 shows the 'dorsolateral prefrontal circuit' and 'anterior cingulate circuit' relevant to the present discussion. These are both examples of the 'complex circuits' referred to in Chapter 10. The functions of these circuits are presently unknown but the participation of major limbic brain regions in the anterior cingulate circuit suggests that this circuit has some role in the control of behaviour and motivation. For the present discussion, what is important, however, is that in both circuits there is control at both the cortical and striatal levels by dopamine via the mesocortical and mesostriatal dopamine pathways (Chapter 5). If the effect of chronic antipsychotic medication is to alter the balance of dopamine actions in favour of prefrontal and cingulate cortical actions, then this will

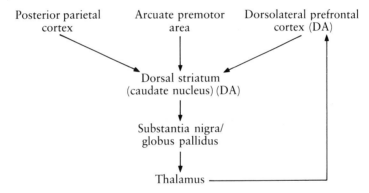

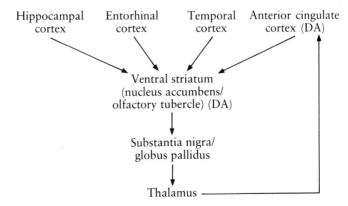

Figure 13.4 Dorsolateral prefrontal and anterior cingulate circuits. DA denotes that the brain region is under control by dopamine.

alter the general activities of both the dorsolateral prefrontal circuit and the anterior cingulate circuit. Because the functions of these circuits are not known, it is difficult to be precise about the outcome of this, but it should be noted that several temporal lobe structures participate in the anterior cingulate circuit. There are changes in temporal lobe structures in the brains of schizophrenic patients and later I shall argue that these changes may underlie the positive symptoms of schizophrenia. Since these are the symptoms principally treated by antipsychotic drugs, it may be that altering the activity of a neuronal pathway in which these temporal lobe structures participate may counteract the changes in brain activity caused by the temporal lobe alterations.

Side effects of antipsychotic drugs

As well as their antipsychotic effect, some of the drugs have a marked sedative effect which can be useful and may be related to their blockade of adrenergic and histamine receptors. The principal undesirable side effects are motor effects although hypotension and tachycardia related to blockade of adrenergic receptors and effects such as dry mouth, reduced sweating, and blurred vision are also seen with some drugs owing to blockade of muscarinic acetylcholine receptors.

The unwanted motor side effects are referred to as extrapyramidal side effects (EPSEs) (Marsden and Jenner 1980) and for some drugs these include early dystonia (muscle spasm) and akathisia (motor restlessness). A common early side effect which can begin in the first few days of drug treatment is the development of a parkinsonian syndrome with many of the symptoms of Parkinson's disease (Chapter 10). This is entirely consistent with the blockade of D_2 dopamine receptors in the striatum which is functionally equivalent to the loss of dopamine seen in Parkinson's disease.

Persistent parkinsonian side effects are seen in 20–40 per cent of patients treated with antipsychotic drugs; the prevalence of such side effects shows a similar age profile to Parkinson's disease itself (Marsden and Jenner 1980). This suggests that the antipsychotic drugs, by interfering with dopamine function in the basal ganglia, are highlighting similar tendencies to those brought out by the Parkinson's disease process. A plausible explanation consistent with the theories proposed in Chapter 10 is that there is a spectrum of loss of the mesostriatal dopamine neurones in different patients and that either advancing loss of these same cells or reducing dopamine transmission by an antipsychotic drug can bring on parkinsonian symptoms in patients who have already lost a substantial proportion of mesostriatal neurones.

A more serious problem is the syndrome of tardive dyskinesia. This presents after months or years of antipsychotic drug administration and can be persistent on discontinuation of antipsychotic medication and resistant to treatment (Kane and Smith 1982; Jeste and Wyatt 1982). About 20 per cent of patients treated with such drugs show this syndrome which consists of abnormal involuntary movements, usually of the tongue and lips e.g. smacking of the lips, chewing, and tongue protrusion, but less commonly of the limbs, thorax, and trunk. It was initially thought that the syndrome was associated with a dopamine receptor supersensitivity (up-regulation, Chapter 6) caused by the antipsychotic drugs. This idea is now thought to be incorrect (Fibiger and Lloyd 1984).

There is some interest in understanding the basis of tardive dyskinesia as it seems to be a problem only for a proportion of patients. Risk factors for the development of the syndrome, apart from drug treatment, seem to be increasing age, the presence of negative symptoms of schizophrenia and cognitive dysfunction, and demonstrable brain pathology as assessed by ventricular enlargement. This suggests that the development of tardive dyskinesia may be associated with the schizophrenic disorders where there is more atrophy of the brain.

It has also been noted that there is a significant but low incidence of abnormal involuntary movements in schizophrenics who have not taken antipsychotic drugs and that this proportion rises sharply if very severely affected chronic patients are examined. It has therefore been suggested that there is a tendency for abnormal involuntary movements to appear in patients with chronic schizophrenia where there is evidence of structural changes in the brain (the type II syndrome of Crow (1980, 1985) which will be discussed in detail later) and that the antipsychotic drugs act as catalysts to bring out or exacerbate such movements in patients who have the chronic form of the disease with severe brain structural changes. There is an interesting parallel here with the parkinsonian side effects. In both instances it seems that the antipsychotic drugs may be in part bringing out an underlying tendency. What that tendency is in the case of tardive dyskinesia is not known but it is tempting to speculate that it relates to changes in pathways in the basal ganglia involved in controlling movement and in particular in the suppression of unwanted movements. In the chapters on Parkinson's disease and Huntington's disease (Chapters 10 and 11), it was shown that normal motor function depends on a balance between two striatal output pathways (the 'direct' and 'indirect' pathways). Imbalance between these could lead to either hypokinetic (Parkinson's disease) or hyperkinetic (Huntington's disease, ballism, and L-DOPA-induced dyskinesias) disorders. It is tempting to suggest that the abnormal movements of tardive dyskinesia are related to some imbalance in the striatal output pathways as in the hyperkinetic disorders; a few scattered observations of basal ganglia pathology in schizophrenia support this.

Fibiger and Lloyd (1984) have proposed that the exacerbation of abnormal movements in tardive dyskinesia by antipsychotic drugs is due to their actions on striatal output pathways. Gunne *et al.* (1984) have shown in primates rendered dyskinetic by prolonged antipsychotic drug treatment that there are reductions in GABA neuronal activity in several basal ganglia regions. Although a complete scheme cannot be provided at present these observations are not inconsistent with the abnormal movements of tardive dyskinesia being related to an imbalance in striatal output.

Despite the problems with antipsychotic drugs, their introduction into clinical practice has resulted in a dramatic reduction in the number of patients chronically institutionalized in mental hospitals and has reduced the length of stay for those who are admitted. This must be seen as a major advance in health care.

Non-physical treatments

An important facet of schizophrenia is disordered social functioning for the patient, either in the positive symptoms of delusions and hallucinations or in the negative symptoms of withdrawal from social contact. It therefore seems sensible to integrate drug treatments with social and psychological interventions and, where drugs may not be of great value, for example in treating the negative symptoms shown more by the chronic patient, social and psychological intervention may be crucial. It is also to be expected that the prominent psychological symptoms of schizophrenia should be amenable to psychological treatment in addition to drug therapy.

Non-physical treatments are based around either avoiding the kind of circumstances that might lead to a relapse or are based on psychological treatment of symptoms. Psychosocial factors seem important in precipitating schizophrenic attacks (see Table 13.3), for example stressful life events may be precipitating factors. Both positive events, e.g. moving to a better house, and negative events, e.g. being mugged, are important. Therefore attempts at reducing psychological stress may be useful but difficult to achieve. There has been much interest in what has been termed 'expressed emotion' (Leff *et al*. 1989; Leff 1978). This refers to close personal relationships of the patient which may be critical, hostile, or emotionally over-involved.

There is good evidence that the emotional climate (the level of 'expressed emotion') in the patient's home affects the risk of relapse. In these studies the relatives of patients were interviewed while the patient was recovering from a relapse. Patients receiving antipsychotic medication, who were discharged to relatives who had been less critical and less over-involved, remained well for considerably longer than those returning to homes with higher levels of 'expressed emotion' (Parker and Hadzi-Pavlovic 1990). Another important predictor of relapse was found to be the duration of face to face contact with relatives. The lower the time spent in the company of key relatives, the lower was the chance of relapse. Later studies have suggested that 'expressed emotion' can be reduced by educating relatives about the illness and teaching the relatives and patients simple problem-solving strategies. These studies suggest that reducing 'expressed emotion' in this way reduces the relapse rate, athough this may be dependent on the structure of the community in which the patient and his family live.

For the chronic patient the situation is different and an impoverished social environment such as used to be found in some mental hospitals can exacerbate the social withdrawal of chronic schizophrenia. Therefore attempts at social stimulation may aid rehabilitation. Psychological intervention has been used in acute and chronic patients directed at management of symptoms and reduction of social withdrawal. Attempts have been made using behavioural treatments to reduce hallucinations by reducing discussion of them or to reduce delusions by providing arguments against them. Also social skills training has been used in an attempt to provide social skills suitable for everyday life that may have been lost.

Theories of the aetiology of schizophrenia

It is clearly of great interest and importance to attempt to explain the basis of schizophrenia. Not only should this help in devising potential new treatments or controlling the incidence but it should help in gaining more insight into basic brain function. The symptoms and the syndromes of schizophrenia are, however, complex and correspondingly complex theories may therefore be required to explain them. Explanations based on deficits of a single neurotransmitter may be too crude. Complexity has, however, never been an inhibitory factor for theoreticians and I shall consider some of the more current ideas below.

For some years there was a general feeling that schizophrenia did not include so-called 'organic' brain changes and it was considered a purely 'functional' disease. In the late 1970s, however, use of more sophisticated techniques for examining brain structure *in vivo* showed clearly for the first time that there were brain changes manifesting as ventricular enlargement in many, but not all, patients.

It was then proposed (Crow 1980) that patients with an acute disorder showing mainly positive symptoms and chronic patients with mainly negative symptoms corresponded to distinct but potentially overlapping syndromes of schizophrenia termed type I and type II (Table 13.5). In this theory the cerebral atrophy of schizophrenia therefore might underlie the negative symptoms of schizophrenia (type II syndrome) whereas the florid or psychotic symptoms might involve dopamine neuronal systems (type I syndrome). Type I and type II patients could be seen, as well as patients with mixed symptoms. Type I patients could show remission of symptoms or could progress to type II but patients with type II symptoms would rarely show remission since the type II syndromes with organic changes would be irreversible.

Subsequent, more extensive imaging work has shown that ventricular enlargement does not show a correlation with any clinical measure of the patient's state except incidence of involuntary movements and impaired performance in neuropsychological tests. Ventricular enlargement is seen in both acute patients soon after presentation and in chronic patients. It appears, therefore, that ventricular enlargement is part of the disease process without being an indicator of the progression of the patient. Ventricular enlargement is also not specific for schizophrenia and is seen in other psychotic patients such as those with affective disorders.

Table 13.5   The type I/type II categorization of Crow in its 1980 formulation

	Type I	Type II
Characteristic symptoms	hallucinations, delusions, and thought disorder (positive symptoms)	affective flattening, poverty of speech, and loss of drive (negative symptoms)
Type of illness in which most commonly seen	acute schizophrenia	chronic schizophrenia, the 'defect' state
Response to antipsychotic drugs	good	poor
Outcome	reversible	irreversible?
Intellectual impairment	absent	sometimes present
Postulated pathological process	increased dopamine receptors	cell loss and structural changes in the brain

The two syndromes are shown with their key features. It should be noted that the postulated pathological processes are not wholly supported by information discussed in this chapter.

It seems that measurements of ventricular enlargement reflect a loss of brain tissue but do not localize the atrophy very well. In schizophrenia, ventricular enlargement is probably a reflection of more specific changes in the temporal lobe with some emphasis on the left side of the brain. It is a presumption here that such changes can account for the symptoms of schizophrenia and I shall justify this in the next section. Since the ventricular enlargement in schizophrenia is not progressive and seems to be present at the beginning of the disease, it therefore may represent some developmental abnormality. There are some indications of neurochemical changes in post-mortem brains from schizophrenics outlined earlier and the alterations in dopamine and glutamate systems could reflect these developmental changes in the brain.

Crow (1985) has now revised his type I/type II classification (Table 13.6) to suggest that the type II symptoms include involuntary movements and are associated with changes in the temporal lobe. These would be the movements exacerbated by antipsychotic drugs and appearing as tardive dyskinesia. The type I and type II syndromes can be relatively independent or can coexist and are thought to be different manifestations of the same pathogen rather than separate disease entities.

What might lead to these symptoms and changes in the brain? Two broad aetiological factors will be considered, i.e. genetic and environmental factors. As outlined earlier, there is good evidence for an important but not overwhelming genetic influence in schizophrenia. With respect to environmental factors, the inheritance data for schizophrenia support an important role for environmental influences in the incidence of schizophrenia. In addition, the elevated winter seasonal birth rate for schizophrenia is also consistent with environmental factors and there has been interest in the idea that

Table 13.6 The type I/type II categorization of Crow in its 1985 formulation

	Type I	Type II
Characteristic symptoms	delusions and hallucinations (positive symptoms)	flattening of affect; poverty of speech (negative symptoms)
Response to antipsychotic drugs	good	poor
Outcome	potentially reversible	irreversible?
Intellectual impairment	absent	sometimes present
Abnormal involuntary movements	absent	sometimes present
Postulated pathological process	increased D_2 dopamine receptors	cell loss in temporal lobe structures (hippocampus, amygdala, and parahippocampal gyrus)

The two syndromes are shown with their key features. It should be noted that the postulated pathological processes are not wholly supported by information discussed in this chapter.

this could represent perinatal or *in utero* influences such as viral infections or obstetric complications. There is indeed evidence that obstetric complications (birth injury) may be a predisposing factor in schizophrenia. It is therefore of interest that some studies on ventricular enlargement in schizophrenia have also highlighted obstetric complications as possible causative factors in addition to genetic factors. There is also circumstantial evidence that maternal infection with influenza during pregnancy can increase the risk of the offspring to suffer schizophrenia (Barr *et al.* 1990; Mednick *et al.* 1990; O'Callaghan *et al.* 1991).

Thus schizophrenia appears to have important genetic and environmental components in its aetiology. One way to view this is in a multifactorial polygenic–environmental threshold model whereby when a threshold of influences is reached, schizophrenia results. These influences could be either genetic or environmental and an important question concerns the extent to which these interact. I shall consider two theories that have attempted to address this question.

Murray *et al.* (1985) have suggested that there may be familial and sporadic cases of schizophrenia. Familial cases have a predominant genetic influence although environmental factors may be important. Sporadic cases are largely environmentally caused, for example by obstetric complications leading to early brain damage and a developmental abnormality. In support of their theory it has been shown in studies on twins that schizophrenics with no evidence of a family history of the disease do show ventricular enlargement, which would be subsequent to an environmental insult, whereas ventricular enlargement may be less evident in those cases where there is a positive family history and where genetic influences would presumably predominate. Also some studies have shown that in schizophrenia with no family history of psychiatric disorder there is greater evidence for obstetric complications (O'Callaghan *et al*. 1990). More recent studies on ventricular enlargement have, however, failed to show a correlation with the absence of a family history.

Others have argued that there are actually very few sporadic (non-genetic) cases of schizophrenia (McGuffin *et al*. 1987) and that schizophrenia represents a continuum from more genetic cases to less genetic cases with environmental influences bearing on this. The challenge then is to define the genes and the environmental factors that lead to schizophrenia and to define whether the same brain changes occur in response to the different factors.

Crow (1988*a,b*, 1990) has suggested that the basis of schizophrenia is entirely 'genetic' and that the approximately 50 per cent concordance rate for monozygotic twins may reflect mutations or some poorly understood developmental change affecting one twin more than the other. He has argued that psychoses including the different syndromes of schizophrenia and affective disorders (Chapter 14) form a continuum. A particular gene which undergoes a high rate of mutation determines the expression and form of the psychosis. He suggests that the gene is found on the pseudoautosomal region of the sex chromosome and this gene is also responsible for development of cerebral dominance, that is the normal difference in structure between the left and right hemispheres of the brain. Aberrant expression of this cerebral dominance gene then leads to schizophrenia and this is seen as lateralized changes in the temporal lobes.

Recent work on monozygotic twins discordant for schizophrenia has also shifted the emphasis more generally in theories of schizophrenia towards the importance of genetic factors. The risk of schizophrenia in the offspring of the discordant twins was about the same whether or not the twin had schizophrenia (Gottesman and Bertelsen 1989). Therefore the genetic tendency to schizophrenia can be unexpressed but still be passed on to children. This may mean that genetic factors are much more important than previously suspected. It also can explain why the concordance rate for monozygotic twins is rather low. It does, however, require that there be factors that alter the expression of the genetic tendency. What these factors are remain to be determined but they must represent features of the environment.

The model for schizophrenia that best fits all the findings is a multifactorial polygenic–environmental threshold model. Single dominant genes or environmental factors can infrequently lead to the disorder. The vast majority of cases, however, are due to a combination of genetic influences and environmental stressors whose combined influence takes the patient over a threshold for the occurrence of schizophrenia symptoms.

The above models invoke in part changes in brain development. The idea that schizophrenia is a neurodevelopmental disorder has become very popular recently and has been discussed in several reviews (see for example: Murray and Lewis 1987; Weinberger 1987; Lewis 1989; Jones and Murray 1991). A neurodevelopmental model is consistent with the neuropathological findings in schizophrenia which provided no evidence of an ongoing degenerative process. Evidence of changes in neuronal ordering were, however, seen. The idea has therefore arisen that schizophrenia is due to altered development of a particular part of the brain, the temporal lobe. This develops slightly differently in the brains of schizophrenics due to genetic influences (brain development is specified by a number of genes) or to environmental influences (obstetric complications or viral infections) as suggested above. The development of the brain is not covered in this book but it depends on a number of processes including cell proliferation, cell migration, and cell elimination. If these processes were altered in some way, development might be different and evidence of neuronal disorder in temporal lobe structures has been reported in schizophrenics (Jakob and Beckmann 1988; Conrad *et al.* 1991), consistent with changes in neuronal migration.

Such a model can also provide a rationalization for the age of onset of schizophrenia, that is late adolescence and early adulthood. The developmental change in one part of the brain may lead to the taking on of functions by other parts of the brain. If the developmentally affected or functionally altered parts of the brain do not normally reach their full potential and function until late adolescence or early adulthood, then a developmental problem present from birth would not manifest itself as clear symptoms until that part of the brain reached functional maturity. Adolescence and early adulthood are times of great psychological stress and strain so it does seem likely that certain higher brain regions would not attain full function until then, hence the delay in appearance of frank symptoms.

This model would also predict that there may be abnormalities of personality and behaviour prior to the occurrence of florid psychotic symptoms and there is some evidence for this. It has also been suggested that there is a continuum between 'normal' people and overt schizophrenics with people in between exhibiting varying amounts of schizoid traits. These might be people with subthreshold genetic/environmental loadings.

There have also been extensive attempts to explain schizophrenia in purely psychological terms. These reflect partly the different approaches to the disorder and partly reactions to the reductionist 'chemical' explanations which have been provided. To what extent these theories can be applied together with theories based on alterations in brain development is unclear and a detailed discussion is beyond the scope of this book. In considering psychological theories of schizophrenia it is important to distinguish effects on the causation of schizophrenia from effects on the course of the illness.

In the 1960s there were strong movements directed towards the idea that schizophrenic patients were not abnormal, rather it was their environment that was abnormal and their response to this abnormal environment was perfectly normal (the 'anti-psychiatry' movement). Such ideas do not have much currency at present. Nevertheless, it is still instructive to consider very briefly some psychological theories of schizophrenia. Both Freud and Klein proposed theories based on altered psychological development. Freud suggested that schizophrenia was due to withdrawal of the libido from external objects and that abnormal beliefs were generated to make sense of external objects. Klein, however, suggested that schizophrenia had its origins in childhood. The failure of the infant to pass through certain early developmental stages led to later schizophrenia. Neither of these theories takes account of the more modern observations on inheritance of schizophrenia and the brain structural changes.

Others have stressed the role of the family as a dominant factor. For example, disordered communication within the family could be important whereby vague or ambiguous messages are communicated. Alternatively there may be disturbances of the normal hierarchies and distinctions within the family. The role of the family in precipitating schizophrenia was stressed strongly in the 1960s by R. D. Laing who highlighted the problem for certain individuals within a confined family. These individuals found themselves in a situation termed (by Bateson) a 'double-bind'—they received from the other members of the family overt positive signals and covert negative signals. Schizophrenia, an apparent private fantasy world, was the only defence.

Although these ideas have not received any support in controlled trials, there is evidence that family interactions in schizophrenia are often impaired and, as outlined earlier, the level of 'expressed emotion' can be important in determining relapse for a schizophrenic although this is not confined to family relationships. Life events may also contribute to the stress preceding a schizophrenic attack. Therefore there is no scientific evidence that psychological factors can on their own give rise to schizophrenia, but there is evidence that psychological factors can affect the course of the illness and may contribute to the occurrence of schizophrenic episodes in susceptible individuals.

In summary, there is now evidence that the occurrence of symptoms of schizophrenia can depend on the combined influence of a variety of factors. A liability is built up in a particular individual dependent on inherited genetic factors and a variety of environmental influences. Effects of these genetic and environmental influences on brain development seem to be important and psychosocial stress must interact with these developmental changes presumably by altering brain chemistry in the susceptible individual.

This theory of the aetiology of schizophrenia combines biological influences and psychological influences to explain a largely psychological disorder. It is convenient to consider these 'biological' and 'psychological' influences separately but this should not be taken to imply a dualistic splitting of body and mind. The symptoms of schizophrenia are psychological when viewed at one level of description but must have a basis in biochemical changes in the brain when viewed at another level. The two levels of description are complementary views of the same entity in line with the discussion in Chapter 8. Schizophrenia is therefore both biological and psychological.

Disordered brain function in schizophrenia

Can we make any sense out of this complex set of information in terms of understanding the symptoms of schizophrenia in relation to the changes occurring in the brain? The principal brain changes, as outlined, are fairly specific neuronal reductions in certain temporal lobe regions such as the hippocampus, amygdala, and parahippocampal gyrus and there is some evidence for altered frontal lobe (prefrontal cortex) function. It is not known at present to what extent these changes are observed in all patients but I shall assume a patient with such changes. I shall also assume that the symptoms of schizophrenia can be accounted for solely in terms of the (developmental) changes in the brain. Psychosocial stress, although it can contribute to the occurrence of symptoms, does so via its effects on the brain which already contains these changes.

One clue to what might be happening comes from patients with temporal lobe epilepsy. Some patients with temporal lobe epilepsy also develop a schizophrenic-like state with prominent positive symptoms. In these patients the epileptic focus tends to be in the left temporal lobe. This suggests that the alterations in temporal lobe structure seen in schizophrenic patients might underlie the positive symptoms (Trimble 1990). Further support for this comes from studies of the electrical stimulation of the temporal cortex, amygdala, and hippocampus where hallucinations and perceptual distortions can be invoked. One theory has been proposed (Frith 1987; Frith and Done 1988) suggesting that the brain changes seen in schizophrenia, particularly in the temporal lobe structures, lead to a defect in the internal monitoring of actions and that this gives rise to the positive symptoms. In this theory it is suggested that all our actions are monitored by the brain and self-initiated actions are labelled by the brain as 'self'. If there is a defect in internal monitoring, then self-generated actions may be wrongly labelled as 'non-self'. To the individual this could be very confusing; his actions would not be seen as part of his 'self' and apparent delusions and hallucinations could result.

It is suggested that the brain structures responsible for monitoring are found in what is termed the septo-hippocampal system (septum and hippocampal formation) (Gray 1987). This system will be discussed again in relation to depression (Chapter 14) and anxiety (Chapter 15) but it is considered that this receives information from the prefrontal cortex about behavioural planning and goal setting. The subiculum (in the hippocampal formation) then compares the internally generated plans with current sensory information on actual outcomes of behaviour. Depending on the matching, various possibilities arise as will be discussed more in Chapters 14 and 15. The hippocampus has other important functions, including a role in memory (Chapter 12) but a comparator function may also be important for the categorization of memories and recognition of familiar situations.

For our present purpose it is sufficient to suggest that in schizophrenia there may be defective transfer of this information from the prefrontal cortex to the monitoring system (subiculum). This may lead to mislabelling of internally generated behaviour which is misinterpreted as externally controlled or generated. If the internally generated behaviour is an action then delusions about certain behaviours may result (delusions of control). If thoughts are occurring and are mislabelled as non-self then these could appear as internal voices (aural hallucinations). In this way the positive symptoms of schizophrenia could result. The pathways linking the prefrontal cortex and the hippocampus are via the entorhinal cortex of the parahippocampal gyrus and the cingulate cortex and there is evidence for some alterations in these regions of the brain in schizophrenia. We can therefore make plausible suggestions for the basis of the positive symptoms based on changes in the temporal lobes of the patients which would interfere with the septo-hippocampal monitor function. Antipsychotic drugs reduce positive symptoms in this theory by reducing the number of self-generated acts.

These ideas, however, do not fit well with the present formulation of the type I/type II classification of schizophrenia (Crow 1985) which invokes changes in the temporal lobes in the type II patients with predominantly negative symptoms. It may be, however, that the temporal lobe changes give rise to alterations in the function of other parts of the brain, as will be discussed below.

It is important to mention at this point an alternative view of disordered brain function in schizophrenia. This refers to explanations of the positive symptoms in terms of disturbances in the function of the two hemispheres of the brain. Normal human function depends on the cooperative interaction of the left hemisphere, which is important for language and is thought to process information more logically or analytically, and the right hemisphere which has a greater visuospatial ability and tends to process information more globally. A number of theories of brain function in schizophrenia have been proposed based on disturbed interhemispheric interaction and, if the normal integration of reality depends on a certain interhemispheric balance, then apparent disturbances of reality as in the positive symptoms of schizophrenia could result from impairments of interhemispheric balance. It is of interest that there are now suggestions, from a number of studies, of lateralized defects in the brains of schizophrenics (temporal lobe size, dopamine in the amygdala) and these could give a biological basis to interhemispheric imbalance.

What about the other principal symptoms seen in schizophrenia, namely the negative symptoms such as lowered mood and poverty of speech? It has been suggested that these are symptoms associated with defective frontal lobe function (Weinberger 1987, 1988; Frith and Done 1988), other 'frontal' symptoms, such as poor insight and deficient problem solving, having been noted in schizophrenics. Although not strictly negative symptoms, the neurological 'soft signs' such as reduced motor coordination which are often seen in schizophrenics can also be attributed to frontal lobe deficits. There is evidence, from neuropathological and neurochemical studies and from measurements of cerebral blood flow and metabolism, for abnormalities of frontal lobe and particularly prefrontal cortex structure and function. Therefore frontal lobe dysfunction could underlie the negative symptoms of schizophrenia. The frontal lobes are important for many higher order functions such as behavioural planning so that a defect in their function would have wide ranging effects. It has also been suggested that certain positive symptoms such as thought disorders may be associated more with frontal lobe dysfunction (Liddle 1987; Robbins 1990). It is of some interest that in the cases of both Huntington's disease and Parkinson's disease (Chapters 10 and 11) there are some of the symptoms of frontal lobe dysfunction. Neither is a frontal lobe disorder at least in the early stages, but the extensive connections of the frontal lobes with the basal ganglia, where there are changes in these diseases, may lead to more minor signs of frontal lobe dysfunction.

A question of some interest, particularly in relation to theories of the aetiology of schizophrenia, is whether the positive and negative symptoms reflect different pathologies. I have presented information above consistent with the generation of the different symptoms by alterations in function in different parts of the brain. Nevertheless, patients frequently exhibit both kinds of symptoms and it was implicit in the theories of aetiology considered in the previous section that a common pathological process could be responsible for both kinds of symptoms.

Perhaps the key to this lies in the extensive neuronal connections between the frontal and temporal lobes. A pathological (neurodevelopmental) process in the temporal lobes may be common to all schizophrenic illnesses. Ventricular enlargement would then be a gross reflection of this temporal pathology. Temporal lobe dysfunction could then give rise to frontal lobe dysfunction as the two brain regions are extensively interconnected. The predominant symptoms seen then would depend on the relative severity of the structural and functional changes in the frontal and temporal lobes. The type II patients in the classification of Crow (1985) who show predominantly negative symptoms may have considerable functional deficits in frontal lobe function owing to alterations in temporal lobe structure. In the next chapter I shall invoke changes in the fronto-temporal systems in some kinds of affective disorders.

In this section on disordered brain function, dopamine has not yet been mentioned, whereas this neurotransmitter featured strongly in previous discussions on drug treatment and aetiology. It was argued earlier that antipsychotic drug action could be understood in terms of the blockade of dopamine (D_2) receptors. Long term antipsychotic therapy leads to general inhibition of dopamine function and a change in the balance in the different dopamine neuronal populations in favour of relatively less inhibition of the neurones innervating the prefrontal and cingulate cortices. Therefore, the effects of dopamine on different target areas will be altered in favour of effects on prefrontal and cingulate cortices and, as suggested earlier, this might be important in altering activity in certain circuits ('dorsolateral prefrontal' and 'anterior cingulate' circuits) in which these brain regions participate.

In terms of the theories of disordered brain function in schizophrenia presented here based on defective septo-hippocampal monitoring, the 'anterior cingulate circuit' includes several temporal lobe structures closely linked to the hippocampus. Also the prefrontal cortex is important for providing information on behavioural plans to the septo-hippocampal monitoring system and the cingulate cortex is important in the transfer of this information. As suggested, there may be a defect in septo-hippocampal monitoring in schizophrenia giving rise to the positive symptoms. Therefore, alterations in the activities of the 'anterior cingulate circuit' or in the activities of the cingulate or prefrontal cortices owing to a change of dopamine control after chronic antipsychotic therapy may be important in suppressing the positive symptoms. It is difficult to be precise about how this could come about but it could be via improving the transfer of information to the monitoring system by alteration of activity in the prefrontal and cingulate cortices so that 'self-labelling' is improved. Alternatively, it could represent a suppression of self-initiated acts so that poor 'self-labelling' is less important.

The theory that antipsychotic drugs act via blockade of dopamine receptors has led to 'dopamine hypotheses' of schizophrenia whereby schizophrenia is suggested to be due to an overactivity of dopamine neuronal systems. It is possible to envisage schemes whereby disordered dopamine control of prefrontal or cingulate cortex function gives rise to defective septo-hippocampal monitoring. Nevertheless, as outlined earlier in this chapter, there is at present little firm neurochemical evidence for overactive dopamine systems that cannot also be ascribed to an effect of antipsychotic medication.

Recommended reading

Abou-Saleh, M. T. (ed.) (1990). Brain imaging in psychiatry. *British Journal of Psychiatry*, **157** (suppl. 9), 5–101.

American Psychiatric Association (1987). *Diagnostic and statistical manual of mental disorders*, DSM III-R. Washington DC.

Andreasen, N. C. (1988). Brain imaging: application in psychiatry. *Science*, **239**, 1381–8.

Claridge, G. (1985). *Origins of mental illness*. Blackwell, Oxford.

Crow, T. J. (ed.) (1987). Recurrent and chronic psychoses. *British Medical Bulletin*, **43**, 479–773.

Gelder, M., Gath, D., and Mayou, R. (1989). *Oxford textbook of psychiatry* (2nd edn). Oxford University Press.

Gerlach, J. and Casey, D. E. (1988). Tardive dyskinesia. *Acta Psychiatrica Scandinavica*, **77**, 369–78.

Gottesman, I. I. (1991). *Schizophrenia genesis. The origins of madness*. Freeman, New York.

Kerwin, R. W. (1989). How do the neuropathological features of schizophrenia relate to preexisting neurotransmitter and aetiological hypotheses? *Psychological Medicine*, **19**, 563–7.

Leff, J. (1992). Over the edge: stress and schizophrenia. *New Scientist*, **133**, 30–3.

McGuffin, P., Farmer, A., and Gottesman, I. I. (1987). Is there really a split in schizophrenia? The genetic evidence. *British Journal of Psychiatry*. **150**, 581–92.

Reynolds, G. P. (1989). Beyond the dopamine hypothesis. The neurochemical pathology of schizophrenia. *British Journal of Psychiatry*, **155**, 305–16.

Roberts, G. W. (1990). Schizophrenia: the cell biology of a functional psychosis. *Trends in Neurosciences*, **13**, 207–11.

Roberts, G. W. (1991). Schizophrenia: a neuropathological perspective. *British Journal of Psychiatry*, **158**, 8–17.

Special Report: Schizophrenia (1987). *Schizophrenia Bulletin*, **13**, 1–171.

Waddington, J. L. (1987). Tardive dyskinesia in schizophrenia and other disorders: associations with ageing, cognitive dysfunction and structural brain pathology in relation to neuroleptic exposure. *Human Psychopharmacology*, **2**, 11–22.

Wing, J. K. (1978). *Schizophrenia: towards a new synthesis*. Academic Press, London.

14 Affective disorders (depression and mania)

In sooth I know not why I am so sad:
It wearies me; you say it wearies you:
But how I caught it, found it, or came by it,
What stuff 'tis made of, whereof it is born,
I am to learn;
And such a want-wit sadness makes of me,
That I have much ado to know myself.

Shakespeare, *The Merchant of Venice*

The feeling of depression (Fig. 14.1) is a common experience for many people at one or more times in their lives and frequently reflects a normal human reaction to events around us. For some people, however, depression can be so severe as to disrupt their lives, leading to severe behavioural changes and sometimes suicide. Others may experience episodes of mania in addition to depression. Certain notable individuals have suffered from depression, for example Winston Churchill suffered bouts of melancholy which he referred to as his 'black dog' (Moran 1966).

In this chapter I shall consider the group of disorders termed depression, depressive illness, or affective disorders, the latter term referring to disorders of the affect or mood. In considering these disorders we are looking at a spectrum of illness from fairly minor neuroses to severe psychoses.

Clinical description

Affective disorders present in a variety of forms with different symptoms. I shall describe first some of the typical features shown by a patient with a depressive disorder of moderate severity and then the differences seen in patients with severe depressive disorder, mild depressive disorder, and mania. These symptom groupings are not meant to imply any major categorization but this will be considered below.

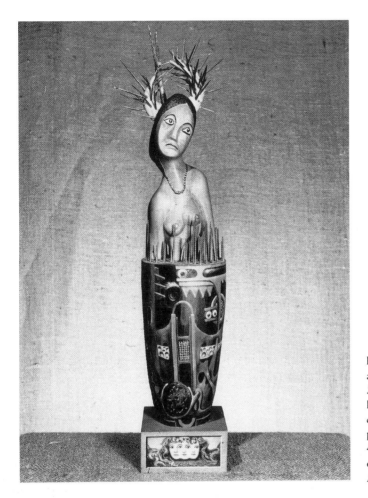

Figure 14.1 Depression in art. Robert Klippel: *Madame Sosostris 1947–48* (a Pre-Raphaelite satire). Wood carved by Robert Klippel, oil paintings by James Gleeson, 49.5 × 10 × 1.0. Art Gallery of New South Wales, Australia.

Moderate depressive disorder

Typical symptoms shown by a moderately depressed patient are:

1. *Depressed mood.* The mood of the patient is one of misery and does not improve under circumstances that would normally be expected to improve mood. The patient will frequently show little interest or enjoyment for activities that are normally enjoyable and may sometimes express fears of a total loss of feeling. The patient may also show reduced energy and a characteristic mournful appearance with 'depressed' facial expression and posture.
2. *Pessimistic thoughts.* The patient experiences pessimistic thoughts about the present, future, and past which include feelings of worthlessness, failure, and lack of self-confidence. The patient may feel a sense of hopelessness which can lead to suicide.

3. *Changes in motor activity.* The patient may exhibit psychomotor retardation with a reduction of body movements, and slowing of speech and thought. Alternatively some patients exhibit agitation with restlessness and an inability to relax.
4. *Anxiety.* Patients may experience the psychological manifestations of anxiety together with the autonomic (somatic) signs (see Chapter 15).
5. *Physiological 'somatic' symptoms.* Patients commonly complain of sleep disturbance, loss of appetite and consequent loss of weight, constipation, loss of libido, tiredness, and muscular pain.

Severe depressive disorders

In severe depressive disorders the symptoms described above occur but with greater intensity. In addition certain symptoms more typical of a psychosis can be seen and the patient loses contact with reality. Thus a patient may suffer from delusions based around his pessimism towards the past, present, and future. Pessimistic thoughts extend to delusional ideas (e.g. the belief that the future is entirely hopeless, the belief that the patient has cancer, or the belief that the world will end tomorrow). There can also be disturbances of perception which may extend to hallucinations. These are typically auditory and may involve voices discussing the pessimistic ideas outlined above. These auditory hallucinations are usually of a critical and derogatory nature and are 'affectively based' (i.e. consistent with the depressed mood).

Mild depressive disorders

Frequently a patient with a mild depressive disorder presents with the symptoms outlined earlier for the moderate disorder but the symptoms are experienced with reduced intensity. There are often, however, a group of other symptoms that are found more frequently in the mild cases which might globally be referred to as neurotic, e.g. anxiety, obsessional symptoms, or phobias. Some workers believe that this type of disorder is distinct and have termed it neurotic depression. In their mildest form these disorders merge with the minor emotional disorders described under anxiety in Chapter 15.

Mania

Some patients show episodes of manic symptoms as well as depressive episodes. The manic and depressive episodes can occur in any temporal sequence but usually the manic episodes are less frequent. The symptoms exhibited are to some extent the opposite of the depressive symptoms so that patients will be overactive with rapid speech and thoughts, exhibit expansive optimistic ideas, need reduced sleep, show increased appetite and sexual desires. Patients may also show delusions or experience hallucinations.

Therefore in the severe depressive disorders and in patients who experience mania there is overlap with some typical symptoms of schizophrenia. This point will be discussed again later in the chapter.

Course of the affective illnesses

The course of the illnesses is very variable. Patients can return entirely to normal functioning after severe depressive episodes but in some cases recurrent major episodes may be experienced and there may be residual symptoms between the episodes. Some patients may experience a mild but chronic depressive disorder. Where mania is experienced, depressive and usually less frequent manic episodes are interdispersed. Clear-cut episodes of mania or depression are seldom single and relapses are the rule. Patients still die of metabolic complications of starvation and the refusal to drink.

Classification of affective disorders

There has been much effort expended in attempts to classify affective disorders into different groups. This has some importance as, if different forms of affective disorder existed, these could have different aetiologies and then different treatments could be required. I shall consider some of these attempts at sub-classification.

Primary and *secondary* depressions have been noted where the latter are secondary to another illness such as schizophrenia or glandular fever. This classification has descriptive value but the symptoms, the course of the illness, and the treatments do not seem to differ. *Neurotic* and *psychotic* depressions have been proposed based on certain symptoms exhibited by the patients (mild and severe depressive disorders respectively as outlined above). There is no agreement as to whether these do represent different disorders, different points on a continuum of symptoms, or a single disorder with certain discrete features. This classification has become intertwined with another based on an assumed aetiology which divides depressive disorders into *reactive* and *endogenous* groups. The former is said to occur in response to a clear external cause and is said to have symptoms characteristic of the mild depressive disorder outlined above. The latter, according to this classification, cannot be assigned to an external precipitating factor and shows symptoms of moderate severity. Although the reactive-endogenous classification has been very popular it is perhaps an over-simplification as no disorder of this kind is truly reactive or endogenous and recent studies have shown that whereas adverse life events do frequently precede depressive episodes, these life events precede endogenous depression as much as other kinds (Bebbington *et al.* 1988). Nevertheless, certain clinical studies still do divide patients on the basis of symptom patterns that are assumed to be characteristic: 'endogenous symptoms' being loss of appetite, weight loss, constipation, reduced libido, amenorrhoea, and early morning waking: 'reactive symptoms' being anxiety, irritability, and phobias. I shall make reference to this later.

One classification that has proven very useful is the *unipolar/bipolar* distinction. Whereas the former patients only show episodes of depressive symptoms, the latter patients have periods of depression interspersed with periods of mania. Support for such a distinction comes from family studies where relatives of bipolar patients who develop depressive illness are more likely to develop a bipolar illness whereas for unipolar patients their depressed relatives are more likely to develop a unipolar illness. I shall return to this when I consider the genetics of depressive illness.

In summary, classification of affective disorders has proven difficult and contentious. The unipolar/bipolar distinction seems to be widely accepted and is included in current classifications such as the DSM III-R of the American Psychiatric Association (1987). This distinguishes bipolar disorders from depressive disorders (no manic symptoms). Within the latter category are major depression (single episode or recurrent, mild or severe, with or without psychotic symptoms) and dysthymia (depressive neurosis). Dysthymia is a chronic but mild depressive disorder. This modern classification of affective disorders omits many of the older attempts at categorization. Nevertheless some current literature continues to use terms such as endogenous depression as opposed to neurotic depression. In the classification of DSM III-R these would probably qualify as major depression and dysthymia respectively and such a categorization is supported by recent work which concludes that these are separate disorders (Andrews *et al.* 1990*a*; Duggan *et al.* 1990).

Tyrer (1985) has argued that there is a group of patients who suffer from a general neurotic syndrome. These patients have variable symptoms; sometimes they will be primarily anxious whereas at other times they will show a neurotic depression and they may also exhibit some phobias. The symptoms may depend on the patient's circumstances. There is some support for this proposal from controlled studies (Andrews *et al.* 1990*b*).

Epidemiology of affective disorders

The lifetime risk for major depression (unipolar) is about 6 per cent whereas for bipolar disorder it is about 1 per cent. When less severe depressive illnesses are included, the lifetime risk rises to about 10 per cent (Regier *et al.* 1988; Weissman *et al.* 1988). The mean age of onset for bipolar disorder is earlier than for unipolar disorder and tends towards adolescence or early adult life, although some depressive episodes can occur later in life. The incidence of unipolar disorders is greater (about double) for females than for males, whereas the incidence of bipolar disorders does not show a sex bias. There is a tendency, similar to that reported for schizophrenia (Chapter 13), for patients with bipolar severe depressive illness to be born in the winter months.

The incidence of clinically significant but minor depressive episodes in the community may be rather higher than these figures given above imply. One study, albeit in an un-representative inner city area, reported lifetime rates of depressive episodes of 46 per cent for men and 72 per cent for women (Bebbington *et al.* 1989). Some of these episodes were probably untreated and many were treated only by a general practitioner; but the study serves to indicate the general occurrence of depressive symptoms in the popula-tion.

There is good evidence for genetic influences on the incidence of severe affective dis-orders. For example, the first degree relatives of patients with bipolar severe depressive illness have a 19 percent risk of also suffering from an affective disorder whereas for first degree relatives of patients with unipolar severe depressive illness the risk is 10 per cent. These figures should be compared with the risks in the general population cited earlier. As this familial clustering could simply reflect shared environmental factors, studies have been performed on the incidence of affective disorders in twin pairs. These studies have shown concordance rates of 50–70 per cent for monozygotic twin pairs where one twin has a severe affective disorder, whereas for dizygotic twin pairs the concordance rate is 13–20 per cent. These data represent amalgamated cases of severe bipolar and unipolar disorders but studies of the separate disorders show a greater genetic loading for the bipolar disorder. In addition, there is a tendency for affected twins to have the same disorder, i.e. either unipolar or bipolar, but there are also examples of crossover. The importance of genetic influences is further supported by limited studies of the occurrence of severe affective disorder in twins reared apart and in adoptive parents and children. Although these results highlight the importance of genetic factors, the concordance rates show that environmental factors are also of great importance.

In fact, examination of the occurrence of the less severe forms of depressive illness shows that genetic factors are much less important for these kinds of affective disorders and crude estimates of the genetic and environmental loadings have been made based on twin studies (Table 14.1) dividing environmental factors into those shared between individuals, for example family influences, and those not shared.

Overall therefore the incidence of affective disorder seems to show a continuum of liability with a liability threshold for occurrence with both genes and environment contributing. The number of genes involved is unknown, neither is it known whether dif-ferent genes are involved in different groups of patients.

The strong implication of inherited factors in the predisposition to certain kinds of affective disorder has prompted work on the linkage of the disorders to DNA markers using the techniques of restriction fragment length polymorphism (RFLP) analysis (outlined in Chapter 11). Bipolar disorder should be a good candidate for such studies owing to its relatively greater genetic loading and there was much excitement when

RFLP analysis picked up a linkage between bipolar disorder and a marker on chromosome 11 in the Amish community in the USA (Egeland *et al.* 1987). This has, however, not been replicated in other communities and the original workers have now retracted their finding (Kelso *et al.* 1989; Owen and Mullan 1990). Some studies have reported linkage to markers on the X chromosome (Baron *et al.* 1987) but if there is a linkage with markers on the X chromosome then this is only likely to hold for a minority of cases (McGuffin and Katz 1989). The situation is thus very unclear and the considerable problems with such analyses (Merikangas *et al.* 1989) require caution in the interpretation of future reports.

Table 14.1 Factors influencing the occurrence of affective disorders

	Genetic factors	Common environment	Non-shared environment
Bipolar depressive illness	0.86	0.07	0.07
Major affective disorder (unipolar)	0.52	0.30	0.18
Neurotic depression	0.08	0.54	0.38

The figures are taken from McGuffin and Katz (1989) and represent crude estimates, expressed as fractions of the total liability, of the contributions of different factors to the liability to depressive illness. The data are derived from twin studies and common environment refers to environmental factors shared with a patient's relatives.

We may obtain some indication of the kinds of environmental factors that might be important by examining predisposing, precipitating, or vulnerability factors. With respect to predisposing factors there has been much discussion about the effects of childhood experience, for example maternal deprivation, and parental relationships. Although these influences must play a part in shaping the personality, there is no consistent evidence that they predispose specifically for depression in later life. It seems likely, however, that certain personality traits will render individuals more vulnerable to stress and subsequent depression; personality disturbances have been shown to be present in patients suffering from depressive illnesses (Andrews *et al.* 1990*a*, *b*; Duggan *et al.* 1990).

With regard to precipitating factors, the occurrence of significant adverse life events, for example bereavement or separation, have been discussed as precipitating factors for depression. There is some evidence to support this but other mental illnesses can also result. Nevertheless there does seem to be some linkage and this poses the question as to why certain individuals are more vulnerable to these life events. This may be related to the personality as hinted above or circumstances as outlined below. There is no consensus as to whether affective disorders showing typical 'neurotic/reactive' symptoms are associated more with preceding life events than are those with typical 'endogenous' symptoms. Recent studies have shown that adverse life events precede either kind of depressive illness equally frequently (Bebbington *et al.* 1989).

Studies of vulnerability factors have given some clues to the susceptibility of certain individuals to experience depression. Some of these factors which have been identified are: the lack of a confiding relationship, looking after young children, not working outside the home, and loss of mother by death or separation before the age of 11. These are factors which may render individuals more susceptible to the effects of life events but in themselves do not precipitate depression. It is then suggested that some of these factors or long periods of adverse circumstance may render depression more likely in response to an adverse life event.

Finally in this discussion we must not forget the tendency for the season of birth to be towards the winter months for patients who have bipolar disorder. As in the case of schizophrenia this could indicate the importance of some environmental factor such as a viral infection.

To summarize, the evidence suggests a mixture of genetic and environmental influences conspiring to produce affective disorders with different components of each being important for the different affective disorders.

Neuropathological observations

Affective disorders have not attracted the intense research effort that has been applied to schizophrenia (Chapter 13) aimed at finding gross or more specific changes in the brains of patients suffering such disorders. Nevertheless, there are some data, which will be reviewed below, that point to such changes. First, it is worth asking whether we could expect to see clear changes in the brains of patients with affective disorders. For some patients their affective illness is episodic with complete remission between episodes. In that case major lesions would not be expected, but alterations in brain chemistry might be anticipated during an episode. For a chronic and particularly a psychotic affective disorder, we might expect to be able to locate a discrete brain alteration. The more recent findings in schizophrenia give us confidence on this point. Also, as for schizophrenia, the issue of diagnosis and patient categorization is important. Consistent correlations between brain state and disease may not be seen unless patient selection is very carefully made.

Neuropathological studies on post-mortem brain tissue from patients who were depressed in life are scarce (Jeste *et al.* 1988) but a recent study showed some changes in the cerebral cortex of elderly depressed patients (Bowen *et al.* 1989). The findings were interpreted in terms of losses of cerebral cortical cells in certain parts of the frontal and temporal lobes although effects of the treatments the patients received could not be ruled out. The use of computerized axial tomography (CAT) scanning has shown some brain alterations which are very similar to those reported in schizophrenia. Ventricular enlargement is seen in 10–30 per cent of patients with affective disorder relative to controls. This is seen in unipolar and bipolar disorders and although the differences are sometimes greater in the more psychotic patients, this is not a consistent finding. The possibility cannot be eliminated that the changes are due to the drug treatments patients have received but a more satisfying account which concurs with the current feelings about similar alterations in schizophrenia would be that ventricular enlargment is a rather gross indication of more specific changes in the brain. The similarity with the neuropathological changes seen in schizophrenia is strengthened from recent magnetic resonance imaging observations showing reduced temporal lobe size in patients with bipolar affective disorder (Altshuler *et al.* 1991). Whether the changes are developmental in origin, as may be the case for schizophrenia, is not clear.

Studies of potential brain dysfunction in depression using regional cerebral glucose metabolism have provided suggestive evidence for reduced left frontal lobe function (Jeste *et al.* 1988; Baxter *et al.* 1989). Studies of regional cerebral blood flow have provided preliminary indications of left anterior and right posterior cerebral cortex changes in some unipolar depressed patients. Other evidence for the involvement of different sides of the brain in depression comes from patients with brain damage where left frontal–temporal and right parietal–occipital lesions can lead to depression.

Also, disorders of the right side of the brain have been implicated in psychological studies on depressed patients and corroborative evidence comes from patients with temporal lobe epilepsy. When affective psychoses occur in patients with temporal lobe epilepsy the epileptic focus tends to be on the right side of the brain.

This information does not provide a very consistent picture but there is some suggestion of frontal lobe dysfunction and many of the observations, but not all, bear a resemblance to those seen for patients with schizophrenia.

Neurochemical observations

An area of intensive activity in the study of affective disorders has been the measurement of neurotransmitters, their metabolites, their receptors, and their synthetic enzymes in body fluids and post-mortem brain tissue. The work has been based on the hypothesis that affective disorders might reflect a fairly circumscribed change in brain chemistry.

It has been very popular to make measurements on blood plasma and urine from depressed patients in order to get an index of brain changes in neurotransmitter metabolism from peripheral measurements. The levels of neurotransmitters and metabolites in urine and blood are generally a poor reflection of these activities in brain so the data obtained are of little value. Of more value may be studies on cerebrospinal fluid and, in the case of the monoamine neurotransmitters, attempts have been made to enhance the sensitivity of these measurements by blocking the exit from the central nervous system to the bloodstream of certain monoamine metabolites with the drug probenecid. Even so, the degree to which cerebrospinal fluid neurochemicals reflect their levels in brain is not clear and this may account for some of the inconsistency in the data obtained.

Much of the work in this area has concentrated on the monoamines, dopamine, noradrenaline, 5-hydroxytryptamine, and their metabolites for reasons which will become clearer below when theories of depression are considered. Although there are some conflicting reports, a reduction in the dopamine metabolite, homovanillic acid, has been reported in cerebrospinal fluid of depressed patients. For noradrenaline no consistent changes in metabolite levels are seen, but for 5-hydroxytryptamine some depressed patients do show a reduced level of the metabolite 5-hydroxyindoleacetic acid (5-HIAA) in cerebrospinal fluid. The tendency for 5-HIAA levels to be low is maintained in depressed patients even after recovery, suggesting that it is not a clear marker of the depressed state. A more consistent reduction in 5-HIAA is seen in patients who have attempted to commit suicide. The basis for these investigations is that many of these patients will have been depressed prior to their attempt but this is not always so. The reduction in 5-HIAA levels may therefore be more of a marker for the suicidal tendency than for depression itself.

Post-mortem brain studies ought theoretically to provide a better measure of the changes in the brains of depressed patients although there are significant problems working with post-mortem human brain material (Chapter 9). Studies have frequently concentrated, for the reasons outlined above, on patients who have committed suicide, but not all these patients will have been depressed prior to their suicide. No consistant changes in dopamine, noradrenaline, or their metabolites are seen and although earlier studies suggested a reduction in 5-hydroxytryptamine function, this has also not been replicated. Measurements of receptors have also provided inconsistent data but an increased number of β-adrenergic receptors and 5-HT$_1$ and 5-HT$_2$ 5-hydroxytryptamine receptors has been reported in several studies (Arora and Meltzer 1989) and in some cases the changes are regionalized to the prefrontal cortex (Arango *et al.* 1990). Other work also shows similar changes in 5-hydroxytryptamine receptors in non-suicidal, severely depressed patients (McKeith *et al.* 1987). Drug effects have not been taken into account and some patients would have been taking antidepressant drugs. These drugs would, however, have tended to reduce receptor number (see below). On balance, therefore, there is some evidence for change in 5-hydroxytryptamine systems in depression.

Studies on changes in cholinergic and peptidergic systems in depressive illness are as yet too limited to draw any firm conclusions. In mania there have been a number of studies performed measuring monoamines and their metabolites but no consistent neurochemical alterations were recorded.

Endocrine parameters as indices of central neurochemical changes

A considerable body of work has been performed measuring endocrine parameters in depressed patients on the basis that these may reflect primary disturbances in depression or may provide an accessible measure of central receptor function (Checkley 1980). The most popular of these tests is the so called 'dexamethasone suppression test' (Glassman 1987). This is seen as a failure to show the normal suppression of cortisol output in response to administration of dexamethasone, a synthetic corticosteroid. 30–70 per cent of patients with major affective disorder fail to show this suppression but there is a greater frequency in the more psychotically depressed patients. The suppression, however, is not a specific marker for depression and is also seen in patients with mania and dementia. The dexamethasone suppression test does not therefore shed light on the primary changes in depressive illness. A hypothesis based on dysfunction in the hypothalamus has been proposed to explain some of the changes seen (Charlton and Ferrier 1989).

The other main area of application of these neuroendrocrine tests has involved agents that will specifically stimulate particular neurotransmitter receptors. These are administered to patients and subsequent changes in hormone levels are determined. The hope in using these tests is that the response to the applied drug will reflect central receptor activation or at least uncover a defect in receptors in depression. A large number of different tests have been applied (Checkley 1980) but I shall consider only two. Administration of the α_2-adrenergic receptor agonist clonidine leads to an increase in growth hormone release and this response has been reported to be impaired in some depressed patients (Mitchell *et al.* 1988). The blunted clonidine response is, however, not specific for depression and the response does not normalize when the patient recovers. Whether this implies that the blunted clonidine response is a marker for some aspects of depression or vulnerability is not clear. The site of action of clonidine seems to be on post synaptic α_2-adrenergic receptors in the hypothalamus and the extent to which changes in hypothalamic receptor sensitivity can be generalized to the rest of the brain is also unclear. Later in this chapter the importance of presynaptic α_2-adrenergic autoreceptors in the treatment of depression will be considered.

Administration of L-tryptophan, the precursor of 5-hydroxytryptamine, to normal and depressed patients elicits an increase in prolactin levels. It is thought that this reflects changes in the activity of 5-hydroxytryptamine neurones projecting from the raphe to the hypothalamus (Cowen 1980) and so changes in the L-tryptophan response may reflect changes in central 5-hydroxytryptamine neurones. Indeed the L-tryptophan response is reported to be blunted in depressed patients (Charney *et al.* 1984*b*) and administration of antidepressants enhances the reduced response (Heninger *et al.* 1984). Although this provides a convenient means of assessing central 5-hydroxytryptamine activity, and although the changes seem consistent with theories of depression outlined later, how far it is possible to extrapolate to all central 5-hydroxytryptamine neurones and how specific the test is for depression are both unclear.

Treatments for affective disorders

It should be clear by now that the model I am assuming for occurrence of affective disorders is a multifactorial one with genetic and environmental influences contributing in different proportions to the different forms of disorder. Treatment may be achieved by physical intervention (drugs and electroconvulsive therapy), psychological treatments, or a mixture of these as will be described below.

In Chapter 9 I tried to show how psychological ('mind type') and neurochemical descriptions of brain function were descriptions of the same entity but at different levels of function. If this argument is valid then it supports the idea that both psychological and physical treatments ought to be applicable to the treatment of a disorder like depressive illness. The two forms of treatment are then likely to be effecting changes in the same or closely related brain systems. Therefore both psychological and physical treatments should be considered in the treatment of depressive illness.

It is also important to bear in mind that for some patients a spontaneous remission will occur in time and the various treatments may aid or hasten recovery but do not provide a cure in themselves. Also there are significant effects on the patients' condition from simply providing care such as hospitalization. We might call this a placebo effect but it encompasses all the social and psychological influences involved in the act of caring. On top of this the different treatments have their effect although this is sometimes quite small.

Let us now consider the different treatments and finally attempt a comparison.

Psychological treatments

As mentioned earlier, the effects of treatment itself which may include psychiatric support or temporary hospitalization are significant and can account for a large part of the apparent placebo effect. More specific psychological interventions can be of additional support.

Psychotherapy in various forms (psychodynamic (addressing the underlying conflicts that create poor self-esteem and depressive vulnerability), or interpersonal (exploring personal relationships)) has been used extensively for the treatment of affective disorders and there has been much discussion of the value of the approach and the results. Generally it seems that the psychotherapies are as effective as drug therapy in treating much depressive illness except when it is very severe. Psychotherapy may also be effective if combined with antidepressant drugs.

Cognitive behaviour therapy has also been applied to the treatment of affective disorders with the aim of altering the way patients think about their problems. The rationale here is that depression is seen to be a cognitive problem with secondary affective changes. The patient has negative thought patterns and therapy consists of challenging these. This treatment also seems of more use in the milder depressive illnesses where it achieves improvement of the depressive symptoms and it is of less use in the more severe illnesses although it is effective in both cases (Thase *et al.* 1991).

In comparisons with drug treatments psychotherapy was found to be as good as the drug in some studies with a beneficial synergy in some cases if both are used. Cognitive therapy also achieves results similar to drug treatments in some trials. A recent major trial comparing drugs, psychotherapy, and cognitive therapy (Elkin *et al.* 1989) in mild to moderate depression showed that the three treatments were equally effective for mild depressive illness but no better than 'placebo'. Both drugs and psychological treatment were better, however, for more severely depressed patients. It should be noted, however, that in this trial the 'placebo' treatment included clinical management comprising considerable contact with a psychiatrist. This may explain the apparent equal efficacy of 'placebo', drugs, and psychological treatments for the mildly depressed patients and echoes the points made earlier.

A drawback with the psychological approaches is the time taken to administer treatment which makes these treatments less cost effective than drugs but it seems that cognitive behaviour therapy is associated with a reduced risk of relapse compared with use of antidepressant drugs.

Drug treatments

Monoamine oxidase inhibitors

In Chapter 5 the importance of the enzyme monoamine oxidase and its two forms A and B in the metabolism of the monoamines, noradrenaline, dopamine, and 5-hydroxy-tryptamine was described. Inhibitors of this enzyme are effective antidepressant drugs as well as having anxiolytic effects (Chapter 15). The monoamine oxidase inhibitors tend to be more effective for milder, more neurotic kinds of depression and appear to be of limited value in severe depressive illness.

Monoamine oxidase inhibitors became unpopular because of some reports of their toxicity, because certain controlled trials showed limited efficacy, and because of side effects. The principal side effect is termed the 'cheese reaction'. This is the hypertensive crisis in patients who have ingested certain foods while taking the drugs. The common factor among the foods (for example cheese, wine, and yeast extract) is a high concentration of tyramine. The tyramine is no longer metabolized (in the gut and liver) by the inhibited monoamine oxidase and displaces noradrenaline from peripheral vascular adrenergic nerve endings, precipitating the hypertensive crisis. The recognition that monoamine oxidase inhibitors may be useful for specific indications, e.g. atypical depression and anxiety, and the advent of newer drugs, some of which have a lower propensity for the 'cheese reaction' (see below), has led to a renewed interest in these compounds (Nutt and Glue 1989*b*).

The earlier monoamine oxidase inhibitors, e.g. phenelzine, iproniazid, and tranylcypromine, are equally potent at inhibiting both forms of monoamine oxidase (A and B, Chapter 5). It seems, however, that inhibition of the A form is important for antidepressant action (Sandler 1981). Another feature of these earlier drugs is their irreversible inhibition of the monoamine oxidase enzyme. Their inhibition is prolonged and only relieved with synthesis of new enzyme. Newer drugs have now been developed which are reversible inhibitors of monoamine oxidase A, e.g. brofaromine, and moclobemide. Clinical trials suggest that these have antidepressant effects.

It seems an obvious conclusion to draw that these drugs exert their antidepressant actions by inhibiting monoamine oxidase and increasing nerve terminal or synaptic concentrations of monoamines, but this hypothesis needs to be questioned on several levels. Which monoamine is more important? This is far from clear and there are no clues from the actions of the drugs as neither monoamine oxidase A or B is fully selective for particular monoamines and neither form of the enzyme is found only in a single population of monoamine neurones (Chapter 5). It is known that monoamine oxidase must be at least 80 per cent inhibited in order to achieve an antidepressant effect but do monoamine levels at the synapse actually increase? Monoamine oxidase is an intracellular enzyme so that effects on monoamine levels will initially be intracellular. Also, the high degree of regulation of noradrenergic and dopaminergic nerve terminal neurotransmitter synthesis and release via autoreceptors render it unlikely that there will be large increases in neurotransmitter concentration in the synapse. Decreased nerve terminal metabolism of the two monoamines owing to inhibition of monoamine oxidase will, however, lead to decreased monoamine synthesis so that monoamine turnover will be reduced. Similar remarks should apply to 5-hydroxytryptamine. In addition to these considerations there is a discrepancy between the acute inhibition of monoamine oxidase, which occurs in a few days, and the appearance of the antidepressant effect, which takes up to three weeks to appear. The drugs have reached their equilibrium plasma levels well before this time and the simplest explanation of this discrepancy is that the acute inhibition of monoamine oxidase leads to a subsequent longer term change. The situation is reminiscent of the effects of antipsychotic drugs (Chapter 13) and explanations of this will be considered below when certain other antidepressant drugs are considered.

Tricyclic antidepressant drugs

This is a large group of compounds so called because of their common three ring structure. Table 14.2 gives some examples of typical drugs. They are the most popular antidepressant drugs on the market and are useful for treating a wide range of depressive

Table 14.2 Structures of some antidepressant drugs and their relative abilities to inhibit noradrenaline, 5-hydroxytryptamine, and dopamine reuptake

Drug	IC_{50} (μM) for inhibition of uptake of		
	Noradrenaline	5-Hydroxytryptamine	Dopamine
Tricyclic drugs			
Desipramine	0.0015	2.0	8.7
Imipramine	0.02	0.24	12.5
Clomipramine	0.044	0.015	3.8
Second generation drugs			
Maprotiline	0.02	12.0	8.6
Fluoxetine	10.0	0.055	—
Iprindole	2.6	10.0	7.9
Mianserin	0.084	11.0	19.0

The data are the concentrations of drug required to produce 50% inhibition of amine reuptake into rat brain synaptosomes (IC_{50}) and are from Randrup and Braestrup (1977) and Green and Costain (1981). Low IC_{50} values indicate potent inhibition.

states as well as for preventing relapse. The antidepressant effect takes several weeks to reach a maximum and there is no evidence for any differences between the drugs in their onset of action. The principal side effects of the drugs are anticholinergic (blurred vision and dry mouth), anti-adrenergic (α_1) (postural hypotension) and antihistamine (H_1) (sedation and drowsiness) owing to their varying potencies as antagonists at these receptors. These receptor antagonist properties are unlikely to be responsible for the antidepressant effects as specific antagonists of these receptors are not antidepressants. The property of the tricyclic drugs that is usually cited as the basis of the antidepressant effect is their ability to inhibit potently the reuptake of monoamines in to the nerve terminal (Chapter 5). It is frequently then assumed that this inhibition of reuptake leads to an increased synaptic level of the monoamine. This is likely to be an over-simplification and so it will be considered in more detail.

The different tricyclic drugs have different abilities to inhibit reuptake of dopamine, noradrenaline, and 5-hydroxytryptamine and some selectivity data are given in Table 14.2. These data tend to place the emphasis more on noradrenaline and 5-hydroxytryptamine for which reuptake is more strongly inhibited and different drugs show a preference for inhibition of reuptake of one or other of these monoamines. As was the case for the inhibition of monoamine oxidase, the strict control of neurotransmitter release and synthesis for the monoamines brings into play compensatory mechanisms when normal nerve terminal activity is disturbed in this way. Indeed, acutely the tricyclic antidepressants decrease monoamine synthesis and turnover, presumably reflecting the normal nerve terminal regulatory mechanisms as well as effects on presynaptic auto-receptors of the increased synaptic levels of monoamine. In line with this, noradrenergic neurones and in some studies 5-hydroxytryptamine neurones show a decreased firing rate in the presence of an acute dose of tricyclic antidepressant; this again may reflect autoreceptor stimulation. There may therefore be some increase but not a large increase in the synaptic concentrations of the monoamines when tricyclic antidepressants are administered acutely.

As with the monoamine oxidase inhibitors there is a delay of 2–6 weeks before clinical antidepressant effects are seen, whereas the acute biochemical changes occur quite quickly. This suggests that there is an adaptive change occurring subsequent to the acute biochemical effect. This will be considered in more detail below.

Second generation antidepressant drugs

The monoamine oxidase inhibitors and tricyclic antidepressant drugs were compounds not specifically designed as antidepressants but found to have such an activity. A new 'second generation' of antidepressant drugs (Table 14.2) has appeared where at least some of the drugs have been designed to model aspects of the presumed therapeutic actions of previous antidepressant drugs. Also some drugs have been introduced with completely different structures and pharmacological effects.

Based on the well recognized abilities of the tricyclic antidepressant drugs to inhibit noradrenaline and 5-hydroxytryptamine reuptake, albeit not very selectively, a group of compounds has been introduced that are quite selective inhibitors of the reuptake of either noradrenaline (e.g. maprotiline) or 5-hydroxytryptamine (e.g. fluoxetine). Their selectivity is shown in Table 14.2. These drugs are effective antidepressants with a slow onset of action and in some cases are as good clinically as the tricyclic drugs without some of the side effects, as the tendency to antagonize adrenergic, histamine, and muscarinic cholinergic receptors is less. Maprotiline is structurally quite similar to the tricyclic drugs except that an additional bridge has been added to the molecule. It is likely to produce synaptic changes similar to those produced by the tricyclic drugs except that the effects will be largely confined to noradrenaline metabolism. Fluoxetine has been shown to increase extraneuronal levels of 5-hydroxytryptamine and turnover of 5-hydroxytryptamine is also reduced as predicted above for the tricyclic drugs (Freeman 1988).

It is of some interest that these more selective inhibitors of monoamine uptake are effective antidepressants and in this light is is surprising that cocaine, which is a good inhibitor of noradrenaline uptake, is not an effective antidepressant. This may suggest that there are added complexities to the ability of a substance to be an antidepressant and I shall consider this again later.

A number of other compounds with differing pharmacological properties have also been introduced as antidepressants and I shall consider in detail only two of these, iprindole and mianserin. Iprindole is atypical in that it does not inhibit monoamine oxidase and has little effect on the uptake of any of the monoamines. Mianserin does inhibit noradrenaline reuptake *in vitro* selectively, but the effect is rather weak and this is not seen *in vivo*; in addition is is a very potent 5-hydroxytryptamine ($5HT_{1C}$ and $5HT_2$) receptor antagonist, and a potent α_2-adrenergic and histamine H_1 receptor antagonist (Pinder 1985). It has a low propensity for anticholinergic side effects which may be an advantage, whereas it causes sedation via its antihistamine effects. It is thought that its effects on presynaptic α_2-adrenergic receptors may be important for its clinical effects with blockade of these presynaptic α_2-adrenergic receptors leading to increased noradrenaline release.

L-Tryptophan

There are a number of reports suggesting that the amino acid L-tryptophan has anti-depressant activity. The results of trials with this substance are variable but given that it is a natural body constituent it has practical safety advantages. It is assumed that L-tryptophan administration leads to increased brain 5-hydroxytryptamine levels but whether this in turn leads to increased 5-hydroxytryptamine function is unclear as intraneuronal metabolism might be expected to direct the extra 5-hydroxytryptamine away from synaptic release. The combination of L-tryptophan and a monoamine oxidase inhibitor has given clearer antidepressant results and it has been suggested that L-tryptophan potentiates the action of the monoamine oxidase inhibitors. It may be that the monoamine oxidase inhibitor prevents intraneuronal destruction of 5-hydroxytryptamine. The interpretation is, however, not simple as tryptamine levels will also rise and these may disturb catecholamine function.

Electroconvulsive therapy (ECT)

Although this is not a drug treatment, it is considered here as it is a physical intervention. ECT consists of passing an electric current through the brain of the patient in order to induce a convulsion. There has been much debate over the efficacy and ethics of this form of treatment but a series of trials have shown that it does have an antidepressant effect (Kendell 1981). The patients for whom ECT would be suitable are the more severely depressed 'endogenous' patients with psychotic symptoms such as depressive delusions (Paykel 1989). These patients frequently do not respond to tricyclic antidepressants and ECT has been shown to be superior to the drugs for severely depressed patients. ECT also seems to exert its therapeutic effect more quickly than do the drugs so is of use in the more rapid management of patients with suicidal tendencies. The effects of ECT do not last long and a significant relapse rate is seen. Also there is some evidence for memory loss after ECT. Nevertheless, ECT does have a place for the treatment of severely depressed patients.

The mechanism of action of ECT is not understood. Attempts have been made to probe this by giving similar electric shocks to normal animals. Postsynaptic effects of the monoamine neurotransmitters dopamine, noradrenaline, and 5-hydroxytryptamine were enhanced in behavioural tests. Whether this has any relevance to the clinical effects in humans is unclear. These kinds of experiments will be considered again below.

Lithium carbonate

This simple substance has been shown to be effective in the control of acute mania and also is of use in the prophylaxis of both bipolar and unipolar recurrent affective disorders (Schou 1989). It can therefore be viewed as a mood stabilizing agent and, in common with the other drugs discussed here, it has a slow onset of its clinical effects. It has a fairly low therapeutic index (i.e. the ratio of toxic to therapeutic levels is only 1.5–2).

There has been much discussion over the mechanism of action of lithium, perhaps reflecting our ignorance of its true effects. Whether it has different mechanisms of action for its anti-manic and anti-depressant effects is unclear but discussion has centred on alterations in neuronal systems dependent on 5-hydroxytryptamine and acetylcholine (see for example Wood and Goodwin 1987; Price *et al.* 1989, 1990). Some evidence has been provided for enhancing effects of lithium on 5-hydroxytryptamine neurone function which could be relevant to antidepressant effects, but the biochemical mechanisms involved are complex. Recently two promising biochemical sites of action of lithium have been identified which could be responsible for changes in synaptic function. One site of action of lithium is as an inhibitor of the enzymes of inositol phospholipid metabolism, notably inositol-1-phosphatase (Fig. 14.2) (Chapter 6; Drummond 1987). Inhibition of this enzyme will lead to an accumulation of inositol-1-phosphate. In peripheral tissues this is unlikely to be a major problem as there is ample inositol in the circulation to provide for new synthesis of inositol phospholipids, but in the brain inositol is only available by *de novo* synthesis from glucose via inositol-1-phosphate, dietary inositol not being able to cross the blood–brain barrier. Thus, in the brain, inhibi-

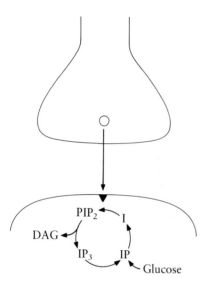

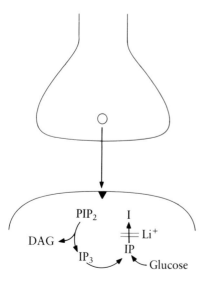

Figure 14.2 Effect of Li$^+$ on inositol phospholipid metabolism in neurones—one possible mechanism for the therapeutic action of Li$^+$ in bipolar affective disorders. In the upper diagram a receptor linked to phospholipase C is shown which, when activated by its neurotransmitter, leads to breakdown of phosphatidylinositol bisphosphate (PIP$_2$) to the two second messengers diacylglycerol (DAG) and inositol trisphosphate (IP$_3$) (Chapter 6). IP$_3$ can be metabolized to inositol monophosphate (IP) which itself is broken down to yield free inositol. Resynthesis of PIP$_2$ requires free inositol and in the brain this can only be supplied by recycling inositol within the neurone or by *de novo* synthesis from glucose via IP. In the lower diagram Li$^+$ is shown inhibiting the IP monophosphatase and blockade of this enzyme will, for active presynaptic neurones and hence postsynaptic receptors, lead to depletion of PIP$_2$ and loss of receptor signalling function as the pathways providing building blocks for resynthesis of PIP$_2$ are inhibited.

tion of inositol-1-phosphatase prevents synthesis of new inositol and the inositol within cells which are actively metabolizing inositol phospholipids will gradually be converted to inositol-1-phosphate. These will be neurones with receptors coupled to phospholipase C as their transduction mechanism (Chapter 6) and receiving active stimulation from their neurotransmitter which may be a reflection of the disturbed mood. The uncompetitive nature of the inhibition of the monophosphatase by lithium ensures that only at neurones with active receptors will lithium have a major effect (Berridge *et al.* 1989). In these neurones, phosphatidylinositol bisphosphate levels will drop and the receptors dependent on phospholipase C will become inactive. It is presumed that this prevents the actions of a neurotransmitter responsible for the mood swings. The hypothesis has the advantage that it explains why lithium would be selective for the brain, but it does not give any clues as to which neurotransmitters might be involved in mania or the mood stabilizing properties of lithium except that these would be linked to phospholipase C.

The other potential site of action of lithium is its ability to interfere with receptor–G-protein interaction in *in vitro* test systems (Avissar *et al.* 1988; Baraban *et al.* 1989). It is thought that this is via a site on the G-protein itself and this leads to reduced responses of neurotransmitter stimulation of adenylyl cyclase and phospholipase C. It is not easy to see how this hypothesis provides any selectivity of action either for the brain or for any particular neurotransmitter and it may provide a mechanism for the toxicity of lithium. At present, therefore, lithium is a rather poorly understood drug although there are emerging indications of its mechanism of action.

Comparison of treatments for depressive illness

There are a number of treatments available for patients with depressive symptoms. For the milder depressive illnesses, especially where neurotic symptoms are observed, monoamine oxidase inhibitors, tricyclic antidepressants (and their second generation counterparts), and psychological treatments, in different forms, can be useful. For the more severe cases, the tricyclic antidepressants (and second generation drugs) may be useful, although psychological treatments have some efficacy. For psychotic patients, however, ECT may be a final recourse. Antipsychotic drugs can be of use in the control of hallucinations and delusions. For bipolar patients lithium offers a successful treatment.

The effects of long term (chronic) antidepressant treatment on neurochemical parameters in animals

A unifying strand for most of the physical treatments considered above is the slow onset of the antidepressant effect which takes up to three weeks to reach a maximum. This contrasts with the known biochemical consequences of the treatments which are essentially immediate, so the clinical efficacy of the treatments cannot be equated with the biochemical effects described so far. This discrepancy does not seem to relate to pharmacokinetic effects as the drugs reach their equilibrium plasma levels within a few days as shown by effects on monoamine oxidase or monoamine reuptake in experimental animals (although see Speight (1987) for a contrasting view). Therefore some other slower change must be occurring upon chronic administration as a result of the acute biochemical effect. These considerations have stimulated much experimental work where animals are treated acutely or chronically with various antidepressant drugs and either neurochemical parameters in brain or functional tests are measured. The underlying purpose of much of the work is to find a unifying neurochemical hypothesis for the antidepressant effect which can then be extrapolated to an aetiological theory. This approach may be entirely unwarranted and may constrain theoretical and experimental work unnecessarily as will be discussed later. The field is very confusing and there is much disagreement, but I shall attempt to extract some generalizations.

Table 14.3 summarizes some of the main observed effects showing alterations in the levels of certain neurotransmitter receptors upon chronic treatment with antidepressants. Although there are clear trends in the kinds of change observed, it is difficult to be certain of the significance of the changes as in most cases it is not clear whether the receptors measured are presynaptic or postsynaptic. It is perhaps better to look at the overall activity of either noradrenergic or 5-hydroxytryptamine systems upon chronic treatment as a guide to functional changes. Here it seems that the activities of both noradrenergic and 5-hydroxytryptamine synaptic systems are potentiated after chronic but not acute antidepressant treatment. This may be the only unifying strand that can be teased out of a very complex picture. I shall return to consider the mechanisms of such changes later.

Table 14.3 Effects of chronic antidepressant treatment on brain receptors in experimental animals

Treatment	Changes in receptor number			
	Adrenergic		5-hydroxytryptamine	
	α_2	β	5-HT$_1$	5-HT$_2$
Tricyclic drugs	↓	↓	—	↓
Monoamine oxidase inhibitors	↓	↓	↓	↓
Iprindole	—	↓	?	↓
Fluoxetine	—	—	↓	—
ECT	↓	↓	—	↑

(Crews and Smith 1978; Garattini and Samanin 1988; Cowen 1990; Green and Costain 1981; Charney *et al.* 1981; Meltzer 1990). A dash denotes no effect; ? denotes that this has not been determined.

Theories of the aetiology of affective disorders

In the preceding sections of this chapter it was established that there are genetic and environmental influences on the occurrence of affective disorders. The genetic component varies from greater than 80 per cent for bipolar illness to less than 10 per cent for mild depressive illness. It is not clear whether the same genetic factors are involved in different forms of the illness and it seems more likely that, overall, several genes will be found to be associated with the occurrence of affective disorders. Recombinant DNA studies should eventually identify these genes although, as outlined earlier, the identification is likely to be a major undertaking.

Environmental factors are also important and by this I mean season of birth effects, predisposing, precipitating and vulnerability factors as outlined earlier. The combination of genetic and environmental influences is then realized in a 'liability threshold model' which allows for the appearance of affective disorders when a threshold of influences (genetic and environmental) is exceeded. The different affective disorders may then form a kind of continuum with the more genetic bipolar disorders at one end and the more environmentally determined mild depressive disorders at the other end (Fig. 14.3).

If we accept the continuum model of Fig. 14.3 then it is necessary to ask how genetic and environmental influences give rise to the affective disorder. A genetic influence could specify a particular pattern of brain development or a neurochemical change that leads to or predisposes to affective disorder. Genetic influences may contribute to personality or to the psychological type, rendering the person vulnerable to precipitating influences such as stressful life events. Environmental (predisposing) influences could be expressed by their effects on early brain development which might lead to the development of a particular personality vulnerable to precipitating influences. Environmental influences such as the vulnerability factors discussed earlier may alter brain function rendering the

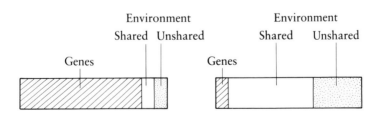

Figure 14.3 Liability–threshold model of affective disorder. The diagram shows the putative influences (liabilities) (genes and shared and unshared environmental factors) that lead to the occurrence of an affective disorder and how these might be partitioned in bipolar severe depressive illness and mild depressive disorders. Each bar is designed to show the relative proportions of the different influences (Table 14.1) which together exceed the threshold for the occurrence of affective disorders. Several genes may be involved and different genes may contribute to different disorders.

individual more susceptible to an adverse life event. Precipitating adverse life events may then interact with these other influences via their effects on brain function.

Although descriptions of this kind are satisfying at a superficial level, they do not provide a detailed understanding. There is in fact little hard information about the way genetic and environmental influences conspire to cause affective disorders but I shall attempt to summarize what information there is below. The discussion will be restricted to depression and depressive symptoms and will not consider mania.

Neuropathological changes in depression

As outlined earlier there is some evidence for structural changes in the brains of some depressed patients as shown by ventricular enlargement. This is likely to be a non-specific indicator of more subtle changes but these have not yet been fully identified. There is some evidence for changes in the structure and function of the frontal and temporal lobes of certain depressed patients. These changes are reminiscent of the changes seen in schizophrenia so there may be some subtle structural alterations in the brain of a depressive patient. These would then perhaps predispose the patient to development of a depressive illness. It is of course important to determine whether the brain changes are seen in all kinds of depressive illness. It is not known whether the changes seen reflect degeneration of neurones or a developmental difference as may be the case for schizophrenia.

Neurochemical hypotheses of depression

Because it has been difficult to show consistent neuropathological changes in the brains of depressed patients, a very active area for theories of depression has been neuro-chemistry. Numerous neurochemical theories of depression have been proposed (Baldessarini 1975; Charney *et al.* 1981; Tyrer and Marsden 1985). As in the case of schizophrenia, these theories are frequently theories of drug action extended in reverse to the disease. Thus the proponents argue that if an antidepressant drug leads to a particular neurochemical change then perhaps depression is due to the opposite change. Without hard evidence this is a very dangerous theoretical route to follow and it really is most important to separate theories of drug action from theories of aetiology. This is frequently not carefully done. There is no *a priori* reason to link the two, for example a biochemical change elicited by the drug could counteract a change in another system altogether and it is this latter system that is actually responsible for the clinical disorder.

Also, affective disorders are characterized by complex groups of symptoms so to attempt to explain their occurrence by a generalized deficit in one neurotransmitter may be too simplistic. Related to this point is the desire by some workers to find common biochemical mechanisms of action for different kinds of antidepressant treatment (leading on to an all-embracing theory of depression) which may be unnecessary and too simplistic. Indeed, if neurochemical explanations of depression are possible there may be neurochemically distinct subgroups of patients.

If a neurochemical hypothesis of depression were sustainable, then it is presumed that the neurochemical change would be specified genetically via a change in a neuro-transmitter system, or via altered brain development in turn specified genetically or environmentally. It is also possible that psychological stress could lead to a temporary change in brain neurochemicals leading to the depressed symptoms.

I shall consider two broad neurochemical hypotheses of depression, the cholinergic hypothesis and the monoamine hypothesis.

Cholinergic hypothesis

This hypothesis (Janowsky *et al.* 1972) suggests that cholinergic and catecholamine systems are reciprocally related and that imbalance between them leads to mood changes. A relative predominance of cholinergic activity results in depression whereas relative catecholaminergic predominance leads to mania. The support for this idea comes from the anticholinergic properties of many antidepressant drugs and the mood elevating properties of certain antiparkinsonian, anticholinergic drugs. This theory was developed before a detailed understanding of the neurochemistry of antidepressant drugs was available. For example, many antidepressant drugs are only weakly anti-cholinergic (Golds *et al.* 1980) and there is no good evidence for changes in cholinergic systems in depression. However, a cholinergic predominance could be achieved by a reduction in catecholaminergic activity and that is the subject of the next theory.

Monoamine hypothesis

This has been the most influential neurochemical hypothesis of depressive illness. Again it is really a theory of drug action applied in terms of aetiology. This hypothesis arose from observations on the effects of two drugs on patients in the 1950s. The alkaloid reserpine, used to treat hypertension, was found to precipitate depression in a proportion of patients. Subsequently reserpine was shown to deplete the levels of the monoamine neurotransmitters dopamine, 5-hydroxytryptamine, and noradrenaline in rat brain. Conversely the drugs iproniazid and isoniazid, used for the treatment of patients suffering from tuberculosis, were found to lift the depression of these chronically ill patients. Iproniazid and isoniazid were later shown to be inhibitors of the enzyme monoamine oxidase and so were probably preventing monoamine degradation in brain.

These observations of monoamine depletion leading to depression and monoamine preservation leading to mood elevation generated the 'monoamine hypothesis' (Fig. 14.4). This can be stated: 'depression may be due to lowered actual or functional monoamine neurotransmitter concentrations at brain synapses and treatment of depression may be achieved by restoring the monoamine levels or actions to normality'. The

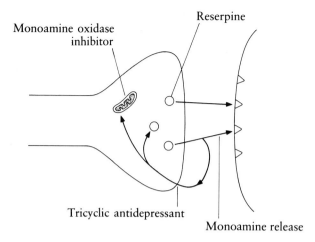

Figure 14.4 Development of the monoamine hypothesis of affective disorders. The diagram shows a monoamine synapse and the effects of certain drugs on its activity. Reserpine depletes the levels of the monoamines by interfering with their storage in vesicles. Monoamine oxidase inhibitors reduce metabolism of the monoamines and tricyclic antidepressants inhibit the reuptake process from the synaptic cleft.

involvement of brain monoamines in the control of mood and certain aspects of behaviour such as motivation and reinforcement was consistent with this (see for example Crow 1973; Tye *et al.* 1977; Le Moal and Simon 1991). The realization that the tricyclic antidepressant drugs inhibited monoamine reuptake into nerve terminals and so might increase synaptic levels of the monoamines provided further impetus for the hypothesis. The hypothesis did not specify a particular monoamine and 'noradrenergic' or '5-hydroxytryptamine' variants of the hypothesis have been championed in various laboratories.

It is important to emphasize that the hypothesis is a theory of drug action extended to aetiology: there is in fact no direct justification for this extension. It could be for example that alteration of the activities of monoamine synapses counteracts some other alteration in brain function. Nevertheless, the hypothesis has spawned a vast amount of work, much of which has been summarized earlier, aimed at probing whether there is a monoamine deficit in depression and if so in which monoamine system.

The specificities of the antidepressant drugs point towards noradrenaline and 5-hydroxytryptamine as candidate monoamines but not definitely to either one. The effects of the combination of L-tryptophan and a monoamine oxidase inhibitor as antidepressant have been taken as support for the idea that raising 5-hydroxytryptamine levels can alleviate depression, but in fact this treatment may also alter catecholamine levels.

Measurements of monoamines, metabolites, and receptor levels in human brain and body fluids has given some suggestions that 5-hydroxytryptamine activities may be reduced in some depressive patients (see earlier discussion) although this may be more a marker for aggression rather than depression. Also there are changes in 5-hydroxytryptamine receptor numbers in post-mortem brains from depressed patients. Other support for an involvement of 5-hydroxytryptamine in depressive symptoms comes from the seasonal affective disorder suffered by some people during the winter months (Wurtman and Wurtman 1989). Patients with this disorder show disturbances of 5-hydroxytryptamine metabolism. Thus there is only weak support for the monoamine hypothesis which comes under further attack from more recent observations. These are:

1. It is not clear from what has been described earlier in this chapter whether the monoamine oxidase inhibitors and the tricyclic antidepressants actually do increase the net synaptic levels of monoamines. The drugs clearly do disturb synaptic monoamine metabolism but, because of the strict regulation of synthesis and release, the net functional monoamine levels may not change greatly. In the case of the tricyclic antidepressants the reduction in neuronal firing rate in response to acute administration is evidence for some increase in neurotransmitter release but this is unlikely to be large.

2. Different drugs, especially the newer ones, all with established antidepressant action, have different propensities for inhibiting either noradrenaline or 5-hydroxytryptamine reuptake, so there does not appear to be any clear relation between neurochemical effects on a particular monoamine and mood changes. In fact there are antidepressant drugs such as iprindole which have antidepressant activity but which do not alter monoamine levels at the synapse. Also, cocaine, which inhibits noradrenaline reuptake, is not an effective antidepressant.

3. The effects of monoamine oxidase inhibitors and tricyclic antidepressants on their target sites are essentially immediate and yet the clinical effects of the drugs take several weeks to reach a maximum. This is not a problem of penetration into the brain as, for the tricyclic antidepressants, blockade of monoamine reuptake and alterations in monoamine synthesis have been demonstrated in experimental animals quite quickly after the drugs are administered. This discrepancy between biochemical and therapeutic effects is similar to that noted for antipsychotic drugs (Chapter 13) and suggests that there are longer term changes triggered by the drugs.

These problems with the 'monoamine hypothesis' have led to a large body of research aimed at devising alternative hypotheses that take account of the time discrepancy and the properties of the newer antidepressant drugs. Much of the work has centred on experiments with animals treated with antidepressants chronically (reviewed earlier) although some data have also been obtained with humans where the neuroendocrine tests have been used as indicators of central monoamine function.

Firstly there are new theories based around *changes in noradrenergic systems*. Slow changes in noradrenergic receptors and systems have been noted earlier upon treatment of animals with antidepressant drugs. For example, the number of brain α_2-adrenergic receptors is decreased by chronic antidepressant treatment (Table 14.3) and in a peripheral model of noradrenergic synapses it has been shown that synaptic efficacy is increased after chronic but not acute administration of a range of antidepressant drugs (Crews and Smith 1980); this is seen whether the drugs affect noradrenaline reuptake (tricyclics) or not (iprindole). Evidence has been presented that the change in synaptic efficacy is due to changes in the control of neurotransmitter release by presynaptic α_2-adrenergic receptors. This could be achieved by a blockade of noradrenaline reuptake (for the tricyclic drugs) leading to raised levels of noradrenaline in turn leading to α_2-adrenergic receptor down-regulation (Fig. 14.5). This would be a slow process as it

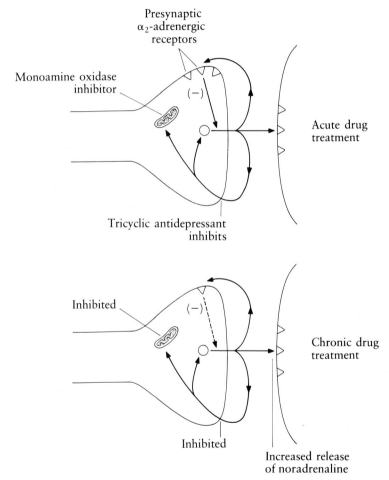

Figure 14.5 α_2-adrenergic receptor down-regulation mechanism for antidepressant action. In the upper diagram a tricyclic antidepressant inhibits noradrenaline reuptake back into the nerve terminal or a mono-amine oxidase inhibitor prevents noradrenaline metabolism. The increased synaptic levels of noradrenaline lead to a slow α_2-adrenergic receptor down-regulation so that gradually the presynaptic autoreceptor control of release is reduced and increased release results (lower diagram). The regulatory mechanisms of the synapse will prevent major changes in the system. If changes in postsynaptic receptors are either insignificant or unimportant then an increase in synaptic efficacy may result.

would require changes in rates of receptor synthesis and degradation. It would therefore be seen only upon chronic drug administration. The net increase in synaptic efficacy suggests that any postsynaptic receptor changes are not great enough to counteract the increased noradrenaline release. There is also evidence for presynaptic α_2 adrenergic receptor desensitization in humans following chronic antidepressant treatment (Charney *et al.* 1983).

These ideas provide a plausible mechanism of action for some antidepressant drugs that takes account of the time delay in clinical action. The observations then beg the question, does depression result from supersensitive presynaptic α_2-adrenergic receptors leading to reduced noradrenaline release? In humans with depression there is no evidence for supersensitive presynaptic α_2-adrenergic receptors (Heninger *et al.* 1988) and besides, as outlined before there is no good evidence for disturbed noradrenergic function in depression.

Another very clear effect of chronic antidepressant treatment in animals for a range of different antidepressant drugs is a down-regulation of brain β-adrenergic receptors that is observed whether the drug used affects noradrenaline reuptake or not. The change in β-adrenergic receptor number is only seen on chronic administration of the drugs. The basis of these changes was felt to be the increased synaptic noradrenaline concentration leading to slow receptor down-regulation (Fig. 14.6). The observation led to a new hypothesis of depression (Sulser *et al.* 1978) namely that the (presumed) postsynaptic β-adrenergic receptor population was increased in depression and the antidepressant drugs act to return this level to normal. This is of course the opposite of a standard monoamine hypothesis.

If this theory were correct, a prediction would be that administration of a brain-penetrating β-adrenergic agonist to a depressed person would exacerbate their depression; there is no evidence for this. Also, the acute administration of an antidepressant drug that raises noradrenaline levels should exacerbate the depression and again there is no evidence for this. Post-mortem brain studies show changes in β-adrenergic receptors in some but not all studies.

Therefore although a reduction in β-adrenergic receptor number may be a contributing factor to the mechanism of action of antidepressant drugs (Hollister 1986), there is little support for a β-adrenergic receptor supersensitivity in depression. In fact, if a classical noradrenaline monoamine hypothesis is considered with reduced noradrenaline levels, this could lead to β-adrenergic receptor up-regulation and then the action of antidepressants would be to reduce the β-adrenergic receptor number. In any case there is no good evidence for changes in noradrenergic systems but the increases in β-adrenergic receptor number following antidepressant drug administration do not predicate new hypotheses.

Alternatively *effects on 5-hydroxytryptamine systems* have formed the basis of other 'monoamine hypotheses'. As outlined earlier, chronic but not acute treatment of animals

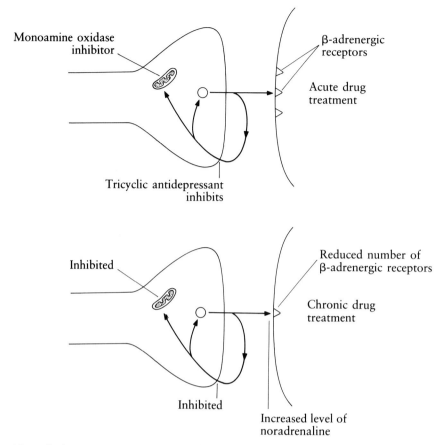

Figure 14.6 β-adrenergic receptor down-regulation hypothesis of antidepressant action. In the upper diagram a tricyclic antidepressant drug is shown inhibiting noradrenaline reuptake into the presynaptic terminal and a monoamine oxidase inhibitor prevents noradrenaline metabolism. The increased levels of noradrenaline (Figure 14.5) lead to a gradual down-regulation of β-adrenergic receptors (lower diagram). How other substances lead to β-adrenergic receptor down-regulation is unclear.

with a range of antidepressant drugs leads to an increase in the efficacy of 5-hydroxytryptamine synapses (Chaput *et al.* 1986). This provides a rationale for the delayed effects of antidepressants in that they induce a slow increase in 5-hydroxytryptamine synaptic efficacy. The mechanism of this change is not clear but could involve a slow down-regulation of presynaptic 5-hydroxytryptamine autoreceptors as suggested for α_2-adrenergic receptors; there is some evidence in support of such receptor alterations (De Montigny and Blier 1991) (Fig. 14.7). Neuroendocrine measures of 5-hydroxytryptamine receptor action in humans also support an increase in synaptic efficacy due to antidepressant treatments (see earlier discussion).

If antidepressants lead to a slow increase in the efficacy of 5-hydroxytryptamine sys-

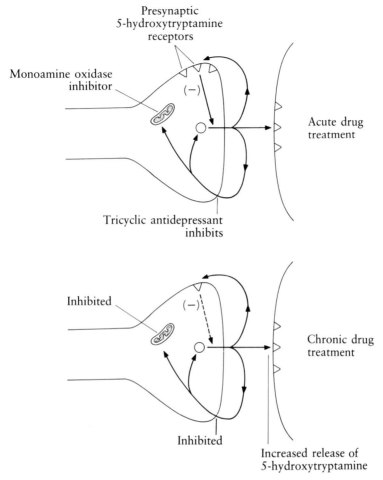

Figure 14.7 *5-hydroxytryptamine receptor down-regulation mechanism for antidepressant action. The upper diagram shows a tricyclic antidepressant inhibiting 5-hydroxytryptamine reuptake into the presynaptic terminal and a monoamine oxidase inhibitor preventing 5-hydroxytryptamine metabolism. The raised levels of 5-hydroxytryptamine lead to gradual down-regulation of presynaptic 5-hydroxytryptamine receptors so that the normal inhibitory autoreceptor control of 5-hydroxytryptamine release is reduced (lower diagram). If postsynaptic receptor changes are insignificant or unimportant then an increase in synaptic efficacy will result. In fact there is some evidence for increased postsynaptic receptor sensitivity. (Blier and De Montigny 1980; Chaput et al. 1986.)*

tems, what evidence is there that depression is due to reduced 5-hydroxytryptamine function? There is in fact some minor evidence in favour of hypotheses of depression based around reduced 5-hydroxytryptamine function as discussed earlier. The observations of increased 5-hydroxytryptamine receptor number in post-mortem brains of depressed individuals could then be accounted for by decreased 5-hydroxytryptamine synaptic action. However, in studies on experimental animals rather large depletions of

5-hydroxytryptamine were required to effect increases in receptor number (Heal *et al.* 1985) and there is little evidence that large changes in the concentration of this neurotransmitter occur in depressed humans.

In summary, therefore, these studies do little to provide new neurochemical hypotheses of depression with the 5-hydroxytryptamine hypothesis remaining but with little solid support. These studies do, however, provide plausible mechanisms of antidepressant drug action that account for the slow onset of clinical efficacy based on slow changes in noradrenergic and 5-hydroxytryptamine synaptic efficacy.

Psychological theories of depression

There have also been extensive attempts to explain depression in psychological terms. Freud suggested that depression arises due to the early experience of the loss of a person important to the patient. The loss is experienced as anger and disappointment which is turned inwards instead of being directed at the lost object; depression results as a form of repressed anger. Klein has suggested that depression has its roots in childhood development. In particular she identified the 'depressive position' which is a stage of learning so that the infant gains the confidence that when his mother leaves him, she will return even if he has been angry. This stage must be successfully passed through and if not the child may develop depression in later life.

In behavioural theories of depression it has been suggested that depressed individuals are relatively insensitive to signals of positive reinforcement that might influence their behaviour. Therefore they are insensitive to signals of reward and susceptible to aversive stimuli. This is a model based on theories of operant conditioning, and the lack of positive reinforcement (reward) for the individual leads to the depression. The neuronal basis of reward and punishment is thought to depend on monoamine (dopamine, 5-hydroxytryptamine, and noradrenaline) neuronal systems (Crow 1973; Tye *et al.* 1977; Le Moal and Simon 1991) and as described above there have been a number of monoamine hypotheses of depression. These at least parallel the behavioural theories of depression but the actual evidence for persistent changes in monoamine neuronal systems in depressed patients is not impressive.

Alternatively, cognitive models have been suggested. For example, Beck has suggested that depressives maintain a negative view of themselves and their present and future circumstances and this negative view is maintained because of certain early experiences. Brown and Harris have provided an alternative model based around hopelessness. Hopelessness is produced by loss events, and certain vulnerability factors (see the earlier discussion in this chapter) intensify the response to the loss event. If the loss is experienced as very extreme it may be denied and depression may result. A third cognitive model is the learned helplessness model. This derived from animal experiments where first the animals were subjected to unavoidable electric shocks. When subsequently the animals were released and allowed to learn an escape response, many of the animals had difficulty in learning how to do so. They also were passive and appeared dejected and it was suggested that they had learnt that they were helpless. In the human situation, a person attempts to control events but cannot and generalizes the inability to control into a learned helplessness that is experienced emotionally as depression. In the animal model, changes in certain brain neurotransmitters (dopamine and noradrenaline) are seen, providing some evidence that psychological stress can induce long-term changes in brain neurochemicals. This parallels in part the neurochemical hypotheses of depression, although the evidence for persistent changes in these monoamines in depressed patients is poor.

Claridge (1985) has discussed these ideas and in particular why only some individuals are prone to depression whereas many of us will experience loss of various kinds in our lives. He suggested that it is the individual's 'nervous type' that renders someone vulnerable to depression. This takes us back to the idea of a biological vulnerability to depression which may be similar to the idea of personality types mentioned before. In this way we can begin to bring together the psychological theories and the neuropathological and neurochemical theories of depression.

In summary, therefore, the theories of the aetiology of depression point to minor structural changes in the brains of some patients, inconsistent changes in neurotransmitter (5-hydroxytryptamine) function, and a number of psychological influences. Individuals may vary in their response to certain life events rendering them more or less susceptible to depression. In the next section I shall discuss brain function in depression and provide a framework to bring these different ideas together.

As was the case for schizophrenia (Chapter 13), 'biological' and 'psychological' explanations of depression have been separated here for convenience of description. This does not imply a dualistic splitting of body and mind—the expression of the largely psychological feeling of depression must ultimately be due to some change in brain chemistry or constitution and can be treated either by psychological or chemical intervention. The brain and a disorder like depression are not to be described in either psychological or biological terms: they are both psychological and biological.

Disordered brain function in depression

It is very difficult given the present state of knowledge to construct theories of disordered brain function in depression. It is still not clear how different forms of depression are related, so it may not be possible to provide an all-embracing theory of brain dysfunction. There is some evidence for neuropathological changes in the brains of patients suffering from some forms of depression and these may be the more severe forms. The neuropathological changes resemble those changes seen in schizophrenia, implying some relationship between depression and schizophrenia. In fact Crow (1986) has suggested that unipolar depression, bipolar depression, and schizophrenia constitute a continuum of psychotic illness related to the expression of particular gene sequences in the human genome (Chapter 13). It seems less likely that the milder forms of depression are associated with neuropathological changes but nevertheless there are symptoms common to both mild and severe depressive illness.

One way to unify depressive illnesses and perhaps schizophrenia is to see them in terms of changes in the function of the septo-hippocampal monitoring system. I described this in relation to schizophrenia (Chapter 13) and will do so again in the next chapter in relation to anxiety (Chapter 15). This system has been discussed extensively by Gray (1987) and is thought to be responsible for comparing internally generated plans with actual outcomes, the subiculum in the hippocampal formation seeming to perform the actual comparator role. He has proposed that activation of the septo-hippocampal monitoring system, for example by a mismatch between predicted and actual behavioural outcomes, generates anxiety when the outcome is likely to be unpleasant. Although this may be an oversimplification of the mechanisms involved in anxiety (see Chapter 15), I shall use this simplified formulation here. Continued mismatch or stress, especially where it appears uncontrollable, leads to continued activation of the septo-hippocampal system as well as changes in certain other brain structures such as the hypothalamus, which receives the outputs of the septo-hippocampal system, and the ventral striatum (nucleus accumbens, Fig. 13.4). The ventral striatum also has neuronal links with the hippocampus and appears to be important for adding motivational influences (incentive and reward) to behaviours. The continued activity in these structures leads in experimental animals to depletion of neurotransmitters (noradrenaline and dopamine) and it is suggested that this depletion results in some of the symptoms of depression. This parallels in part the monoamine hypotheses of depression described earlier although the evidence for persistent changes in these monoamines in depressed humans is sparse.

The evidence for this proposal is not very strong, but it is not unreasonable to propose the involvement of the septo-hippocampal monitoring system in the generation of feelings like depression. In at least some cases of depression the symptoms seem to result from conflict between planned behaviour and actual outcomes in a manner that is unpleasant and seems prolonged and out of control. This situation would be recognized as a mismatch in the septo-hippocampal monitor but, because of its excessive and persistent nature, it has additional neurochemical effects and generates feelings different from simple anxiety.

With these ideas mild depression with a strong anxiety component and perhaps more severe depressions can be seen to be realized via the septo-hippocampal system. These would be depressions that are a result of external circumstances but there is individual variation in the response to circumstances and the experience of anxiety and depression. This variation may result from different sensitivities of the septo-hippocampal system to the mismatch between predicted and actual behavioural outcomes. This may in turn relate back to the earlier discussions about biological variability. These forms of depression would then constitute psychological reactions to circumstance in susceptible individuals, but we can also conceive of depressions caused by actual changes in the structure of the brain. For example, neuropathological changes in temporal or frontal lobe function could disturb septo-hippocampal monitoring leading to feelings of depression but also to certain psychotic symptoms as described for schizophrenia. Indeed Bowen *et al.* (1989) have suggested that the neuropathological changes they observed in frontal and temporal regions of post-mortem brains from depressed patients could indicate degeneration of neurones linking the two regions, which would disturb the input of information to the septo-hippocampal system. Since the septo-hippocampal system receives a 5-hydroxytryptamine innervation, it is also possible to imagine disturbed 5-hydroxytryptamine function, for which there is some evidence, leading to disturbed septo-hippocampal monitoring and feelings of depression.

Finally, is it possible to account for the activities of the antidepressant drugs within such a framework? Overall the principal unifying strand of antidepressant drug function was their ability to alter the activities of noradrenergic and 5-hydroxytryptamine systems. The septo-hippocampal system receives both noradrenergic and 5-hydroxytryptamine innervation so it is possible that antidepressant drugs act to alter the control of the septo-hippocampal system by noradrenergic and 5-hydroxytryptamine inputs. Therefore we can conceive of depression as being a result of altered septo-hippocampal function, either due to external circumstances or due to constitutional changes in the brain. The altered function can be reset by changing noradrenergic or 5-hydroxytryptamine control of the system. Antidepressant treatments achieve this by effecting slow changes in synaptic efficacy as described above. Psychological treatments presumably effect changes in the same or closely related brain systems.

Recommended reading

Akiskal, H. S. and McKinney, W. T. (1975). Overview of recent research in depression. *Archives of General Psychiatry*, **32**, 285–305.

Baldessarini, R. J. (1975). The basis for amine hypotheses of affective disorder. *Archives of General Psychiatry*, **32**, 1087–93.

Bebbington, P. (1985). Three cognitive theories of depression. *Psychological Medicine*, **15**, 759–69.

Claridge, G. (1985). *Origins of mental illness*. Blackwell, Oxford.

Cowen, P. J. (1990). A role for 5-HT in the action of antidepressant drugs. *Pharmacology and Therapeutics*, **46**, 43–51.

Crow, T. J. (ed.) (1987). Recurrent and chronic psychoses. *British Medical Bulletin*, **43**, 479–773.

Finberg, J. P. M. (1987). Antidepressant drugs and down-regulation of preynaptic receptors. *Biochemical Pharmacology*, **36**, 3557–662.

Garattini, S. and Samanin, R. (1988). Biochemical hypotheses of antidepressant drugs: a guide for clinicians or a toy for pharmacologists. *Psychological Medicine*, **18**, 287–304.

Gelder, M., Gath, D., and Mayou, R. (1989). *Oxford textbook of psychiatry* (2nd edn). Oxford University Press.

Gilman, A. G., Goodman, L. S., Rall, T. W., and Murad, F. (1985). The pharmacological basis of therapeutics (7th edn). Macmillan, New York.

Green, A. R. and Costain, D. (1981). *Pharmacology and biochemistry of psychiatric disorders*. Wiley, Chichester.

Hare, E. H. (1987). Epidemiology of schizophrenia and affective psychoses. *British Medical Bulletin*, **43**, 514–30.

Joyce, P. R. and Paykel, E. S. (1989). Predictors of drug response in depression. *Archives of General Psychiatry*, **46**, 89–99.

Karasu, T. B. (1990). Towards a clinical model for psychotherapy for depression I: systematic comparison of three psychotherapies. *American Journal of Psychiatry*, **147**, 133–47.

Karasu, T. B. (1990). Towards a clinical model for psychotherapy for depression II: an integrative and selective treatment approach. *American Journal of Psychiatry*, **147**, 269–78.

Kendell, R. E. (1976). The classification of depression: a review of contemporary confusion. *British Journal of Psychiatry*, **129**, 15–28.

McGuffin, P. and Katz, R. (1989). The genetics of depression and manic-depressive disorder. *British Journal of Psychiatry*, **155**, 294–304.

Meltzer, H. (1989) Serotonergic dysfunction in depression. *British Journal of Psychiatry*, **155** (suppl. 8), 25–31.

Miller, E. and Cooper, P. J. (eds) (1988) *Adult abnormal psychology*. Churchill Livingston, Edinburgh.

Mitchell, R. (1975). *Depression*. Penguin Books, Harmondsworth.

Nutt, D. and Glue, P. (1989). Monoamine oxidase inhibitors: rehabilitation from recent research? *British Journal of Psychiatry*, **154**, 287–91.

Paykel, E. S. (1989). Treatment of depression: the relevance of research for clinical practice. *British Journal of Psychiatry*, **155**, 754–63.

Paykel, E. S. and White, J. L. (1989). A European study of views on the use of monoamine oxidase inhibitors. *British Journal of Psychiatry*, **155** (suppl. 6), 9–17.

Sugrue, M. F. (1983). Do antidepressants possess a common mechanism of action? *Biochemical Pharmacology*, **32**, 1811–17.

Tyrer, P. and Marsden, C. A. (1985). New antidepressant drugs: is there anything new they tell us about depression? *Trends in Neurosciences*, **8**, 427–31.

Van Praag, H. M. (1982). Depression. *Lancet*, ii, 1259–64.

15 *Anxiety*

The only thing we have to fear is fear itself

Franklin D. Roosevelt

Everyone has some idea of what anxiety is like and it seems to be a normal, perhaps protective, human response to novel or stressful situations. The circumstances that provoke anxiety are generally those where there is expectation of danger or distress or where there is a need for a special effort. Although it may be a normal reaction, and at moderate levels may be highly motivating, severe anxiety and its effects on performance can be crippling for certain individuals. For example, it is thought that a significant number of people engaged in the performing arts turn to anti-anxiety drugs or alcohol to help with this. Anxiety symptoms are also widespread in the general population: in 1985 in the UK about 8 per cent of the population took a benzodiazepine anti-anxiety drug in the preceding year (Dunbar *et al.* 1989).

It has been estimated that 10 per cent or more of the population will experience some form of more or less severe anxiety reaction requiring medical help during their lives. It is also of some interest that at the time of writing the two best selling drugs in the UK are for treatment of gastric ulcer. It is thought that some of the factors contributing to the development of ulcers are stress and anxiety.

This chapter is concerned with anxiety and the anti-anxiety drugs.

Clinical description

Anxiety and the more specific anxiety syndromes which will be described below are examples of neuroses. Neurotic disorders can occur at three 'levels', individual symptoms, minor neurotic disorders, and specific neurotic syndromes. Individual neurotic symptoms, for example anxiety and depression, are experienced by a very large proportion of the population at one time or another. The minor neurotic (emotional) disorders show lifetime prevalence rates of up to 10 per cent. These kinds of disorder are frequently seen in general practice and patients report anxiety, worry, despondency, and sadness together with somatic symptoms (see below for a description of these in relation to specific anxiety syndromes) and sleep disturbances. These disorders are often reactions to stress or to adjustments in circumstances undergone by the patient, for example, bereavement, migration, or separation.

The specific neurotic syndromes are characterized by groups of associated symptoms and are more frequently seen in the psychiatric clinic. I shall consider these disorders in three groups, generalized anxiety disorder, phobic anxiety disorders, and obsessive compulsive disorder as suggested by Gelder *et al.* (1989).

Specific neurotic syndromes

In each of the three specific neurotic syndromes, certain symptoms are present to greater or lesser extents. Firstly there are psychological symptoms such as awareness of threat, mental tension, difficulty in concentration, unpleasant anticipation and, in some cases, fear. These feelings may be combined with feelings of restlessness, difficulty in relaxation and concentration and disturbances in sleep. Secondly there are the somatic symptoms of anxiety which can largely be accounted for by the activation of the sympathetic nervous system. Examples of these are activation of the cardiovascular system, increased muscular tension (which may lead to muscular tremor), gastrointestinal changes (dry mouth, nausea, sinking feeling in the stomach, and diarrhoea), difficulty in breathing, and increased sweating (leading to increased skin conductance). These latter somatic symptoms are easy to measure and may be used in some forms of treatment involving psychophysiological measures (e.g. biofeedback).

Generalized anxiety disorder is characterized by psychological feelings of anxiety coupled with variable somatic symptoms as described above, occurring without any obvious precipitating stimulus. In some cases symptoms may be exacerbated by situational cues, e.g. social gatherings, but this is not always so. Panic may be a prominent feature but panic attacks may also occur in other neurotic disorders (see below).

Generalized anxiety disorder, and also minor emotional disorders (adjustment and stress reactions, see above) may be a response to a single highly stressful event or situation or a series of such factors, and the reaction may pass as the person regains their normal equilibrium. In some people there may be periodic recurrences of acute attacks whereas in others the anxiety state may become semi-permanent, leading to the disablement of the patient. The dividing line between normal anxiety and 'pathological' anxiety is difficult to define but if the anxiety is perceived as unpleasant, out of control, and impairing function, it may qualify for the 'pathological' label. In addition to this distinction there are large variations in individual responses to anxiety provoking events and situations. The prevalence in the population of generalized anxiety disorder has been estimated as 3–6 per cent.

In *phobic anxiety disorders* the same symptoms are experienced as in generalized anxiety disorder only the symptoms occur in response to or in anticipation of certain situations. In simple phobias there is a fear of a specific object or situation, e.g. spiders, the dark, heights, or thunder and lightning. Social phobias occur where the patient fears situations where he may be observed or criticized. In agoraphobia the patient is anxious when away from home or in crowds or in situations he cannot leave easily. Agoraphobic patients experience panic attacks and anxious cognitions about fainting and loss of control. Panic disorder may be a separate disorder (Gelder 1989; Nutt and Glue 1989*a*). Patients experience recurrent panic attacks characterized by the rapid build-up of severe symptoms such as choking, palpitations, and shortness of breath. Patients also fear a catastrophic outcome such as death or 'going crazy'. The lifetime risk for phobic anxiety disorders is generally about 10 per cent except for panic disorder where the risk is about 1 per cent.

Obsessive–compulsive disorder includes patients who have obsessional thoughts, images, doubts, impulses (for example shouting blasphemies in church), or rituals (for example repeated hand-washing). These disorders are often linked to obsessional personality traits. In many cases anxiety reinforces obsessional behaviour in that responding to the obsession can be seen as a means of avoiding the anxiety provoked by not carrying out the ritual. Anxiety is a prominent symptom in many of these states. The lifetime risk of obsessive–compulsive disorder is 2–3 per cent.

Anxiety is also a prominent symptom in a number of other disorders, notably depressive disorders (Chapter 14). As indicated in Chapter 14, it has been suggested that there is a group of patients suffering from what has been termed general neurotic syndrome (Tyrer 1985). These patients have a varying pattern of symptoms ranging from anxiety at one time to non-psychotic depression at another time depending on their circumstances. They may also exhibit phobic or panic symptoms. This emphasises the overlap between the syndromes of anxiety and depression at certain levels.

Certain factors have been recognized that may contribute to or trigger the development of a neurosis whether of the adjustment and stress reaction kind (minor neurotic disorder) or one of the specific syndromes. Factors such as a stressful working or home environment as well as life events, e.g. childbirth, marriage, or moving home, are considered to be important here. There are also very large variations in individual responses to anxiety-provoking events and situations. This may reflect biological variation which could be due to inherited differences in the reaction to anxiety-provoking situations or effects of the environment, for example the family situation during early life. In either case these factors may influence brain development and hence the development of particular personalities and behaviour patterns.

Some indication of the influence of genetic factors on the prevalence of anxiety disorders has been obtained from the increased prevalence of anxiety disorders in first degree relatives of those suffering from such disorders compared with control families (Murray and Revely 1981; Marks 1986). This could indicate that genetic factors influence the prevalence but shared environmental factors could also account for the increased prevalence. Some studies have been performed comparing the prevalence in monozygotic and dizygotic twin pairs each containing at least one affected twin. For anxiety disorders a higher rate of concordance (about 40 per cent) was seen in the monozygotic pairs compared with the dizygotic pairs (15 per cent or less) (Mahmood *et al.* 1983; Marks 1986). This suggests that there is a moderate genetic influence on the occurrence of these anxiety disorders. Similar concordance data have been reported for the incidence of panic disorder, some phobic disorders and obsessive compulsive disorder in monozygotic and dizygotic twin pairs (Murray and Reveley 1981; Marks 1986). The genetic tendency seems to be related to the inheritance of a personality prone to anxiety disorders as well as the inheritance of specific patterns of behaviour, for example obsessional behaviour. These genetic tendencies will then be influenced by the environmental triggering factors outlined above, and the particular combination of genetic and environmental factors influences the expression of the anxiety disorder.

Neuropathological and biochemical changes in anxiety states

If we take the view that anxiety, at least in its acute manifestations, is a normal response to certain situations, then it seems unlikely that the syndrome will reflect any major brain changes such as loss of nerve cells. This conclusion is reinforced by the observation that for many patients suffering from the specific neurotic disorders, their symptoms remit in time. The variations in responsiveness to life events in different individuals may, however, reflect minor, genetically and environmentally determined differences in brain architecture or chemistry and it may be possible to detect these differences. Also during anxiety attacks there are significant alterations in behaviour which should be matched by alterations in neuronal activity. If these changes are sufficiently marked it may be possible to detect these changes or their sequelae and thus gain clues to the neuronal systems involved.

Some recent studies have attempted to examine brain systems involved in anxiety by using modern imaging studies of cerebral blood flow (see Chapter 7) as an index of changes in brain activity. A group of patients was tested in whom a panic attack can be induced by lactate infusion (Reiman *et al.* 1986). In these patients, cerebral blood flow was measured before and during a panic attack and compared with control patients. During the panic attack the greatest changes in cerebral blood flow were seen in the polar temporal cortex (the tip of the temporal lobe) (Reiman *et al.* 1989*b*). By contrast, before the panic attack, that is in these patients' normal resting state, differences in cerebral blood flow were detected in a different part of the brain. Before the panic attack a specific (asymmetric) abnormality in cerebral blood flow was detected in the parahippocampal gyrus (Reiman *et al.* 1986). These changes in cerebral blood flow in temporal lobe structures are of interest in the light of findings from magnetic resonance imaging studies on patients with panic disorder where temporal lobe abnormalities were detected

(Fontaine *et al.* 1990). Since patients who experience panic attacks may be a distinct group, similar studies on cerebral blood flow were performed on patients experiencing anticipatory anxiety and, as in the case of the patients experiencing panic, changes in cerebral blood flow in their polar temporal cortex were seen (Reiman *et al.* 1989*a*). A possible explanation of these results is that the changes in activity in the parahippocampal gyrus represent a vulnerability to panic attacks whereas the experience of anxiety/panic is realized in part via the polar temporal cortex. The two brain regions are both parts of the limbic association cortex and are linked by neuronal pathways so changes in one region could lead to changes in the other. The polar temporal (paralimbic) cortex is thought to be involved in the evaluation of sensory information, in this case danger.

Rather different observations have been reported in patients with obsessive–compulsive disorder. Using a variety of imaging techniques evidence has been obtained for differences in brain structure relative to controls with the frontal cortex and caudate nucleus being affected (Behar *et al.* 1984; Baxter *et al.* 1987; Luxenberg *et al.* 1988; Garber *et al.* 1989).

Very few neurochemical studies of the kind that have been performed in schizophrenia (Chapter 13) or depression (Chapter 14) have been applied to anxiety, so there is no evidence of any consistent neurochemical alterations. Indirect information on changes in the sensitivity of brain neurochemical systems has been obtained by challenge of patients with drugs and this information will be considered later.

Treatments for anxiety and related neuroses

Anxiety and anxiety disorders are psychological disorders whose occurrence depends on genetic and environmental factors. Treatment should be possible both using psychological approaches and using drugs. This is indeed the case and the use of the two kinds of treatment fits well with the general view of the brain and mind–body integration expressed in this book. It is assumed that the psychological and drug treatments affect the same or related brain systems in effecting treatment.

Psychological approaches

In many cases acute anxiety, manifest as part of an adjustment or stress reaction (minor neurotic disorder), and generalized anxiety disorder can be treated by giving the patient support and reassurance alone. For example, a study of neurotic patients in a general practice setting showed that counselling was as effective as drug (benzodiazepine) therapy (Catalan *et al.* 1984). The patient will nevertheless need to resolve problems in his life that are leading to the anxiety and this may require the help of social workers, family, and friends. Psychotherapy may be useful where there are persistent emotional problems. For patients whose anxiety does not pass quickly there is a high chance that these symptoms will persist for some years.

For some phobias including agoraphobia or obsessive–compulsive disorder, very successful treatment can be achieved by behaviour therapy where the patient is exposed in different ways to the situation or object that elicits fear in a controlled environment (Marks and O'Sullivan 1988). The patient builds up the ability to cope with anxiety-inducing situations. The relapse rate after behaviour therapy is also lower than for drug therapy. Alternatively or additionally, cognitive therapy can be used to interrupt intrusive thoughts and neutralize their effects. Given the emerging problems with the use of drugs these positive results obtained using psychological treatments are very encouraging.

Drug treatments

A number of classes of compound have been reported as useful anti-anxiety agents (anxiolytics) and the principal groups of compounds will be considered here. Understanding their mode of action may shed light on the mechanisms underlying anxiety.

Barbiturates

Compounds of this chemical class, e.g. phenobarbitone, used to be prescribed for anxiety although they have also been used in higher doses as hypnotics. They are no longer prescribed for anxiety because of severe problems with toxicity in overdose and both physical and psychological dependence. Unpleasant withdrawal symptoms are experienced when the dependent individual ceases taking the drug. Also, there are risks of death due to overdosage. These were sufficient reasons for restricting the use of barbiturates but also other drugs such as the benzodiazepines, which were thought to be much safer (although see below) became available, further suppressing prescribing of barbiturates.

Benzodiazepines

This class of compound was first introduced in the early 1960s and benzodiazepines, e.g. diazepam (Valium), are still the drugs of choice as anxiolytics (Fig. 15.1). There are many structural variants available with varied claims of different pharmacological, pharmacodynamic, and pharmacokinetic properties. Indeed the number of benzodiazepines consumed is staggering. In 1981 it was estimated that 30 million prescriptions for benzodiazepines were issued in a year in the UK, with one in five women and one in ten men taking a benzodiazepine for part of a year (Dunbar *et al.* 1989). Usage has declined more recently owing to increasing awareness of the problems of dependence (see below).

Benzodiazepines are also used as hypnotics (especially the rapidly metabolised

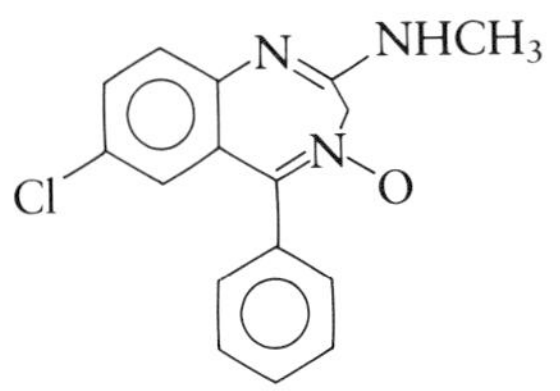

chlordiazepoxide

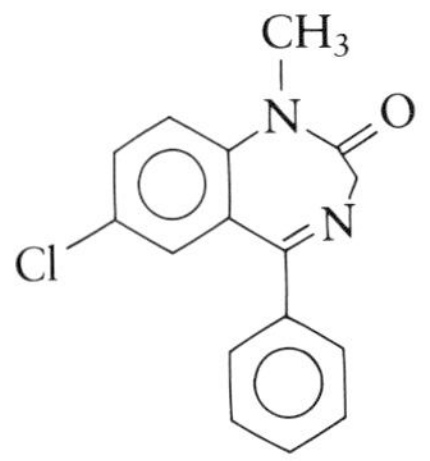

diazapam

Figure 15.1 The structures of some popular benzodiazepines.

compounds), anti-convulsants, and muscle relaxants (for example, as premedication before an operation). Although these are useful properties in some circumstances, they can be the source of undesirable side effects such as sedation, muscle relaxation, and ataxia (when the drugs are taken as anxiolytics (see below)).

Considerable euphoria greeted the introduction of the benzodiazepines as, in addition to their anxiolytic properties, they had a very low toxicity or propensity for other undesirable side effects shown by the barbiturates, e.g. respiratory depression and hypotension. Increasingly, however, it has become apparent that for a significant proportion of patients, benzodiazepines, if taken for more than a few weeks, have problems of side effects and tolerance/dependency (Ashton 1989). The side effects are drowsiness, lack of coordination, and impaired memory and concentration. Some patients complain of 'emotional anaesthesia' or depression and in some patients uncharacteristic behaviour is seen, for example aggressive behaviour, and outbursts of rage and violence. Anterograde amnesia can develop so that the patient may deny the existence of the very problem that causes the anxiety and this may impair psychological adjustment. In animal studies benzodiazepines have been shown to hinder normal adjustment to stressful situations.

The tolerance/dependence on benzodiazepines can also develop quite quickly and some authors believe that the drugs lose their efficacy as anxiolytics after about four weeks due to tolerance (Lader and File 1987; Higgitt *et al.* 1985). There is considerable debate about this issue and this may reflect the differing sensitivities of different patients to the drugs (Taylor 1989; Catalan and Gath 1985). As well as this tolerance/dependence there is an unpleasant withdrawal syndrome if the drug is stopped abruptly. Withdrawal symptoms are apparent if the drug is stopped after only a few weeks of treatment but the symptoms are more prevalent after chronic therapy. Withdrawal symptoms are experienced by about 40 per cent of patients taking benzodiazepines for a moderate length of time and consist of an intensified form of the original anxiety together with panic attacks, perceptual disturbances, and somatic disturbances.

There are, therefore, significant problems with benzodiazepine therapy, particularly as in the past there has been a tendency to treat patients over long periods with the drugs with little personal support to the patient. Nevertheless, the drugs do have an important place in the treatment of anxiety but, because of these problems, it has now been suggested that these drugs should only be prescribed for short term relief of anxiety in a highly stressful situation and then a flexible intermittent dosing regime should be followed. If regular dosing is used it should be for no longer than two weeks and dosage should be reduced gradually, not abruptly (Higgitt *et al.* 1985; Tyrer and Murphy 1987). Taylor (1989) has argued that long term use of benzodiazepines should, however, not be dismissed out of hand and that these drugs can help certain people live relatively normal lives.

For more chronic anxiety, psychological treatments as described above should be considered rather than chronic benzodiazepine treatment and it has been suggested that antidepressant drugs (Chapter 14) may be more effective in these cases as well as in panic and phobic disorders and obsessive–compulsive disorder (see below) (Johnstone *et al.* 1980; Liebowitz 1989; Catalan *et al.* 1984; Kahn *et al.* 1986).

I shall consider the mechanism of action of the benzodiazepines in treating anxiety below.

Antidepressant drugs

Drugs that have been commonly used to treat depression (Chapter 14) are also useful for treating certain forms of anxiety. Tricyclic antidepressants, e.g. imipramine, have been shown to be of use in treating generalized anxiety disorder as well as some panic and phobic disorders (Johnstone *et al.* 1980; Kahn *et al.* 1986; Tyrer *et al.* 1988). These drugs do not have the problems of dependence seen with the benzodiazepines. The monoamine oxidase inhibitors have also been used for treatment of anxiety and phobic states (Liebowitz 1989). Newer monoamine oxidase inhibitors may not suffer from the problems of the older drugs (Chapter 14).

The mechanism of action of these antidepressant drugs in treating anxiety disorders is not clear. They have well established effects on brain monoamine systems which have been discussed in relation to depression (Chapter 14). It seems that both noradrenergic and 5-hydroxytryptamine systems may have roles in regulating anxiety, so the anti-depressant drugs may be exerting their therapeutic effects on these systems. I shall discuss this again below.

Effects of the relatively selective 5-hydroxytryptamine uptake inhibitor clomipramine and the more selective compound fluvoxamine have been reported on obsessive–compulsive disorder (Murphy *et al.* 1989*b*; Goodman *et al.* 1990). There does appear therefore to be some selectivity in the pattern of drug responsiveness, obsessive–compulsive disorder responding selectively to 5-hydroxytryptamine uptake blockade whereas more generalized anxiety, panic, and some phobic states respond to a variety of drugs including selective 5-hydroxytryptamine uptake inhibitors. It has been suggested that the uptake blockers achieve their therapeutic effects via enhancing 5-hydroxytryptamine neurotransmission by reducing autoreceptor control of release (Chapter 14) (De Montigny and Blier 1991). It should not, however, be concluded that obsessive–compulsive neurosis is a disorder of 5-hydroxytryptamine systems. There is no evidence for that conclusion, although 5-hydroxytryptamine systems have been implicated in the control of certain anxiety symptoms as outlined above.

Compounds active at 5-hydroxytryptamine receptors

A novel class of compounds, e.g. buspirone, that act as partial agonists at central 5-hydroxytryptamine (5-HT_{1A}) receptors have been reported to possess anxiolytic potencies similar to benzodiazepines but without the ataxia, muscle relaxant, and sedative properties of benzodiazepines which can be undesirable when they are used for anxiety treatment (File 1987; Taylor 1988). It is too early to know how useful these compounds will be and particularly whether they will be devoid of the tolerance/dependence/withdrawal cycle that typifies other anxiolytics, but preliminary indications suggest that they do not lead to tolerance (Murphy *et al.* 1989*a*, but see also Oswald 1990).

It has been suggested that buspirone acts as a 5-hydroxytryptamine agonist on 5-hydroxytryptamine (5-HT_{1A}) autoreceptors on the cell bodies of 5-hydroxytryptamine neurones in the raphe nucleus, reducing their firing rate.

Alcohol

Alcohol (ethanol), although not a prescribed drug, is widely used and abused and has a variety of effects on humans including a form of anxiolytic effect at low doses. The responses to low doses of alcohol are very variable but can result in release of inhibition so that the individual appears euphoric and relaxed. As the blood alcohol level increases there is some evidence of clumsiness and lack of coordination, and some people may become violent whereas others may become withdrawn. At higher doses, sedative effects predominate and the individual appears 'drunk', with confusion, unsteadiness, and slurred speech. Chronic alcohol consumption can lead to tolerance and dependence, with a severe withdrawal syndrome if ingestion is ceased. Thus, the effects of alcohol are more complex than those of the benzodiazepines, but both substances share the property of a tolerance/dependence/withdrawal syndrome, although it is not known if the mechanisms of tolerance are similar.

'β-blockers'

Compounds that act as antagonists of β-adrenergic receptors ('β-blockers'), e.g. propranolol, have been found to be of use as anxiolytics in both acute stress reactions (e.g. public speaking) and some cases of more persistent generalized anxiety. It seems that these drugs do not act centrally, but instead suppress the peripheral symptoms of anxiety (particularly those mediated through β-adrenergic receptors) which are largely a result of the activation of the sympathetic nervous system. Certainly, the suppression of the peripheral symptoms of anxiety is advantageous especially for example in the performing arts. Whether there is also a link between the central expectation of peripheral symptoms and their occurrence in an anxiety-provoking situation which is broken by the β-blocker is unclear.

A common site of action for benzodiazepines, barbiturates, and alcohol?

Benzodiazepines, barbiturates, and alcohol share a common property—they are all anxiolytics. It seems that this may be due to their actions on a common neurochemical site, the $GABA_A$ receptor. This was described in Chapter 6 as a typical example of a fast ion channel linked receptor where the action of the neurotransmitter GABA is to open a Cl^- channel leading to hyperpolarization and inhibition of neuronal excitation. It seems that the oligomeric receptor–ion channel complex also contains specific separate binding sites for benzodiazepines and barbiturates and that when these are occupied by their respective ligands, the action of GABA at its receptor site is facilitated (Fig. 15.2) and hyperpolarization is enhanced. Alcohol (ethanol) also has as one of its many actions the ability to facilitate GABA action by some interaction with the $GABA_A$ receptor complex (Gonzales and Hoffman 1991; Starke 1991). Although this common action of these drugs on the $GABA_A$ receptor provides a satisfactory explanation of their actions, the $GABA_A$ receptor is distributed widely throughout the brain and questions of specificity of action arise. These will be addressed later.

There has been some interest in examining the mechanism of actions of the benzo-diazepines in inducing tolerance upon prolonged administration. A simple explanation would be that there is a 'down-regulation' (Chapter 6) of the benzodiazepine binding sites. Prolonged administration of benzodiazepines to experimental animals, however, produces inconsistent changes in brain benzodiazepine binding sites. It seems that the effects of prolonged benzodiazepine therapy may be more subtle (Zorumski and Isen-berg 1991).

The existence of a high affinity specific site of action for the benzodiazepine drugs has stimulated much interest and speculation about why there are such sites. A similar question once existed for opiate receptors. Specific high affinity binding sites for opiates like morphine had been discovered in the brain but it was not clear what was their normal function. This led to a search for endogenous ligands for the 'opiate receptors' and eventually the enkephalins were discovered (Kosterlitz 1979). Subsequently a family

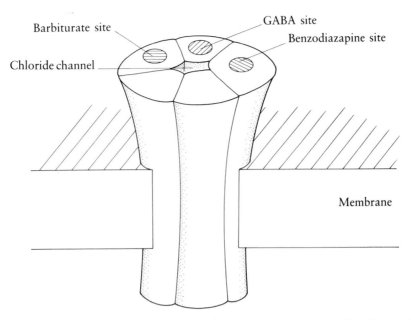

Barbiturate site

GABA site

Benzodiazapine site

Chloride channel

Membrane

Figure 15.2 The structure of the GABA$_A$–benzodiazepine receptor complex. The diagram is highly speculative but shows the five subunits of the receptor forming an oligomer in the membrane. For molecular details see Figs 6.2 and 6.4. The relative positions of the different ligand binding sites are not known.

of endogenous opiates has been recognised. In the case of the benzodiazepines much effort has been expended on finding an 'endogenous benzodiazepine' or endogenous anxiety substance (De Robertis *et al.* 1988). A number of substances have been proposed, none of which has been clearly validated as an endogenous ligand for the benzodiazepine site.

The search for endogenous benzodiazepine-like substances has proceeded on two fronts, the discovery of small organic molecules and the discovery of small proteins. The first substance that was isolated was ethyl-β-carboline carboxylate but it soon became apparent that this was an artefact of the isolation procedure. Subsequently butyl-β-carboline carboxylate has been isolated from brain and shown to have potent actions at the benzodiazepine binding site of the GABA$_A$ receptor and to have anxiogenic potential in animal tests. Benzodiazepines themselves have also been isolated from human brain and shown to be associated with synaptic vesicles. The relevance of these observations to anxiety is not yet clear (Izquierdo 1989).

Two small proteins, diazepam binding inhibitor (DBI, M$_r$ 11 000) (and small fragments of DBI) and endozepine (M$_r$ 10 000) have been isolated from brain and proposed as modulators of the GABA$_A$–benzodiazepine receptor complex, but the widespread non-neuronal localization of these substances makes them poor candidates as endogenous ligands for the benzodiazepine site.

It may well be that there is no endogenous ligand but why there are high affinity saturable specific sites for benzodiazepines then remains a puzzle. As pointed out in Chapter 6 it seems to be a property of fast ion channel linked receptors to contain modulatory sites for drugs, these may fortuitously bind benzodiazepines in the case of the $GABA_A$ receptor. Certain steroids also modulate the $GABA_A$–benzodiazepine receptor complex and since the levels of these may be altered during stress this affords an alternative means of modulating this important site of drug action.

Psychological treatments and drug treatments for anxiety disorders

At the beginning of this section it was suggested that, because anxiety disorders are psychological disorders whose expression was dependent on genetic and environmental factors, it was to be expected that treatment could be achieved using both psychological approaches and drugs. As outlined above, this is indeed the case. It is not known how the psychological treatments impinge upon brain systems. Nevertheless it is my assumption that both psychological treatments and drugs, where effective on the same symptoms, are effecting change in the same or closely related brain systems. This is then consistent with the general philosophy of this book that psychological and neuronal/neuro-chemical descriptions of brain function are descriptions of the same entity but at different levels. No dualistic split of mind and body is implied in describing psycho-logical and drug treatments separately, this is for convenience and clarity.

Theories of aetiology and brain function in anxiety

This section describes some of the theories that have been proposed to account for the occurrence of anxiety neuroses and related conditions.

Anxiety is the emotion felt in anticipation of some unpleasant, unwanted, or threaten-ing outcome. It is a normal emotion felt by everyone at one time or another. Gray (1987) has suggested that the situations where anxiety may be experienced can be categorized as those where the anticipated outcome of an action is either punishment or lack of reward and we can all think of numerous anxiety-provoking events that fit this model. He has also suggested that novel situations can engender anxiety. In this case the very nature of a novel situation renders the anticipated outcome uncertain and therefore potentially threatening. A fourth source of anxiety proposed by Gray comprises certain stimuli to which we have an innate (inherited) anxiety response e.g. heights or snakes. In all these cases, however, the anxiety can be seen as a normal human response to those situations that may serve an adaptive role in the future in avoiding the unpleasant outcome or in coping with similar circumstances. The considerable individual variation in anxiety responses to similar situations shows that there is variation between people in their sensitivity to these anxiety-provoking situations. This in turn reflects variation at the biological level.

In seeking to provide explanations of anxiety I hope to consider cases where the anxiety is a normal reaction and results from a clearly defined situation as described above but also cases where the anxiety seems to occur and persist with no obvious external trigger (generalized anxiety disorder) and the specific syndromes of phobic anxiety disorder and obsessive–compulsive disorder.

Earlier in this chapter I reviewed studies that indicated that for some anxiety disorders there was evidence for a genetic influence on their occurrence. This influence was not overwhelming and it seemed to reflect a tendency towards the development of a neurotic personality as well as the development of specific disorders. This genetic influence on the occurrence of anxiety disorders would then contribute to the individual biological variation in responses to anxiety-provoking situations. There is some evidence for biological variation in respect of the anxiety disorders from the brain imaging studies. Patients who experience panic attacks or obsessive–compulsive disorder do show apparent alterations in certain brain structures as outlined earlier.

Biological variation could also be influenced by environmental factors, for example the family environment, affecting brain development and hence development of the personality; certain environmental factors are also important for triggering anxiety, for example stress and other psychological influences. These different factors must be considered in proposing theories of anxiety and anxiety disorders.

There have been extensive attempts to account for anxiety disorders in psychological terms. Freud first suggested that anxiety resulted from suppressed sexual drive but he later modified this to propose that anxiety was experienced when repressed unconscious motives threatened to intrude into consciousness.

Accounts of anxiety based on animal behaviour have invoked classical conditioning theories. A neutral stimulus eventually can elicit fear by classical conditioning if it is initially paired with a threatening stimulus. This framework has been used to account for phobic neuroses. I shall describe an example to make this clearer. A case has been described of a woman so afraid of cats that she would not go out at night for fear of encountering one. This phobia could be traced to the patient having witnessed, at the age of four, her father drowning a kitten in a bucket of water. Her phobia also generalized to any item closely associated with cats. In terms of classical conditioning, the neutral stimulus, i.e. the cat, came to elicit fear because it had been paired with the threatening stimulus, her father drowning the kitten.

There are, however, some problems with such accounts. For example, many children witness similar events but do not develop phobias. This could be related to biological variation in the sensitivity to aversive stimuli. A more serious problem is that for many phobias there does not seem to be a threatening past event associated with the fear-evoking stimulus, or at least it cannot be remembered.

There are also some problems with this kind of approach in explaining generalized anxiety disorders where anxiety is present in the apparent absence of a threatening situation. One possibility is that some everyday internal physiological event has become conditioned to evoke anxiety. This is very difficult to test.

Cognitive models of anxiety have also been proposed whereby anxiety, whether normal or abnormal, is seen as an appropriate emotional reaction to highly threatening thoughts, often referring to possible future dangers. Anxiety disorders are, according to this scheme, thought disorders. Generalized anxiety disorder would then be seen as a result of the patient having particularly threatening patterns of thinking, the patient exaggerating the probability of the occurrence of negative events. These disturbed thought patterns could be a result of a biological predisposition, exposure to threatening life events and acquired ways of reacting. A cognitive theory of panic has been presented (Clark *et al.* 1988) whereby the patient misinterprets normal autonomic changes, e.g. breathlessness, as signs of impending physical or mental disaster.

A neuropsychological account of anxiety has been extensively developed by Gray (1987). He has taken information from animal experiments which seem to be applicable to humans. The stimuli which evoke anxiety are signals of punishment, signals of lack of reward, novel stimuli, and certain innate fear stimuli. A brain system then exists to detect these potentially threatening stimuli and generate anxiety; Gray has termed this the 'behavioural inhibition system'.

The role of the 'behavioural inhibition system' is to assess the organism's environment for these potentially threatening stimuli. Therefore an important component of the system will be a comparator which can compare actual events or states of the environment with predictions of these (based on plans and anticipation of events) and search for mismatches especially where the mismatch leads to threatening situations (Fig. 15.3). If a mismatch is detected, the 'behavioural inhibition system' is activated, leading in experimental animals to inhibition of current behaviour, increased readiness for action, and increased attention to environmental stimuli. Similar behavioural effects are seen in humans together with the psychological sensation of anxiety. Comparator function may be unnecessary for innate fear stimuli as our response to these may be essentially 'hard wired' into the brain circuitry.

If we accept the concept of a 'behavioural inhibition system' which in humans is responsible for the psychological sensation of anxiety, then it is not unreasonable to propose that the functioning of the system and its sensitivity to the mismatches between actual and predicted events will be determined by genetic influences on brain development and by environmental influences. By environmental influences I mean early experiences in life that could affect the development of the 'behavioural inhibition system' and could presumably permanently affect its functioning. Therefore individuals may vary in the function of their 'behavioural inhibition system' making certain individuals more or less sensitive to anxiety provoking situations.

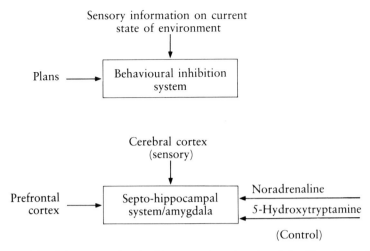

Figure 15.3 Models of the systems involved in generation of anxiety (after Gray 1987). The upper diagram shows the model at a neuropsychological level with the 'behavioural inhibition system' (anxiety generator) responding to the comparison of anticipated outcomes (plans) and actual outcomes (based on sensory information). The lower diagram shows the brain systems thought to perform these roles and also includes the control pathways (noradrenergic and 5-hydroxytryptamine) that can change the sensitivity of the 'behavioural inhibition system'.

This analysis provides a plausible account of individual variation in susceptibility to anxiety-provoking situations. Generalized anxiety disorder would then occur in susceptible individuals with particularly reactive 'behavioural inhibition systems'. In this case it is still necessary to suggest a trigger for the anxiety and one possibility suggested above is that it is some everyday physiological event. Certain phobias, according to Gray, could be due to innate fear responses in highly reactive individuals. Phobias do tend to be directed at particular objects or situations and it may be that we have an innate fear reaction to threatening objects or situations such as snakes or heights. Other phobias, e.g. fear of certain animals, may be normal childhood reactions that have continued into later life. Obsessive–compulsive neurosis according to Gray results from a hyperactive 'behavioural inhibition system' which tags too many environmental stimuli as potentially threatening. The obsessive–compulsive patient then scans his environment to an excessive degree for potential threats and this scanning takes the form of checking rituals. Repetitive hand-washing is a frequent compulsive behaviour and this could result from continual checking for dirt.

Agoraphobia deserves some comment as some agoraphobics experience sporadic panic attacks. It is possible that the agoraphobia results from a fear of having a panic attack in public. If the first time a panic attack occurs is when the patient is outside his home environment, then agoraphobia, or fear of being where a panic attack could occur, may result. This leaves open the source of the panic attack in the first place but one possibility is that panic results from intense fear due to spontaneous neuronal discharge in a brain system involved in generation of this emotion.

It is difficult to reconcile these different psychological accounts of anxiety and anxiety disorders. Gray's account provides a plausible mechanistic scheme for the generation of the emotion of anxiety based on the evaluation and comparison of predicted and actual outcomes of events. Individual responses to anxiety-provoking situations would then depend on biological variation, but this could be modified by learned conditioned behavioural responses and acquired cognitive responses both dependent on prior life experiences.

Grays 'behavioural inhibition system' has been extended to actual brain structures and in the next section I shall consider what these brain structures might be.

The septo-hippocampal system as the 'behavioural inhibition system'

Gray (1987) has proposed that the brain system responsible for the 'behavioural inhibition system' and hence for mediating anxiety is to be found in two linked limbic regions of the brain, the septum and hippocampal formation (the septo-hippocampal system) (Fig. 15.3). The main evidence for this contention comes from the similar effects on the behaviour of experimental animals of anti-anxiety drugs and lesions to the septohippocampal system. Some further evidence, however, comes from the studies on cerebral blood flow outlined above. These highlighted the parahippocampal gyrus (part of the limbic association cortex, Chapter 2 (Fig. 2.9) and Chapter 7) as a potential brain region where altered activity might generate a vulnerability to panic attacks. The parahippocampal gyrus (which contains the entorhinal cortex) forms the major input and output region of the hippocampal formation. During a panic attack or during anticipatory anxiety, however, another region, the polar temporal cortex, showed changes in cerebral blood flow. The polar temporal cortex (also part of the limbic association cortex) is thought to evaluate the relevance of environmental information, for example danger signals, and it is linked to the parahippocampal gyrus. Electrical stimulation of the polar temporal cortex, the parahippocampal gyrus, the hippocampus, and the amygdala (which has neuronal connections to the septo-hippocampal system) elicit syndromes resembling anxiety or fear. There is therefore circumstantial evidence that the septo-hippocampal system and associated brain areas are involved in mediating anxiety and may therefore represent the 'behavioural inhibition system'. The septo-hippocampal system receives information on the current state of the organism (from the sensory regions of the cerebral cortex) via the parahippocampal gyrus (entorhinal cortex) and information on anticipated outcomes (plans) from the prefrontal cortex. Gray has proposed that the comparator function, which compares actual and predicted outcomes of behaviour, is in the subiculum (part of the hippocampal formation). It is important to note, however, that these are not the only functions subserved by the septo-hippocampal system. For example, in Chapter 12 the importance of the hippocampus for certain aspects of memory function was outlined.

In addition to the septo-hippocampal system, Gray has suggested that noradrenergic pathways linking the locus coeruleus to the septo-hippocampal system and 5-hydroxytryptamine pathways linking the raphe to the same system are important in the control of the 'behavioural inhibition system'. In a threatening situation these pathways may be activated to affect several brain regions including the septo-hippocampal system increasing its ability as a comparator. Effects of noradrenergic and 5-hydroxytryptamine pathways on other brain regions are thought to be important for other components of the behavioural inhibition (anxiety) response, e.g. arousal and motor inhibition.

The proposals of Gray (1987) may, however, be an over-simplification. The septo-hippocampal system may only be a part of the 'behavioural inhibition system' and anxiety generator. One additional brain area that seems to be very important is the amygdala. Electrical stimulation of the amygdala can provoke anxiety or fear responses and in experimental animals lesions of the amygdala abolish certain fear responses (Davis 1991). It may, therefore, be that the amygdala and septo-hippocampal system are important for different aspects of the anxiety response. It has been suggested that the amygdala may be important for the detection of fear-provoking signals, for example the presence of a predator for an animal, as well as some innate fear responses. The hippocampus may be more important for anxiety or fear dependent on the context or place and so this mechanism would be important for anxiety in novel environments and may be involved in the development of agoraphobia (Deakin and Graeff 1991; Selden *et al.* 1991).

A further brain region important for this anxiety response is the periaqueductal grey region. This may be important for the realization of certain aspects of anxiety and fear such as 'fight and flight'. Electrical stimulation of the periaqueductal grey region provokes an intense fear/anxiety response. Both the amygdala and periaqueductal grey region are innervated by 5-hydroxytryptamine systems, underlining the importance of this neurotransmitter in the control of anxiety.

If this account of brain systems and anxiety is accepted it can be seen that differences in the development of the amygdala, septo-hippocampal system, periaqueductal grey region, and related structures could account for differences in susceptibility to anxiety-provoking situations. The differences in cerebral blood flow in the parahippocampal gyrus in patients who are susceptible to panic give some support for this. Also, as proposed earlier, panic could be due to spontaneous neuronal discharge in a brain region associated with the amygdala/septo-hippocampal system and the data on blood flow in the polar temporal cortex during a panic attack provide circumstantial evidence for this idea. This region of the cerebral cortex has neuronal connections directly to the amygdala and indirectly to the hippocampus via the parahippocampal gyrus. Panic could also be generated by spontaneous neuronal discharge in other brain regions associated with the anxiety response.

Information that does not fit into this scheme is emerging for obsessive–compulsive disorder. Imaging techniques have shown that alterations in brain structure are found but these are in the frontal cortex and caudate nucleus. Patients with lesions in the basal ganglia can exhibit obsessive–compulsive symptoms (Laplane *et al.* 1989). Obsessive–compulsive disorder does seem to be separate from the other anxiety disorders on the basis of drug therapy in that 5-hydroxytryptamine uptake inhibitors seem to have a selective effect on the disorder.

It is possible that in obsessive–compulsive disorders there is a disturbance in the function of one of the complex (cognitive) cortico-striato-pallido-thalamo-cortical basal ganglia circuits. These have been discussed in relation to Parkinson's disease (Fig. 10.8), Huntington's disease (Chapter 11) and schizophrenia (Fig. 13.4). These circuits do have important roles in the control of behaviour so the observations of frontal cortical and caudate nucleus changes in patients exhibiting obsessive–compulsive disorders are at least consistent with this suggestion (Rapoport 1989, 1990; Volkow and Tancredi 1991).

Effects of drugs on the septo-hippocampal system

It should be possible to account for the actions of anxiolytic drugs using the same ideas outlined above. If the model of anxiety is correct then anxiolytic drugs should influence the activity of the septo-hippocampal (behavioural inhibition) system. There is some evidence for this as effects of drugs that modulate the $GABA_A$ receptor (benzodiazepines) have been described on the hippocampus itself (increasing the inhibitory actions of GABA that limit firing in other hippocampal neurones by a negative feed back loop (see below)). Effects have also been described on the noradrenergic neurones innervating the septo-hippocampal system, decreasing the ability of these neurones to activate the septo-hippocampal system.

One question that arises with such a hypothesis concerns specificity of action. $GABA_A$ receptors are widely distributed in the brain, so how does modulation of the receptor account for a specific action on the hippocampus? One possible explanation is that neurones containing GABA are frequently involved in negative feedback loops. The neurones are activated by firing in other cells and their action is to restrain the activity of the other cells (Chapter 7). If so, when a generalized $GABA_A$ receptor activator such as a benzodiazepine is administered, it will have its action only on those cells that are firing and these may indeed be the ones associated with the septo-hippocampal system when anxiety is perceived. It is also the case that benzodiazepines are not entirely specific and do have significant side effects which can be attributed to their actions on $GABA_A$ receptors in other parts of the brain.

Another group of anxiolytic drugs are those that manipulate 5-hydroxytryptamine systems (antidepressants, 5-hydroxytryptamine uptake inhibitors, and buspirone). Their ability to alleviate anxiety presumably results from actions on the 5-hydroxytryptamine neuronal systems innervating the septo-hippocampal system. This could be due to actions on the raphe, the source of the innervation, but it is also of relevance that the $5-HT_{1A}$ subtype of 5-hydroxytryptamine receptor, thought to be the site of action of buspirone, is concentrated in the hippocampus and parahippocampal gyrus. Further evidence for a role of 5-hydroxytryptamine systems in anxiety comes from the effects of the 5-hydroxytryptamine agonist *m*-chlorophenyl piperazine (mCPP) which can induce anxiety if administered to normal volunteers. This same compound can under various circumstances increase the incidence of panic or obsessive–compulsive disorder in patients susceptible to these conditions (Murphy *et al.* 1989*b*). The precise effects and sites of action of these various compounds that affect 5-hydroxytryptamine function and manipulate anxiety symptoms are at present unclear.

The α_2-adrenergic antagonist yohimbine can also induce panic if administered to patients susceptible to panic attacks (Charney *et al.* 1984*a*) and this supports a role for noradrenergic systems in modulation of anxiety. Stimulation of the locus coeruleus, the source of noradrenergic neurones, can induce in animals a state resembling anxiety and yohimbine is likely to increase locus coeruleus activity by blocking inhibitory auto-receptors. There is therefore evidence for a role of noradrenergic pathways in the regulation of anxiety and these could be the pathways innervating the septo-hippocampal system. The effects of antidepressant drugs on anxiety could also be due to effects on noradrenergic systems in addition to their effects on 5-hydroxytryptamine systems.

The effects of yohimbine on patients susceptible to panic attacks have been interpreted in terms of a noradrenergic theory of panic (see for example Nutt 1989). This theory suggests that panic is due to excessive activity in the noradrenergic projections from the locus coeruleus (Gorman *et al.* 1989) and this could include projections to the septo-hippocampal system. This theory is based on drug effects alone and does not fit well with the observations of specific changes in activity in certain regions of the cerebral cortex outlined above.

Yohimbine does not, however, affect patients with obsessive–compulsive disorder, there being no increase in obsessive–compulsive symptoms in these patients. This is consistent with the point noted earlier in considering drug effects that there may be some neurochemical specificity to such disorders. Thus from the point of view of the drugs that can treat symptoms and those that can precipitate symptoms, obsessive–compulsive disorder seems to be separate from the other anxiety states. Obsessive–compulsive disorder also differs from the other anxiety disorders in that different areas of the brain showed alterations in structure when examined using imaging techniques.

Recommended reading

American Psychiatric Association (1987). *Diagnostic and statistical manual of mental disorders* (3rd edn, revised). American Psychiatric Association, Washington DC.

Ashton, H. (1989). Anything for a quiet life. *New Scientist*, **122**, 52–5.

Braestrup, C. and Nielsen, M. (1982). Anxiety. *Lancet*, **ii**, 1030–4.

Gelder, M., Gath, D., and Mayou, R. (1989). *Oxford textbook of psychiatry* (2nd edn). Oxford University Press.

Gorman, J. M., Liebowitz, M. R., Fyer, A. J., and Stern, J. (1989). A neuroanatomical hypothesis for panic disorders. *American Journal of Psychiatry*, **146**, 148–61.

Gray, J. A. (1987). *The psychology of fear and stress* (2nd edn). Cambridge University Press.

Healy, D. (1991). The marketing of 5-hydroxytryptamine: depression or anxiety. *British Journal of Psychiatry*, **158**, 737–42.

Hoehn-Saric, R. (1982). Neurotransmitters in anxiety. *Archives of General Psychiatry*, **39**, 735–42.

Kidman, A. (1989). Neurochemical and cognitive aspects of anxiety disorders. *Progress in Neurobiology*, **32**, 391–402.

Lader, M. and File, S. E. (1987). The biological basis of benzodiazepine dependence. *Psychological Medicine* **17**, 539–47.

Martin, I. L. (1983). The benzodiazepines and their receptor. In *Cell surface receptors* (ed. P. G. Strange), pp. 50–81. Ellis Horwood, Chichester.

Miller, E. and Cooper, P. J. (eds) (1988). *Adult abnormal psychology*. Churchill Livingstone, Edinburgh.

Nutt, D. J. and Glue, P. (1989). Clinical pharmacology of anxiolytics and antidepressants: a psycho-pharmacological perspective. *Pharmacology and Therapeutics*, **44**, 309–34.

Stephenson, F. A. (1988). Understanding the GABA$_A$ receptor: a chemically gated ion channel. *Biochemical Journal*, **249**, 21–32.

Tyrer, P. and Murphy, S. (1987). The place of benzodiazepines in psychiatric practice. *British Journal of Psychiatry*, **151**, 719–23.

Zorumski, C. F. and Isenberg, K. E. (1991). Insights into the structure and function of GABA-benzo-diazepine receptors: ion channels and psychiatry. *American Journal of Psychiatry*, **148**, 162–73.

16 *The present and the future*

Whether you have read the preceding chapters sequentially or just browsed through, I hope you have noticed that this book divides roughly into two halves. The first half outlines the present state of knowledge on basic brain structure and function with particular emphasis on biochemical aspects, while the second half outlines the present state of knowledge on six disorders of human brain function, again emphasizing a biochemical analysis of the dysfunction with the material in the first half of the book providing a basis for this.

In most of the disorders there were prominent psychological changes and I have tried to outline the biochemical changes that might underlie these. I hope it has been apparent that descriptions of the disorders at both the psychological and biochemical levels are complementary and provide descriptions of the same system but at different levels of analysis. There is no dualistic split of mind and body here, the psychological and biochemical are different but necessary descriptions of the same overall system. This in turn implies that treatments for these disorders may be based on either drugs or psychological intervention. Where both kinds of treatment are effective, as for example in anxiety disorders and affective disorders, it seems likely that the treatments are ultimately affecting the same or closely related brain systems. These ideas are then in line with the philosophy proposed for theories of the mind in Chapter 8 which provides an interface between the two halves of the book.

So much for the present state of knowledge. The question I wish to ask finally is, what is the future for brains? I shall highlight just a few topics that I think will provide significant advances in the study of the brain in the near future.

Drug treatments will advance to provide more selective therapy for brain disorders with fewer side effects. The vast number of receptor isoforms uncovered by gene cloning (Chapter 6) and found to be selectively localized should provide new targets for selective therapeutic agents (Strange 1991*b*). I hope, however, that where effective psychological treatments are also available, such as in the cases of anxiety and depression, these will be used increasingly as their effects are often associated with less risk of relapse than those of drug treatments.

Brain repair has already started—in Chapter 10 the use of fetal brain implants for the treatment of Parkinson's disease was outlined. So far the results of this treatment have been mixed but there is much interest in the possible application of these techniques for treatment of other degenerative diseases, for example Alzheimer's disease and Huntington's disease (Lindvall 1991). A major problem with the approach is that there may be ongoing degeneration which will also affect the implant. Unless very marked effects of the implant on the symptoms of the disease are seen, it seems likely that a better approach would be to aim to understand the basis of the disease and prevent it (see below).

Understanding of brain disorders will increase. In particular it should be possible to identify environmental agents that together with a genetic susceptibility lead to the disorder. If these environmental factors are dietary components, then decisions will need to be made about eliminating them from the diet. Genetic testing of individuals will in time allow those at risk for certain diseases to be identified as outlined for Huntington's disease (Chapter 11). Together with presymptomatic testing (see below) this may enable early intervention for these individuals. In the absence of a suitable intervention technique, the use of genetic testing will, however, raise significant ethical issues.

Methods for analysing the working brain such as PET and SPECT (Chapter 9) will provide more and more detailed pictures of the brain in action. In time this will allow testing of the theories of mind proposed in Chapter 8 to be undertaken. Use of PET and SPECT in individuals at risk for disease will allow presymptomatic testing to be performed to detect early changes in the brain. For presymptomatic testing to be of use, however, it is necessary to have an appropriate intervention and at least for some disorders this may entail assessment and reduction of potential risk factors.

Bibliography

Abramsky, O. and Litvin, Y. (1978). Autoimmune response to dopamine receptor as a possible mechanism in the pathogenesis of Parkinson's disease and schizophrenia. *Perspectives in Biology and Medicine*, **22**, 104–14.

Aktories, K. and Frevert, J. (1987). ADP ribosylation of a 21–24 kDa eukaryotic protein by C3, a novel botulinum ADP-ribosyltransferase, is regulated by guanine nucleotides. *Biochemical Journal*, **247**, 363–8.

Alberts, B., Bray, D., Lewis, J., Raff, M., Roberts, K., and Watson, J. D. (1989). *Molecular biology of the cell* (2nd edn), Garland Publishing, New York and London.

Albin, R. L., Young, A. B., and Penney, J. B. (1989). The functional anatomy of basal ganglia disorders. *Trends in Neurosciences*, **12**, 366–75.

Alexander, G. E. and DeLong, M. R. (1985). Microstimulation of the primate neostriatum: I, physiological properties of striatal microexcitable zones. *Journal of Neurophysiology*, **53**, 1417–32.

Alexander, G. E., DeLong, M. R., and Strick, P. L. (1986). Parallel organisation of functionally segregated circuits linking basal ganglia and cortex. *Annual Review of Neuroscience*, **9**, 357–81.

Almers, W. and Tse, F. W. (1990). Transmitter release from synapses: does a preassembled fusion pore initiate exocytosis. *Neuron*, **4**, 813–18.

Altman, J. (1989). A nose for Alzheimer's disease. *Nature*, **337**, 688.

Altshuler, L. L., Conrad, A., Hauser, P., Li, X., Guze, B. H., Denikoff, K., Tourtelotte, W., and Post, R. (1991). Reduction of temporal lobe volume in bipolar disorder: a preliminary report of magnetic resonance imaging. *Archives of General Psychiatry*, **48**, 482–3.

American Psychiatric Association (1987). *Diagnostic and statistical manual of mental disorders* (3rd edn, revised), American Psychiatric Association, Washington DC.

Anderson, K. D. and Reiner, A. (1990). Extensive cooccurrence of substance P and dynorphin in striatal projection neurons: an evolutionarily conserved feature of basal ganglia organisation. *Journal of Comparative Neurology*, **295**, 339–69.

Anderton, B. H. (1987). Alzheimer's disease: progress in molecular pathology. *Nature*, **325**, 658–9.

Andreasen, N. C., Ehrhardt, J. C., Swayze, V. W., Alliger, R. J., Yuh, W. T. C., Cohen, G., and Ziebell, S. (1990). Magnetic resonance imaging of the brain in schizophrenia. *Archives of General Psychiatry*, **47**, 35–44.

Andrews, G., Stewart, G., Morris-Yates, A., Holt, P., and Henderson, S. (1990a). Evidence for a general neurotic syndrome. *British Journal of Psychiatry*, **157**, 6–12.

Andrews, G., Neilson, M., Hunt, C., Stewart, G., and Kiloh, L. G. (1990b). Diagnosis, personality and the long term outcome of depression. *British Journal of Psychiatry*, **157**, 13–18.

Arango, V., Ernsberger, P., Marzuk, P. M., Chen, J. S., Tierney, H., Stanley, M., Reis, D. J., and Mann, J. J. (1990). Autoradiographic demonstration of increased serotonin $5HT_2$ and β-adrenergic receptor binding sites in the brain of suicide victims. *Archives of General Psychiatry*, **47**, 1038–47.

Arora, R. C. and Meltzer, H. Y. (1989). Serotonergic measures in the brains of suicide victims: $5HT_2$ binding sites in the frontal cortex of suicide victims and control subjects. *American Journal of Psychiatry*, **146**, 730–6.

Ashton, H. (1989). Anything for a quiet life. *New Scientist*, **122**, 52–5.

Aston-Jones, G., Foote, S. L., and Segal, M. (1985). Impulse conduction properties of noradrenergic locus coeruleus axons projecting to monkey cerebrocortex. *Neuroscience*, **15**, 765–77.

Augustine, G. J., Charlton, M. P., and Smith, S. J. (1987). Calcium action in synaptic transmitter release. *Annual Review of Neuroscience*, **10**, 633–93.

Avissar, S., Schreiber, G., Danon, A., and Belmaker, R. H. (1988). Lithium inhibits adrenergic and cholinergic increases in GTP binding in rat cortex. *Nature*, **331**, 440–2.

Azmitia, E. and Gannon, P. (1983). The ultrastructural localisation of serotonin immunoreactivity in myelinated and unmyelinated axons within the medial forebrain bundle of rat and monkey. *Journal of Neuroscience*, **3**, 2083–90.

Baines, A. J. (1990). Ankyrin and the node of Ranvier. *Trends in Neurosciences*, **13**, 119–21.

Bakalyar, H. A. and Reed, R. R. (1990). Identification of a specialised adenylyl cyclase that may mediate odorant detection. *Science*, **250**, 1403–6.

Balch, W. E. (1990). Small GTP-binding proteins in vesicular transport. *Trends in Biochemical Sciences*, **15**, 473–7.

Baldessarini, R. J. (1975). The basis for amine hypotheses of affective disorder. *Archives of General Psychiatry*, **32**, 1087–93.

Baraban, J. M., Worley, P.F., and Snyder, S. H. (1989). Second messenger systems and psychoactive drug action: focus on the phosphoinositide system and lithium. *American Journal of Psychiatry*, **146**, 1251–60.

Barinaga, M. (1990). Neuroscience models the brain. *Science*, **247**, 524–6.

Barnard, E. A., Darlison, M. G., and Seeburg, P. (1987). Molecular biology of the GABA$_A$ receptor: the receptor/channel superfamily. *Trends in Neurosciences*, **10**, 502–9.

Baron, M. and Rainer, J. D. (1988). Molecular genetics and human disease. *British Journal of Psychiatry*, **152**, 741–53.

Baron, M., Risch, N., Hamburger, R., Mandel, B., Kushner, S., Newman, M., Drumer, D., and Belmaker, R. H. (1987). Genetic linkage between X-chromosome markers and bipolar affective illness. *Nature*, **326**, 289–92.

Barr, C. E., Mednick, S. A., and Munk-Jorgensen, P. (1990). Exposure to influenza epidemics during gestation and adult schizophrenia. *Archives of General Psychiatry*, **47**, 869–74.

Bauswein, E., Fromm, C., and Preuss, A. (1989). Corticostriatal cells in comparison with pyramidal tract neurones: contrasting properties in the behaving monkey. *Brain Research*, **493**, 198–203.

Baxter, L. R., Phelps, M. E., Mazziotta, J. C., Guz, B. H., Schwartz, J. M., and Selin, C. E. (1987). Local cerebral glucose metabolic rates in obsessive compulsive disorder. *Archives of General Psychiatry*, **44**, 211–18.

Baxter, L. R., Schwartz, J. M., Phelps, M. E., Mazziotta, J. C., Guze, B. H., Selin, C. E., Gerner, R. H., and Sumida, R. M. (1989). Reduction of prefrontal cortex glucose metabolism common to three types of depression. *Archives of General Psychiatry*, **46**, 243–50.

Beal, M. F., Kowall, N. W., Swartz, K. J., Ferrante, R. J., and Martin, J. B. (1988). Model of Huntington's disease. *Science*, **241**, 475.

Bebbington, P. E., Brugha, T., MacCarthy, B., Potter, J., Sturt, E., Wykes, T., Katz, R., and McGuffin, P. (1988). The Camberwell collaborative depression study. I, Depressed probands: adversity and the form of depression. *British Journal of Psychiatry*, **152**, 754–65.

Bebbington, P., Katz, R., McGuffin, P., Tennant, C., and Hurry, J. (1989). The risk of minor depression before age 65: results from a community survey. *Psychological Medicine*, **19**, 393–400.

Behar, D., Rapoport, J. L., Berg, C. J., Benckla, M. B., Mann, L., Cox, C., Fedro, P., Zah, T., and Wolfman, M. G. (1984). Computerised tomography and neuropsychological test measures in adolescents with obsessive compulsive disorder. *American Journal of Psychiatry*, **141**, 363–9.

Benes, F. M., Davidson, J., and Bird, E. D. (1986). Quantitative cytoarchitectural studies of the cerebral cortex of schizophrenics. *Archives of General Psychiatry*, **43**, 31–5.

Benes, F. M. and Bird, E. D. (1987). An analysis of the arrangement of neurones in the cingulate cortex of schizophrenic patients. *Archives of General Psychiatry*, **44**, 608–16.

Beneviste, H. (1989). Brain microdialysis. *Journal of Neurochemistry*, **52**, 1667–79.

Bennett, V. (1985). The membrane skeleton of human erythrocytes and its implications for more complex cells. *Annual Review of Biochemistry*, **54**, 273–304.

Benovic, J. L., De Blasi, A., Stone, W. C., Caron, M. G., and Lefkowitz, R. J. (1989). β-adrenergic receptor kinase: primary structure delineates a multigene family. *Science*, **246**, 235–40.

Berg, D. K., Boyd, T., Halvorsen, S. W., Higgins, L. S., Jacob, M. H., and Margrotta, J. F. (1989). Regulating the number and function of neuronal acetylcholine receptors. *Trends in Neurosciences*, **12**, 16–21.

Berger, B., Gaspar, P., and Verney, C. (1991). Dopaminergic innervation of the cerebral cortex: unexpected differences between rodents and primates. *Trends in Neurosciences*, **14**, 21–7.

Berridge, M. J., Downes, C. P., and Hanley, M. R. (1989). Neuronal and developmental actions of lithium: a unifying hypothesis. *Cell*, **59**, 411–19.

Betz, H. (1990). Homology and analogy in transmembrane channel design, lessons from synaptic membrane proteins. *Biochemistry*, **29**, 3591–9.

Billah, M. M. and Anthes, J. C. (1990). The regulation and cellar functions of phosphatidylcholine hydrolysis. *Biochemical Journal*, **269**, 281–91.

Birnbaumer, L. (1990). G proteins in signal transduction. *Annual Review of Pharmacology and Toxicology*, **30**, 675–705.

Black, D., Exton-Smith, A. N., Moore-Smith, B., Arnott, M., Hodkinson, H. M., Evans, J. G., Portsmouth, O. H. D., Davison, A. N., Elliott, A. F., Bergmann, K., Jefferys, P. M., Robinson, R. A., and Mason, P. (1981). Organic mental impairment in the elderly. *Journal of the Royal College of Physicians of London*, **15**, 141–67.

Blakemore, C. (1977). *Mechanics of the mind*. Cambridge University Press.

Blair, J., Farrar, G., and Cowburn, J. D. (1990). Alzheimer's disease—some biochemical clues. *Chemistry in Britain*, **26**, 1169–73.

Blier, P. and De Montigny, C. (1980). Effect of chronic tricyclic antidepressant treatment on the serotonin autoreceptor. *Naunyn Schmiedeberg's Archives of Pharmacology*, **314**, 123–8.

Blin, J., Bonnet, A. M., and Agid, Y. (1988). Does levodopa aggravate Parkinson's Disease. *Neurology*, **38**, 1410–16.

Boarder, M. R. (1989). Presynaptic aspects of cotransmission: relationship between vesicles and neurotransmitters. *Journal of Neurochemistry*, **53**, 1–11.

Bondareff, W., Mountjoy, C. Q., Roth, M., Rossor, M. N., Iversen, L. L., and Reynolds, G. P. (1987). Age and histopathologic heterogeneity in Alzheimer's disease. *Archives of General Psychiatry*, **44**, 412–17.

Boulter, J., Hollmann, M., O'Shea-Greenfield, A., Hartley, M., Deneris, E., Maron, C., and Heinemann, S. (1990). Molecular cloning and functional expression of glutamate receptor subunit genes. *Science*, **249**, 1033–7.

Bouvier, M., Collins, S., O'Dowd, B. F., Campbell, P. T., de Blasi, A., Kobilka, B. K., MacGregor, C., Irons, G. P., Caron, M. G., and Lefkowitz, R. J. (1989). Two distinct pathways for cAMP mediated down regulation of the β_2-adrenergic receptor. *Journal of Biological Chemistry*, **264**, 16786–92.

Bowen, D. M. (1990). Treatment of Alzheimer's disease. Molecular pathology versus neurotransmitter-based therapy. *British Journal of Psychiatry*, **157**, 327–30.

Bowen, D. M., Najlerahim, A., Procter, A. W., Francis, P. T., and Murphy, E. (1989). Circumscribed changes in the cerebral cortex in neuropsychiatric disorders of later life. *Proceedings of the National Academy of Sciences of the USA*, **86**, 9504–8.

Brandt, J. and Butters, N. (1986). The neuropsychology of Huntington's disease. *Trends in Neurosciences*, **9**, 118–20.

Breitner, J. C. S. (1990). Life table methods and assessment of familial risk in Alzheimer's disease. *Archives of General Psychiatry*, **47**, 395–6.

Breitner, J. C. S. and Folstein, M. F. (1984). Familial Alzheimer dementia: a prevalent disorder with specific clinical features. *Psychological Medicine*, **14**, 63–80.

Brown, P. (1990). Researchers divided over Alzheimer's and aluminium. *New Scientist*, **127**, 21.

Brown, A. and Birnbaumer, L. (1990). Ionic channels and their regulation by G-protein subunits. *Annual Review of Physiology*, **52**, 197–213.

Brown, R. G. and Marsden, C. D. (1990). Cognitive function in Parkinson's disease: from description to theory. *Trends in Neurosciences*, **13**, 21–9.

Brown, R., Colter, N., Corsellis, A. N., Crow, T. J., Firth, C. D., Tagoe, R., Johnstone, E. C., and Marsh, L. (1986). Postmortem evidence of structural brain changes in schizophrenia. *Archives of General Psychiatry*, **43**, 36–42.

Browning, M. D., Bureau, M., Dudek, E. M., and Olsen, R. W. (1990). Protein kinase C and cyclic AMP dependent protein kinase phosphorylate the β subunit of the purified γ-aminobutyric acid receptor. *Proceedings of the National Academy of the Sciences of the USA*, **87**, 1315–18.

Burns, A., Lewis, G., Jakoby, R., and Levy, R. (1991). Factors affecting survival in Alzheimer's disease. *Psychological Medicine*, **21**, 363–70.

Burns, A., Philpot, M. P., Costa, D. C., Ell, P. J., and Levy, R. (1989). The investigation of Alzheimer's disease with single photon emission tomography. *Journal of Neurology, Neurosurgery and Psychiatry*, **52**, 248–53.

Buss, J. E., Mumby, S. M., Casey, P. J., Gilman, A. G., and Sefton, B. M. (1987). Myristoylated α subunits of guanine nucleotide binding regulatory proteins. *Proceedings of National Academy of Sciences of the USA*, **84**, 7493–7.

Calne, D. B. (1989). Current concepts on the aetiology of Parkinson's disease. *Movement Disorders*, **4** suppl. 1, S11–S14.

Calne, D. B. and Langston, J. W. (1983). Aetiology of Parkinson's disease. *Lancet*, **ii**, 1457–9.

Calne, D. B. and McGeer, P. L. (1988). Tissue transplantation for Parkinson's disease. *Canadian Journal of the Neurological Sciences*, **15**, 364–5.

Calne, D. B., Langston, J. W., Martin, W. R. W., Stoessl, A. J., Ruth, T. J., Adam, M. J., Pale, B. D., and Shulzer, M. (1985). Positron emission tomography after MPTP: observations relating to the cause of Parkinson's disease. *Nature*, **317**, 246–8.

Calne, D. B., Ersen, A., McGeer, E., and Spencer, P. (1986). Alzheimer's disease, Parkinson's disease and motor neurone disease: abiotrophic interaction between ageing and environment. *Lancet*, **ii**, 1067–70.

Carlsson, A., Lindquist, M., and Magnusson, T. (1957). 3,4-dihydroxyphenylalanine and 5-hydroxytryptamine as reserpine antagonists. *Nature*, **180**, 1200.

Carpenter, G. (1987). Receptors for epidermal growth factor and other polypeptide mitogens. *Annual Review of Biochemistry*, **56**, 881–914.

Carpenter, G. A. and Grossberg, S. (1988). The ART of adaptive pattern recognition by a self-organising neural network. *Computer*, **21**, 77–8.

Carpenter, G. A. and Grossberg, S. (1990). ART 3: Hierarchical search using chemical transmitters in self organising pattern recognition architectures. *Neural Networks*, **3**, 129–52.

Carter, C. J., Benavides, J., and Dubois, A. (1989). The biochemistry of Huntington's chorea. In *Disorders of movement* (ed. N. P. Quinn and P. G. Jenner), pp. 469–94. Academic Press, London.

Casey, P. J., Fong, K. W., Simon, M. I., and Gilman, A. G. (1990). G_z a guanine nucleotide binding protein with unique biochemical properties. *Journal of Biological Chemistry*, **265**, 2383–90.

Caspar, D. L. D. (1990). Bacteriorhodopsin—at last! *Nature*, **345**, 666–7.

Catalan, J. and Gath, D. H. (1985). Benzodiazepines in general practice: time for a decision. *British Medical Journal*, **290**, 1374–6.

Catalan, J., Gath, D., Edmonds, G., and Ennis, J. (1984). The effects of non-prescribing of anxiolytics in general practice. *British Journal of Psychiatry*, **144**, 593–602.

Catterall, W. A. (1988). Structure and function of voltage sensitive ion channels. *Science*, **242**, 50–61.

Changeux, J. P. (1985). *Neuronal man*. Oxford University Press.

Chaput, Y., De Montigny, C., and Blier, P. (1986). Effects of a selective 5HT uptake blocker, citalopram on the sensitivity of 5HT autoreceptors: electrophysiological studies in the rat brain. *Naunyn Schmiedeberg's Archives of Pharmacology*, **333**, 342–8.

Charlton, B. G. and Ferrier, I. N. (1989). Hypothalamo-pituitary-adrenal axis abnormalities in depression: a review and a model. *Psychological Medicine*, **19**, 331–6.

Charney, D. S., Menker, D. B., and Heninger, G. R. (1981). Receptor sensitivity and the mechanism of action of antidepressant treatment. *Archives of General Psychiatry*, **38**, 1160–80.

Charney, D. S., Heninger, G. R., and Sternberg, D. E. (1983). Alpha-2 adrenergic receptor sensitivity and the mechanism of antidepressant treatment. *British Journal of Psychiatry*, **142**, 265–75.

Charney, D. S., Heninger, G. R., and Breier, A. (1984a). Noradrenergic function in panic anxiety. *Archives of General Psychiatry*, **41**, 751–63.

Charney, D. S., Heninger, G. R., and Sternberg, D. E. (1984b). Serotonin function and mechanism of action of antidepressant treatment. *Archives of General Psychiatry*, **41**, 359–65.

Checkley, S. A. (1980). Neuroendocrine tests of monoamine function in man: a review of basic theory and its application to the study of depressive illness. *Psychological Medicine*, **10**, 35–53.

Chiu, S. Y., Ritchie, J. M., Rogart, R. B., and Stagg, D. (1979). A quantitative description of membrane currents in rabbit myelinated nerve. *Journal of Physiology* (London), **292**, 149–66.

Claridge, G. (1985). *Origins of mental illness*. Blackwell, Oxford.

Clark, D. M., Salkovski, P. M., Gelder, M., Koehler, C., Martin, M., Anastasiades, P., Hackmann, A., Middleton, H., and Jeavons, A. (1988). Tests of a cognitive theory of panic. In *Panic and phobias 2* (ed. I. Hand and H. U. Wittchen), pp. 149–58. Springer Verlag, Berlin.

Clark, R. B., Friedman, J., Dixon, R. A. F., and Strader, C. D. (1989). Identification of a specific site required for rapid heterologous desensitisation of the β-adrenergic receptor by cAMP-dependent protein kinase. *Molecular Pharmacology*, **36**, 343–8.

Coleman, P. D. and Flood, D. G. (1987). Neuron numbers and dendritic extent in normal ageing and in Alzheimer's disease. *Neurobiology of Ageing*, **8**, 521–45.

Collerton, D. (1986). Cholinergic function and intellectual decline in Alzheimer's disease. *Neuroscience*, **19**, 1–28.

Collinge, J., Owen, F., Poulter, M., Leach, M., Crow, T. J., Rossor, M. N., Hardy, J., Mullan, M. J., Janota, I., and Lantos, P. L. (1990). Prion dementia without characteristic pathology. *Lancet*, **336**, 7–9.

Conrad, A. J., Akebe, T., Austin, R., Forsythe, S., and Scherbet, A. B. (1991). Hippocampal pyramidal cell disarray in schizophrenia as a bilateral phenomenon. *Archives of General Psychiatry*, **48**, 413–17.

Conti-Tronconi, B. M. and Raftery, M. A. (1982). Nicotinic cholinergic receptors. *Annual Review of Biochemistry*, **51**, 491–530.

Cooper, J. R., Bloom, F. E., and Roth, R. H. (1986). *The biochemical basis of neuropharmacology*. Oxford University Press, New York.

Cotzias, G. C., Papavisiliou, P. S., and Gellene, R. (1967). L-Dopa in Parkinson's syndrome. *New England Journal of Medicine*, **281**, 272–8.

Cowburn, R. F., Hardy, J. A., and Roberts, P. J. (1990). Glutamatergic neurotransmission in Alzheimer's disease. *Biochemical Society Transactions*, **18**, 390–2.

Cowen, P. J. (1990). A role for 5-HT in the action of antidepressant drugs. *Pharmacology and Therapeutics*, **46**, 43–51.

Crews, F. T. and Smith, C. B. (1978). Presynaptic alpha receptor subsensitivity after long term antidepressant treatment. *Science*, **202**, 322–4.

Crews, F. T. and Smith, C. B. (1980). Potentiation of responses to adrenergic nerve stimulation in isolated rat atria during chronic tricylic antidepressant administration. *Journal of Pharmacology and Experimental Therapeutics*, **215**, 143–9.

Critchley, M. (1984). History of Huntington's chorea. *Psychological Medicine*, **14**, 725–7.

Crossman, A. R. (1990). A hypothesis on the pathophysiological mechanisms that underlie levodopa or dopamine agonist induced dyskinesia in Parkinson's disease: implications for future strategies in treatment. *Movement Disorders*, **5**, 100–8.

Crossman, A. R., Mitchell, I. J., Sambrook, M. A., and Jackson, A. (1988). Chorea and myoclonus in the monkey induced by gamma aminobutyric acid antagonism in the lentiform complex. *Brain*, **111**, 1211–33.

Crow, T. J. (1973). Catecholamine-containing neurones and electrical self-stimulation: 1. A theoretical interpretation and some psychiatric implications. *Psychological Medicine*, **3**, 66–73.

Crow, T. J. (1980). Molecular pathology of schizophrenia: more than one disease process? *British Medical Journal*, **280**, 66–8.

Crow, T. J. (1985). The two syndrome concept: origins and current status. *Schizophrenia Bulletin*, **11**, 471–86.

Crow, T. J. (1986). The continuum of psychosis and its implication for the structure of the gene. *British Journal of Psychiatry*, **149**, 419–29.

Crow, T. J. (1988*a*). The viral theory of schizophrenia. *British Journal of Psychiatry*, **153**, 564–6.

Crow, T. J. (1988*b*). Sex chromosomes and psychosis. *British Journal of Psychiatry*, **153**, 675–83.

Crow, T. J. (1989). A current view of the type II syndrome: age of onset, intellectual impairment, and the meaning of structural changes in the brain. *British Journal of Psychiatry*, **155** (suppl. 7), 15–20.

Crow, T. J. (1990). The continuum of psychosis and its genetic origins. *British Journal of Psychiatry*, **156**, 788–97.

Crow, T. J., Johnstone, E. C., Longden, A., Owen, F., and Riley, G. (1977). The role of dopamine in the antipsychotic effect and the pathogenesis of schizophrenia. *Proceedings of the Royal Society of Medicine*, **70** (suppl. 10), 15–19.

Crow, T. J., Ball, J., Bloom, S. R., Brown, R., Bruton, C. J., Colter, N., Frith, C. D., Johnstone, E. C., Owens, D. G. C., and Roberts, G. W. (1989). Schizophrenia as an anomaly of development of cerebral asymmetry. *Archives of General Psychiatry*, **46**, 1145–50.

D'Amato, R. J., Lipman, Z. P., and Snyder, S. H. (1986). Selectivity of parkinsonian neurotoxin MPTP: toxic metabolite MPP+ binds to neuromelanin. *Science*, **231**, 987–9.

Davies, S. W. and Roberts, P. J. (1988*a*). Sparing of cholinergic neurones following quinolinic acid lesions of the rat striatum. *Neuroscience*, **26**, 387–93.

Davies, S. W. and Roberts, P. J. (1988*b*). Model of Huntington's disease. *Science*, **241**, 474–5.

Davis, M. (1991). The role of the amygdala in conditioned fear. In *The amygdala: neurobiological aspects of emotion, memory, and mental dysfunction.* (ed. J. Aggleton), pp.255–305. John Wiley, New York.

Deakin, J. F. W. and Graeff, F. G. (1991). 5HT and mechanisms of defence, *Journal of Psychopharmacology* **5**, 305–15.

Deakin, J. F. W., Slater, P., Simpson, M. D. C., Gilchrist, A. C., Skan, W. J., Royston, M. C., Reynolds, G. P., and Cross, A. J. (1989). Frontal cortical and left temporal glutamatergic dysfunction in schizophrenia. *Journal of Neurochemistry*, **52**, 1781–6.

De Camilli, P. and Jahn, R. (1990). Pathways to regulated exocytosis in neurons. *Annual Review of Physiology*, **52**, 625–45.

De Montigny, C. and Blier, P. (1991). Desensitisation of terminal 5HT autoreceptors by 5HT reuptake blockers. *Archives of General Psychiatry*, **48**, 483–4.

De Robertis, E., Pena, C., Paladini, A. C., and Medina, J. H. (1988). New developments in the search for the endogenous ligand(s) of central benzodiazepine receptors. *Neurochemistry International*, **13**, 1–11.

Dexter, D., Carter, C., Agid, F., Agid, Y., Lees, A. J., Jenner, P., and Marsden, C. D. (1986). Lipid peroxidation as cause of nigral cell death in Parkinson's disease. *Lancet*, **ii**, 639–40.

Dexter, D. T., Carter, C. J., Wells, F. R., Javoy-Agid, F., Agid, Y., Lees, A., Jenner, P., and Marsden, C. D. (1989*a*). Basal lipid peroxidation in substantia nigra is increased in Parkinson's disease. *Journal of Neurochemistry*, **52**, 381–9.

Dexter, D. T., Wells, F. R., Lees, A. J., Agid, Y., Agid, F., Jenner, P., and Marsden, C. D. (1989*b*). Increased nigral iron content and alterations in other metal ions occurring in brain in Parkinson's disease. *Journal of Neurochemistry*, **52**, 1830–6.

Dodd, P. R., Hambley, J. W., Cowburn, R. F., and Hardy, J. A. (1988). A comparison of methodologies for the study of functional transmitter neurochemistry in human brain. *Journal of Neurochemistry*, **50**, 1333–45.

Drummond, A. H. (1987). Lithium and inositol lipid linked signalling systems. *Trends in Pharmacological Sciences*, **8**, 129–33.

Duggan, C. F., Lee, A. S., and Murray, R. M. (1990). Does personality predict long term outcome in depression? *British Journal of Psychiatry*, **157**, 19–24.

Dunbar, G. C., Perera, M. H., and Jenner, F. A. (1989). Patterns of benzodiazepine use in Great Britain as measured by a general population survey. *British Journal of Psychiatry*, **155**, 836–41.

Duncan, M. W., Steele, J. C., Kopin, I. J., and Markey, S. P. (1990). 2-amino-3-(methylamino)-propanoic acid in cycad flour: an unlikely cause of amyotrophic lateral sclerosis and parkinsonism–dementia of Guam. *Neurology*, **40**, 767–72.

Duvoisin, R. C. (1989). New strategies in dopaminergic therapy of Parkinson's disease: the use of a controlled release formulation. *Neurology*, **39** (suppl. 2), 4–106.

Duyckaerts, C., Delaere, P., Poulain, V., Brion, J. P., and Hauw, J. J. (1988). Does amyloid precede paired helical filaments in the senile plaque? A study of 15 cases with graded intellectual status in ageing and Alzheimer's disease. *Neuroscience Letters*, **91**, 354–9.

Eagger, S. A., Levy, R., and Sahakian, B. J. (1991). Tacrine in Alzheimer's disease. *Lancet*, **337**, 989–92.

Edelman, G. M. (1987). *Neural Darwinism*. Oxford University Press.

Edelman, G. M. and Mountcastle, V. B. (1978). *The mindful brain*. MIT Press, Cambridge, MA.

Egeland, J. A., Gerhard, D. S., Pauls, D. L., Sussex, J. N., Kidd, K. K., Allen, C. R., Hostelter, A. M., and Housman, D. E. (1987). Bipolar affective disorders linked to DNA markers on chromosome 11. *Nature*, **325**, 783–7.

Elkin, I., Shea, M. T., Watkins, J. T., Imber, S. D. Sotsky, S. M., Collins, J. F., Glass, D. R., Pilkonis, P. A., Leber, W. R., Docherty, J. P., Fiester, S. J., and Parloff, M. B. (1989). National Institute of Mental Health treatment of depression collaborative research program. *Archives of General Psychiatry*, **46**, 971–82.

Ellison, D. W., Beal, M. F., Mazurek, M. F., Malloy, J. R., Bird, E. D., and Martin, J. B. (1987). Amino acid neurotransmitter abnormalities in Huntington's disease and the quinolinic acid model of Huntington's disease. *Brain*, **110**, 1657–73.

Esiri, M. M., Pearson, R. C. A., Steele, J. E., Bowen, D. M., and Powell, T. P. S. (1990). A quantitative study of the neurofibrillary tangles and the choline acetyltransferase activity in the cerebral cortex and amygdala in Alzheimer's disease. *Journal of Neurology, Neurosurgery and Psychiatry*, **53**, 161–5.

Everall, I. P. and Kerwin, R. (1990). The role of nerve growth factor in Alzheimer's disease. *Psychological Medicine*, **20**, 249–51.

Farrer, L. A., Myers, R. H., Cupples, L. A., St George-Hyslop, P. H., Bird, T. D., Rossor, M. N., Mullan, M. J., Plinsky, R., Nee, L., Heston, L., Van Broeckhoven, C., Martin, J. J., Crapper McLachlan, C., and Growden, J. H. (1990). Transmission and age at onset patterns in familial Alzheimer's disease. *Neurology*, **40**, 395–403.

Ferry, G. (1987). New light on Parkinson's disease. *New Scientist*, **113**, 56–60.

Fertuck, H. C. and Salpeter, M. M. (1976). Quantitation of junctional and extrajunctional acetylcholine receptors by electron microscope autoradiography after ^{125}I-α-bungarotoxin binding at mouse neuromuscular junctions. *Journal of Cell Biology*, **69**, 144–58.

Fibiger, H. C. and Lloyd, K. G. (1984). Neurobiological substrates of tardive dyskinesia: the GABA hypothesis. *Trends in Neurosciences*, **7**, 462–4.

File, S. E. (1987). The search for novel anxiolytics. *Trends in Neurosciences*, **10**, 461–3.

Findlay, J. B. C. and Pappin, D. J. C. (1986). The opsin family of proteins. *Biochemical Journal*, **238**, 625–42.

Fodor, J. A. (1983). *The modularity of mind*. Bradford Books, The MIT Press, Cambridge, MA and London, UK.

Fontaine, R., Breton, G., Dery, R., Fontaine, S., and Elie, R. (1990). Temporal lobe abnormalities in panic disorder: an MRI study. *Biological Psychiatry*, **27**, 304–10.

Foote, S. L. and Morrison, J. H. (1987). Extrathalamic modulation of cortical function. *Annual Review of Neuroscience*, **10**, 67–95.

Foote, S. L., Bloom, F. E., Aston-Jones, G. (1983). Nucleus locus coeruleus: new evidence of anatomical and physiological specificity. *Physiological Reviews*, **63**, 844–914.

Frankel, J. P., Lees, A. J., Kempster, P. A., and Stern, G. M. (1990). Subcutaneous apomorphine in the treatment of Parkinson's disease. *Journal of Neurology, Neurosurgery and Psychiatry*, **53**, 96–101.

Freed, W. J. (1990). Fetal brain grafts and Parkinson's disease. *Science*, **250**, 1434.

Freed, C. R., Breeze, R. E., Rosenberg, N. L., Schneck, S. A., Wells, T. H., Barrett, J. N., Grafton, S. T., Huang, S., Edelberg, D., and Rottenberg, D. A. (1990). Transplantation of human fetal dopamine cells for Parkinson's disease. Results at one year. *Archives of Neurology*, **47**, 505–12.

Freeman, H. (1988). Progress in antidepressant therapy. *British Journal of Psychiatry*, **153** (suppl. 3), 1–112.

Freissmuth, M., Casey, P. J., and Gilman, A. G. (1989). G proteins control diverse pathways of transmembrane signalling. *FASEB Journal*, **3**, 2125–31.

Freund, T. F., Powell, J. F., and Smith, A. D. (1984). Tyrosine hydroxylase immunoreactive boutons in synaptic contact with identified striatonigral neurones, with particular reference to dendritic spines. *Neuroscience*, **13**, 1189–215.

Friedland, R. P., Brun, A., and Budinger, T. F. (1985). Pathological and positron emission tomographic correlations in Alzheimer's disease. *Lancet*, i, 228.

Frith, C. D. (1987). The positive and negative symptoms of schizophrenia reflect impairments in the perception and initiation of action. *Psychological Medicine*, **17**, 631–48.

Frith, C. D. and Done, D. J. (1988). Towards a neuropsychology of schizophrenia. *British Journal of Psychiatry*, **153**, 437–43.

Gabizon, R. and Prusiner, S. B. (1990). Prion liposomes. *Biochemical Journal*, **266**, 1–14.

Gallo, J. M. and Anderton, B. H. (1989). Ubiquitous variations in nerves. *Nature*, **337**, 687–8.

Garber, H. J., Ananth, J. V., Chui, L. C., Griswold, V. J., and Oldendorf, W. H. (1989). Nuclear magnetic resonance study of obsessive compulsive disorder. *American Journal of Psychiatry*, **146**, 1001–5.

Garruto, R. M. and Yase, Y. (1986). Neurodegenerative disorders of the Western Pacific: The search for the mechanism of pathogenesis. *Trends in Neurosciences*, **9**, 368–74.

Garruto, R. M., Yanagihara, R., and Gajdusek, D. C. (1988). Cycads and amyotrophic lateral sclerosis/parkinsonism dementia. *Lancet* ii, 1079.

Gelder, M. G. (1989). Panic disorder: fact or fiction? *Psychological Medicine*, **19**, 277–83.

Gelder, M., Gath, D., and Mayou, R. (1989). *Oxford textbook of psychiatry* (2nd edn). Oxford University Press.

Gerfen, C. R. (1984). The neostriatal mosaic. *Nature*, **311**, 461–4.

Gerfen, C. R. (1989). The neostriatal mosaic: striatal patch-matrix organisation is related to cortical lamination. *Science*, **246**, 385–8.

Gerfen, C. R., Engber, T. M., Mahan, L. C., Susel, Z., Chase, T. N., Monsma, F. J., and Sibley, D. R. (1990). D_1 and D_2 dopamine receptor-regulated gene expression of striatonigral and striatopallidal neurons. *Science*, **250**, 1429–32.

Gibb, W. R. G. (1989). Neuropathology in movement disorders. *Journal of Neurology, Neurosurgery and Psychiatry*, special supplement, 55–67.

Gibb, W. R. G. and Lees, A. J. (1988). The relevance of the Lewy body to the pathogenesis of idiopathic Parkinson's disease. *Journal of Neurology, Neurosurgery and Psychiatry*, **51**, 745–52.

Gilman, A. G. (1987). G proteins: transducers of receptor generated signals. *Annual Review of Biochemistry*, **56**, 615–49.

Glassman, A. H. (1987). The dexamethasone suppression test: an overview of its current status in psychiatry. *American Journal of Psychiatry*, **144**, 1253–62.

Goate, A., Chartier-Harlin, M. C., Mullan, M., Brown, J., Crawford, F., Fidani, L., Giufria, L., Haynes, A., Irving, N., James, L., Mant, R., Newton, P., Rooke, K., Roques, P., Talbot, C., Pericack-Vance, M., Roses, A., Williamson, R., Rosser, M., Owen, M., and Hardy, J. (1991). Segregation of a nonsense mutation in the amyloid precursor protein gene with familial Alzheimer's disease. *Nature*, **349**, 704–6.

Golbe, L. I., Iorio, G. D., Bonavita, V., Miller, D. C., and Duvoisin, R. C. (1990). A large kindred with autosomal dominant Parkinson's disease. *Annals of Neurology*, **27**, 276–82.

Goldberg, T. E., Weinberger, D. R., Berman, K. F., Pliskin, N. H., and Podd, M. H. (1987). Further evidence for dementia of the prefrontal type in schizophrenia. *Archives of General Psychiatry*, **44**, 1008–14.

Goldman-Rakic, P. S., Leranth, C., Williams, S. M., Mons, N., and Geffard, M. (1989). Dopamine synaptic complex with pyramidal neurons in primate cerebral cortex. *Proceedings of the National Academy of Sciences of the USA*, **86**, 9015–19.

Golds, P. R., Przyslo, F. R., and Strange, P. G. (1980). The binding of some antidepressant drugs to brain muscarinic acetylcholine receptors. *British Journal of Pharmacology*, **68**, 541–9.

Gonzales, R. A. and Hoffman, P. C. (1991). Receptor gated ion channels may be selective CNS targets for ethanol. *Trends in Pharmacological Sciences*, **12**, 1–3.

Goodman, W. K., Price, L. H., Delgado, P. L., Palumbo, J., Krystal, J. H., Nagy, L. M., Rasmussen, S. A., Heninger, G. R., and Charney, D. S. (1990). Specificity of serotonin reuptake inhibitors in the treatment of obsessive compulsive disorder. *Archives of General Psychiatry*, **47**, 577–85.

Gorman, J. M., Liebowitz, M. R., Fyer, A. J., and Stein, J. (1989). A neuroanatomical hypothesis for panic disorder. *American Journal of Psychiatry*, **146**, 148–61.

Gotham, A. M., Brown, R. G., and Marsden, C. D. (1988). Frontal cognitive function in patients with Parkinson's disease on and off levodopa. *Brain*, **111**, 299–321.

Gottesmann, I. I. and Bertelsen, A. (1989). Confirming unexpressed genotypes for schizophrenia. *Archives of General Psychiatry*, **46**, 867–72.

Grafstein, B. and Forman, D. S. (1980). Intracellular transport in neurones. *Physiological Reviews*, **60**, 1167–283.

Gray, J. A. (1987). *The psychology of fear and stress* (2nd edn). Cambridge University Press.

Graybiel, A. M. (1990). Neurotransmitters and neuromodulators in the basal ganglia. *Trends in Neurosciences*, **13**, 244–54.

Green, A. R. and Costain, D. (1981). *Pharmacology and biochemistry of psychiatric disorders*. Wiley, Chichester.

Guiroy, D. C., Miyazaki, M., Multlaup, G., Fischer, P., Garruto, R. M., Beyreuther, K., Masters, C. L., Simms, G., Gibbs, C. J., and Gajdusek, C. (1987). Amyloid of neurofibrillary tangles of guamanian parkinsonism dementia and Alzheimer's disease share identical amino acid sequence. *Proceedings of the National Academy of Sciences of the USA*, **84**, 2073–7.

Gunne, L. M., Haggstrom, J. E., and Sjoquist, B. (1984). Association with persistent neuroleptic induced dyskinesia of regional changes in brain GABA synthesis. *Nature*, **309**, 347–9.

Gusella, J. F. (1989). Location cloning strategy for characterising genetic defects in Huntington's disease and Alzheimer's disease. *FASEB Journal*, **3**, 2036–41.

Guyenet, P. G. and Aghajanian, G. K. (1978). Antidromic identification of dopaminergic and other output neurones of the rat substantia nigra. *Brain Research*, **150**, 69–84.

Hailey, A. (1985). *Strong medicine*. Pan Books, London.

Harding, A. E. (1991). Neurological disease and mitochondrial genes. *Trends in Neurosciences*, **14**, 132–8.

Hardy, J. (1988). Molecular biology and Alzheimer's disease: more questions than answers. *Trends in Neurosciences*, **11**, 293–4.

Harrison, P. J., McLaughlin, D., and Kerwin, R. W. (1991). Decreased hippocampal expression of a glutamate receptor gene in schizophrenia. *Lancet*, **337**, 450–2.

Hausdorff, W. P., Caron, M. G., and Lefkowitz, R. J. (1990). Turning off the signal: desensitisation of β-adrenergic receptor function. *FASEB Journal*, **4**, 2881–9.

Haxby, J. V., Grady, C. L., Koss, E., Horwitz, B., Heston, L., Schapiro, M., Friedland, R. P., and Rapoport, S. I. (1990). Longitudinal study of cerebral metabolic asymmetries and associated neuropsychological patterns in early dementia of the Alzheimer type. *Archives of Neurology*, **47**, 753–60.

Heal, D. J., Philipot, J., Molyneux, S. G., and Metz, A. (1985). Intracerebroventricular administration of 5,7-dihydroxytryptamine to mice increases both head-twitch response and the number of cortical $5HT_2$ receptors. *Neuropharmacology*, **24**, 1201–5.

Henderson, R., Baldwin, J. M., Ceska, T. A., Zemtin, F., Beckmann, E., and Downing, K. H. (1990). Model for the structure of bacteriorhodopsin based on high resolution electron cryomicroscopy. *Journal of Molecular Biology*, **213**, 899–929.

Heninger, G. R., Charney, D. S., and Sternberg, D. E. (1984). Serotonergic function in depression. *Archives of General Psychiatry*, **41**, 398–402.

Heninger, G. R., Charney, D. S., and Price, L. H. (1988). α_2-adrenergic receptor sensitivity in depression. *Archives of General Psychiatry*, **45**, 718–26.

Herve, D., Pickel, V. M., Joh, T. H., and Beaudet, A. (1987). Serotonin axon terminals in the ventral tegmental area of the rat: fine structure and synaptic input to dopaminergic neurons. *Brain Research*, **435**, 71–83.

Heuser, J. E. and Reese, T. S. (1981). Structural changes after transmitter release at the frog neuromuscular junction. *Journal of Cell Biology*, **88**, 564–80.

Heuser, J. E., Reese, T. S., Dennis, M. J., Jan, Y., Jan, L., and Evans, L. (1979). Synaptic vesicle exocytosis captured by quick freezing and correlated with quantal release. *Journal of Cell Biology*, **81**, 275–300.

Higashida, H. and Brown, D. A. (1986). Two polyphosphatidylinositide metabolites control two K^+ currents in a neuronal cell. *Nature*, **323**, 333–5.

Higgitt, A. C., Lader, M. H., and Fonagy, P. (1985). Clinical management of benzodiazepine dependence. *British Medical Journal*, **291**, 688–90.

Hirokawa, N., Sobue, K., Kanda, K., Harada, A., and Yorifuji, H. (1989). The cytoskeletal architecture of the presynaptic terminal and molecular structure of synapsin I. *Journal of Cell Biology*, **108**, 111–26.

Hirsch, E., Graybiel, A. M., and Agid, Y. A. (1988). Melanized dopaminergic neurons are differentially susceptible to degeneration in Parkinson's disease. *Nature*, **334**, 345–8.

Hodgkin, A. L. and Huxley, A. F. (1952). A quantitative description of membrane circuits and its application to conductance and excitation in nerve. *Journal of Physiology* (London), **117**, 500–44.

Holt, T. A. and Phillips, J. (1988). Bovine spongiform encephalopathy. *British Medical Journal*, **296**, 1581–2.

Hollister, L. E. (1986). Current antidepressants. *Annual Review of Pharmacology and Toxicology* **26**, 23–37.

Hornykiewicz, O. (1973). Dopamine in the basal ganglia. *British Medical Bulletin*, **29**, 172–8.

Hsu, Y. P. P., Powell, J. F., Sims, K. B., and Breakfield, X. O. (1989). Molecular genetics of the monoamine oxidases. *Journal of Neurochemistry*, **53**, 12–18.

Hubel, D. H. and Wiesel, T. N. (1979). Brain mechanisms of vision. *Scientific American*, **241**(3), 130–44.

Hughes, A. J., Bishop, S., Lees, A. J., Stein, G., Webster, R., and Bovingdon, M. (1991). Rectal apomorphine in Parkinson's disease. *Lancet*, **337**, 118.

Hyman, B. T., Hoesen, G. W. V., Damasio, A. R., and Barnes, C. L. (1984). Alzheimer's disease: cell specific pathology isolates the hippocampus. *Science*, **225**, 1168–70.

Ikebe, S., Tanaka, M., Ohno, K., Sato, W., Hattori, K., Kondo, T., Mizuno, Y., and Ozawa, T. (1990). Increase in deleted mitochondrial DNA in the striatum in Parkinson's disease and senescence. *Biochemical and Biophysical Research Communications*, **170**, 1044–8.

Ishiura, S. (1991). Proteolytic cleavage of the Alzheimer's disease amyloid A4 precursor protein. *Journal of Neurochemistry*, **56**, 363–9.

Ito, M. (1984). *The cerebellum and neural control*. Raven Press, New York.

Izquierdo, I. (1989). A game with shifting mirrors. *Trends in Pharmacological Sciences*, **10**, 473–6.

Jakob, H. and Beckmann, H. (1989). Gross and histological criteria for developmental disorders in brains of schizophrenics. *Journal of the Royal Society of Medicine*, **82**, 466–9.

Janowsky, D. S., El-Yousef, M. K., Davis, J. M., Hubbard, B., and Sekerke, H. J. (1972). Cholinergic reversal of manic symptoms. *Lancet*, **i**, 1236–7.

Janssen, P. A. J. and Van Beven, W. F. M. (1978). Neuroleptics as antagonists of apomorphine induced sterotyped behaviour in rats. *Handbook of Psychopharmacology*, **10**, 1–36.

Jeste, D. V. and Wyatt, R. J. (1982). Therapeutic strategies against tardive dyskinesia: two decades of experience. *Archives of General Psychiatry*, **39**, 803–16.

Jeste, D. V., Lohr, J. B., and Goodwin, F. K. (1988). Neuroanatomical studies of major affective disorders. *British Journal of Psychiatry*, **153**, 444–59.

Jimenez Castellanos, J. and Graybiel, A. M. (1987). Subdivisions of the dopamine containing A8–A9–A10 complex identified by their different mesostriatal innervation of striosomes and extrastriosomal matrix. *Neuroscience*, **23**, 223–42.

Jinnai, K. and Matsuda, Y. (1979). Neurons of the motor cortex projecting commonly on the caudate nucleus and the lower brainstem in the cat. *Neuroscience Letters*, **13**, 121–6.

Joachim, C. L., Mori, H., and Selkoe, D. J. (1989). Amyloid β-protein deposition in tissues other than brain in Alzheimer's disease. *Nature*, **341**, 226–30.

Johnson, W. G., Hodge, S. E., and Duvoisin, R. (1990). Twin studies and the genetics of Parkinson's disease—a reappraisal. *Movement Disorders*, **5**, 187–94.

Johnstone, E. C., Cunningham-Owens, D. G., Frith, C. D., McPherson, K., Dowie, C., Riley, G., and Gold, A. (1980). Neurotic illness and its response to anxiolytic and antidepressant treatment. *Psychological Medicine*, **10**, 321–8.

Johnstone, E. C., Owens, D. G. C., Crow, T. J., Frith, C. D., Alexandropolis, K., Bydden, G., and Colter, N. (1989). Temporal lobe structure as determined by nuclear magnetic resonance in schizophrenia and bipolar affective disorder. *Journal of Neurology, Neurosurgery and Psychiatry*, **52**, 736–41.

Jones, E. G. and Powell, T. P. S. (1970). An anatomical study of converging sensory pathways within the cerebral cortex of the monkey. *Brain*, **93**, 793–820.

Jones, E. G. and Hendry, S. H. C. (1986). Colocalisation of GABA and neuropeptides in neocortical neurones. *Trends in Neurosciences*, **9**, 71–6.

Jones, P. and Murray, R. M. (1991). The genetics of schizophrenia is the genetics of neurodevelopment. *British Journal of Psychiatry*, **158**, 615–23.

Kahn, R. J., McNair, D. M., Lipman, R. S., Cori, L., Richels, K., Downing, R., Fisher, S., and Frankenthaler, L. M. (1986). Imipramine and chlordiazepoxide in depressive and anxiety disorders, II, Efficacy in anxious outpatients. *Archives of General Psychiatry*, **43**, 79–85.

Kane, J. M. and Smith, J. M. (1982). Tardive dyskinsia: prevalence and risk factors, 1959–79. *Archives of General Psychiatry*, **39**, 473–81.

Kane, J. M., Honigfeld, G., Singer, J., and Meltzer, H. Y., and the Clozaril collaborative study group (1988). Clozapine for the treatment—resistant schizophrenic. *Archives of General Psychiatry*, **45**, 789–96.

Kapoor, R., Turjanski, N., Frankel, J., Kleedorfer, B., Lees, A., and Stern, G. (1990). Intranasal apomorphine: a new treatment for Parkinson's Disease. *Journal of Neurology, Neurosurgery and Psychiatry*, **53**, 1015.

Kawata, M., Matsui, Y., Kondo, J., Hishida, T., Teranishi, Y., and Takai, Y. (1988). A novel small molecular weight GTP binding protein with the same putative effector domain as the ras proteins in bovine brain membranes. *Journal of Biological Chemistry*, **263**, 18965–71.

Kay, D. W. K. (1989). Genetics, Alzheimer's disease and senile dementia. *British Journal of Psychiatry*, **154**, 311–20.

Kelso, J. R., Ginns, E. I., Egeland, J. A., Gerhard, D. S., Goldstein, A. M., Bale, S. J., Pauls, D. L., Long, R. T., Kidd, K. K., Conte, G., Housman, D. E., and Paul, S. M. (1989). Reevaluation of the linkage relationship between chromosome 11p loci and the gene for bipolar affective disorder in the Old Order Amish. *Nature*, **342**, 238–42.

Kendell, R. E. (1981). The present status of electroconvulsive therapy. *British Journal of Psychiatry*, **139**, 265–83.

Kennedy, M. B. (1988). Synaptic memory molecules. *Nature*, **335**, 770–2.

Kenny, A. J. and Maroux, S. (1982). Topology of microvillar membrane hydrolases of kidney and intestine. *Physiologial Reviews*, **62**, 91–128.

Kerwin, R. W. (1989). How do the neuropathological changes of schizophrenia relate to pre-existing neurotransmitter and aetiological hypotheses. *Psychological Medicine*, **19**, 563–7.

Kerwin, R. W., Patel, S., Meldrum, B. S., Czudek, C., and Reynolds, G. P. (1988). Asymmetrical loss of glutamate receptor subtype in left hippocampus in schizophrenia. *Lancet*, i, 583–4.

Kimelberg, H. K. and Norenberg, M. D. (1989). Astrocytes. *Scientific American*, **260**(4), 44–52.

Kish, S. J., Chang, L. J., Mirchandani, L., Shannak, K., and Hornykiewicz, O. (1985). Progressive supra-nuclear palsy: relationship between extrapyramidal disturbances, dementia and brain neurotransmitter markers. *Annals of Neurology*, **18**, 530–6.

Kish, S. J., Shannak, K., and Hornykiewicz, O. (1988). Uneven pattern of dopamine loss in the striatum of patients with idiopathic Parkinson's disease. *New England Journal of Medicine*, **318**, 876–90.

Koller, W., Vetere-Overfeld, B., Gray, C., Alexander, C., Cin, T., Dolezal, J., Harsarein, R., and Tanner, C. (1990). Environmental risk factors in Parkinson's disease. *Neurology*, **40**, 1218–22.

Kosterlitz, H. (1979). The best laid schemes o' mice an' men gang aft agley. *Annual Review of Pharmacology and Toxicology*, **19**, 1–12.

Krupinski, J., Coussen, F., Bakalyar, H. A., Tang, W., Feinstein, P. G., Orth, K., Slaughter, C., Reed, R. R., and Gilman, A. G. (1989). Adenylyl cyclase amino acid sequence: possible channel or transporter like structure. *Science*, **244**, 1558–64.

Kuffler, S. W., Nicholls, J. G., and Martin, A. R. (1984). *From neuron to brain* (2nd edn). Sinauer Associates, Inc., Sunderland, MA.

Kwatra, M. M., Benovic, J. L., Caron, M. G., Lefkowitz, R. J., and Hosey, M. M. (1989). Phosphorylation of chick heart muscarinic cholinergic receptors by β-adrenergic receptor kinase. *Biochemistry*, **28**, 4543–7.

Lader, M. H. and File, S. E. (1987). The biological basis of benzodiazepine dependence. *Psychological Medicine*, **17**, 539–47.

Landis, D. M. D., Hall, A. K., Weinstein, L. A., and Reese, T. S. (1988). The organisation of cytoplasm at the presynaptic active zone of a central nervous synapse. *Neuron*, **1**, 201–9.

Langston, J. W. (1985). Mechanism of MPTP toxicity: more answers, more questions. *Trends in Pharmacological Sciences*, **6**, 375–8.

Laplane, D., Levasseur, M., Pillon, B., Dubois, B., Baulec, M., Mazoyer, B., Tran Dinh, S., Sette, G., Danze, F., and Baron, J. C. (1989). Obsessive compulsive and other behavioural changes with bilateral basal ganglia lesions. *Brain*, **112**, 699–725.

Lapper, S. R. and Bolam, J. P. (1991). The anterograde and retrograde transport of neurobiotin in the central nervous system of the rat: comparison with biocytin. *Journal of Neuroscience Methods*, **39**, 163–74.

Lasek, R. (1988). Studying the intrinsic determinants of neuronal form and function. In *Intrinsic determinants of neuronal form and function* (ed. R. Lasek and M. M. Black), pp. 1–60. A. R. Liss, New York.

Lasek, R. J., Garner, J. A., and Brady, S. T. (1984). Axonal transport of the cytoplasmic matrix. *Journal of Cell Biology*, **99**, 212S–221S.

Lassen, N. A., Ingvar, D. H., and Skinhoj, E. (1978). Brain function and blood flow. *Scientific American*, **239**(4), 50–9.

Leff, J. (1978). Social and psychological causes of the acute attack. In *Schizophrenia towards a new synthesis* (ed. J. K. Wing), pp. 139–66. Academic Press, London.

Leff, J., Berkowitz, R., Shavit, N., Strachan, A., Glam, I., and Vaughn, C. (1989). A trial of family therapy v. a relatives group for schizophrenia. *British Journal of Psychiatry*, **154**, 58–66.

Lefkowitz, R. J. and Caron, M. G. (1988). The adrenergic receptors: models for the study of receptors coupled to guanine nucleotide regulatory proteins. *Journal of Biological Chemistry*, **263**, 4993–6.

Le Moal, M. and Simon, H. (1991). Mesocortical dopaminergic network: functional and regulatory roles. *Physiological Reviews*, **71**, 155–234.

Lewin, R. (1985). Clinical trial for Parkinson's disease. *Science*, **230**, 527–8.

Lewis, S. W. (1989). Congenital risk factors for schizophrenia. *Psychological Medicine*, **19**, 5–13.

Lewis, D. A., Campbell, W. J., Terry, R. D., and Morrison, J. H. (1987). Laminar and regional distributions of neurofibrillary tangles and neuritic plaques in Alzheimer's disease: a quantitative study of visual and auditory cortices. *Journal of Neuroscience*, **7**, 1799–808.

Leysen, J. E. and Niemegeers, C. J. E. (1985). Neuroleptics. *Handbook of neurochemistry*, (2nd edn). Vol. 9, (ed. A., Lajtha), pp. 331–61. Plenum Press, New York.

Liddle, P. F. (1987). Schizophrenic syndromes, cognitive performance and neurological dysfunction. *Psychological Medicine*, **17**, 49–57.

Liebowitz, M. R. (1989). Antidepressants in panic disorders. *British Journal of Psychiatry*, **155** (suppl. 6), 46–52.

Liggett, S. B., Caron, M. G, Lefkowitz, R. J., and Hnatowich, M. (1991). Coupling of a mutated form of the human β_2-adrenergic receptor to G_i and G_s. *Journal of Biological Chemistry*, **266**, 4816–21.

Linden, J. and Delahunty, T. M. (1989). Receptors that inhibit phosphoinositide breakdown. *Trends in Pharmacological Sciences*, **10**, 114–20.

Lindvall, O. (1989). Transplantation into the human brain: present status and future possibilities. *Journal of Neurology, Neurosurgery and Psychiatry*, supplement, 39–54.

Lindvall, O. (1991). Prospects of transplantation in human neurodegenerative diseases. *Trends in Neurosciences*, **14**, 376–84.

Lindvall, O. and Bjorklund, A. (1982). Neuroanatomy of central dopamine pathways: review of recent progress. *Advances in the Biosciences*, **37**, 297–311.

Lindvall, O., Brundin, P., Widner, H., Rehnorona, S., Gustavii, B., Frackowiak, R., Leenders, K. L., Sawle, G., Rothwell, J. C., Marsden, C. D., and Bjorklund, A. (1990). Grafts of fetal dopamine neurons survive and improve motor function in Parkinson's disease. *Science*, **247**, 574–7.

Linsker, R. (1986*a*). From basic network principles to neural architecture: emergence of spatial opponent cells. *Proceedings of the National Academy of Sciences of the USA*, **83**, 7508–12.

Linsker, R. (1986*b*). From basic network principles to neural architecture: emergence of orientation-selective cells. *Proceedings of the National Academy of Sciences of the USA*, **83**, 8390–4.

Linsker, R. (1986*c*). From basic network principles to neural architecture: emergence of orientation columns. *Proceedings of the National Academy of Sciences of the USA*, **83**, 8779–83.

Linsker, R. (1988). Self organisation in a perceptual network. *Computer*, **21**, 105–17.

Linsker, R. (1990). Perceptual neural organisation: some approaches based on network models and information theory. *Annual Review of Neuroscience*, **13**, 257–81.

Lipscombe, D., Kongsamut, S., and Tsien, R. W. (1989). α-adrenergic inhibition of sympathetic neurotransmitter release mediated by modulation of N-type calcium channel gating. *Nature*, **340**, 639–42.

Lohse, M. J., Benovic, J. L., Codina, J., Caron, M. G., and Lefkowitz, R. J. (1990). β-Arrestin: a protein that regulates β-adrenergic receptor function. *Science*, **248**, 1547–9.

Lundberg, J. M. and Hokfelt, T. (1983). Coexistence of peptides and classical neurotransmitters. *Trends in Neurosciences*, **6**, 325–33.

Luxenberg, J. S., Swedo, S. E., Flament, M. F., Friedland, R. P., Rapoport, J., and Rapoport, S. I. (1988). Neuroanatomical abnormalities in obsessive compulsive disorder detected with quantitative X-ray computed tomography. *American Journal of Psychiatry*, **145**, 1089–93.

Maelicke, A. (1988). Structural similarities between ion channel proteins. *Trends in Biochemical Sciences*, **13**, 199–202.

Mahmood, T., Reveley, A. M., and Murray, R. M. (1983). Genetic studies of affective and anxiety disorders. In *The scientific basis of psychiatry* (ed. M. Weller), pp. 266–77. Bailliere-Tindal, London.

Mandel, J. L. (1989). Dystrophin—the gene and its product. *Nature*, **339**, 584–6.

Mann, D. M. A. (1984). Dopamine neurones of the vertebrate brain: some aspects of anatomy and pathology. In *The neurobiology of dopamine systems* (ed. W. Winlow and R. Markstein), pp. 87–103. Manchester University Press.

Manuelidis, E. E., de Figueiredo, J. M., Kim, J. H., Fritch, W. W., and Manuelidis, L. (1988). Transmission studies from blood of Alzheimer disease patients and healthy relatives. *Proceedings of the National Academy of Sciences of the USA*, **85**, 4898–901.

Manyam, B. V. (1990). Paralysis agitans and levodopa in 'Ayurveda': ancient Indian medical treatise. *Movement Disorders*, **5**, 47–8.

Marks, I. M. (1986). Genetics of fear and anxiety disorders. *British Journal of Psychiatry*, **149**, 406–18.

Marks, I. and O'Sullivan, G. (1988). Drugs and psychological treatments for agoraphobia/panic and obsessive–compulsive disorders: a review. *British Journal of Psychiatry*, **153**, 650–8.

Marsden, C. D. and Jenner, P. (1980). The pathophysiology of extrapyramidal side effects of neuroleptic drugs. *Psychological Medicine*, **10**, 55–72.

Martin, J. B. (1984). Huntington's disease. *Neurology*, **34**, 1059–72.

Martin, G. M., Schellenberg, G. D., Wijsman, E. M., and Bird, T. D. (1990). Alzheimer's disease. Dominant susceptibility genes. *Nature*, **347**, 124.

Martinot, J. L., Peron-Magnan, P., Huret, J. D., Mazoyer, B., Baron, J. C., Boulenger, J. P., Loch, C., Maziere, B., Coullard, V., Loo, H., and Synota, A. (1990). Striatal D_2dopaminergic receptors assessed with positron emission tomography and [^{76}Br]bromospiperone in untreated schizophrenic patients. *American Journal of Psychiatry*, **147**, 44–50.

Martyn, C. N., Osmond, C., Edwardson, J. A., Barker, D. J. P., Harris, E. C., and Lacey, R. F. (1989). Geographical relation between Alzheimer's disease and aluminium in drinking water. *Lancet*, i, 59–62.

Marx, J. L. (1987). Animals yield clues to Huntington's disease. *Science*, **238**, 1510–11.

Marx, J. L. (1988). Evidence uncovered for second Alzheimer's gene. *Science*, **241**, 1507–8.

Marx, J. (1990). NGF and Alzheimer's disease: hopes and fears. *Science*, **247**, 408–10.

Mayeux, R. (1990). Therapeutic strategies in Alzheimer's disease. *Neurology*, **40**, 175–80.

McCormick, D. A. (1989). Cholinergic and noradrenergic modulation of thalamocortical processing. *Trends in Neurosciences*, **12**, 215–21.

McEwen, B. S., De Kloet, E. R., and Rostene, W. (1986). Adrenal steroid receptors and actions in the nervous system. *Physiological Reviews*, **66**, 1121–88.

McGeer, P. L., Eccles, J. C., and McGeer, E. G. (1987a). *Molecular neurobiology of the mammalian brain*. Plenum Press, New York.

McGeer, P. L., McGeer, E. G., Itagaki, S., and Mizukawa, K. (1987b). Anatomy and pathology of the basal ganglia. *Canadian Journal of the Neurological Sciences*, **14** (suppl.), 363–72.

McGuffin, P. and Katz, R. (1989). The genetics of depression and manic-depressive disorders. *British Journal of Psychiatry*, **155**, 294–304.

McGuffin, P., Farmer, A., and Gottesman, I. I. (1987). Is there really a split in schizophrenia? The genetic evidence. *British Journal of Psychiatry*, **150**, 581–92.

McKeith, I. G., Marshall, E. F., Ferrier, I. N., Armstrong, M. M., Kennedy, W. N., Perry, R. H., Perry, E. K., and Eccleston, D. (1987). 5HT receptor binding in post-mortem brain from patients with affective disorders. *Journal of Affective Disorders*, **13**, 67–74.

McKenzie, F. R. and Milligan, G. (1990). δ-opioid receptor mediated inhibition of adenylate cyclase is transduced specifically by the guanine nucleotide binding protein G_{i2}. *Biochemical Journal*, **267**, 391–8.

Mednick, S. A., Machon, R. A., Huttunen, M. O., and Barr, C. E. (1990). Influenza and schizophrenia: Helsinki versus Edinburgh. *Archives of General Psychiatry*, **47**, 875–8.

Meldrum, E., Parker, P. J., and Carozzi, A. (1991). The PtdIns-PLC superfamily and signal transduction. *Biochimica et Biophysica Acta*, **1092**, 49–71.

Meller, E., Bohmaker, K., Namba, Y., Friedhoff, A. J., and Goldstein, M. (1987). Relationship between occupancy and response at striatal dopamine receptors. *Molecular Pharmacology*, **31**, 592–8.

Meltzer, H. (1989). Serotonergic dysfunction in depression. *British Journal of Psychiatry*, **155** (suppl. 8), 25–31.

Merikangas, K. R., Spence, M. A., and Kupfer, D. J. (1989). Linkage studies of bipolar disorder: methodological and analytical issues. *Archives of General Psychiatry*, **46**, 1137–41.

Miller, R. J. (1990). Receptor mediated regulation of calcium channels and neurotransmitter release. *FASEB Journal*, **4**, 3291–9.

Miller, C. (1991). 1990: annus mirabilis of potassium channels. *Science*, **252**, 1092–6.

Mitchell, P. B., Bearn, J. A., Corn, T. H., and Checkley, S. A. (1988). Growth hormone response to clonidine after recovery in patients with endogenous depression. *British Journal of Psychiatry*, **152**, 34–8.

Mizuno, Y., Ohta, S., Tanaka, M., Takamiya, S., Suzuki, K., Sato, T., Oya, H., Ozawa, T., and Kagawa, Y. (1989). Deficiencies in complex I subunits of the respiratory chain in Parkinson's disease. *Biochemical and Biophysical Research Communications*, **163**, 1450–5.

Moore, R. Y. (1987). Parkinson's disease—a new therapy? *New England Journal of Medicine*, **316**, 872–3.

Moore, R. Y. and Bloom, F. E. (1978). Central catcholamine neuron systems: anatomy and physiology of the dopamine system. *Annual Review of Neuroscience*, **1**, 129–69.

Moran (1966). *Winston Churchill, the struggle for survival*. Constable, London.

Morris, R. G., Downes, J. J., Sahakian, B., Evenden, J. L., Heald, A., and Robbins, T.W. (1988). Planning and spatial working memory in Parkinson's disease. *Journal of Neurology, Neurosurgery and Psychiatry*, **51**, 757–66.

Mumby, S. M., Heukeroth, R. O., Gordon, J. I., and Gilman, A. G. (1990*a*). G-protein α-subunit expression, myristoylation and membrane association in COS cells. *Proceedings of the National Academy of Sciences of the USA*, **87**, 728–32.

Mumby, S. M., Casey, P. J., Gilman, A. G., Gutowski, S., and Sternweis, P. C. (1990*b*). G protein γ subunits contain a 20 carbon isoprenoid. *Proceedings of the National Academy of Sciences of the USA*, **87**, 5873–7.

Murphy, S. M., Owen, R., and Tyrer, P. (1989*a*). Comparative assessment of efficacy and withdrawal of symptoms after six and twelve weeks treatment with diazepam or buspirone. *British Journal of Psychiatry*, **154**, 529–34.

Murphy, D. L., Zohar, J., Benkelfat, C., Pato, M. T., Pigott, T. A., and Insel, T. R. (1989*b*). Obsessive compulsive disorder as a 5HT subsystem related behavioural disorder. *British Journal of Psychiatry*, **155** (suppl. 8), 15–24.

Murray, R. M. and Lewis, S. W. (1987). Is schizophrenia a neurodevelopmental disorder? *British Medical Journal*, **295**, 681–2.

Murray, R. M. and Reveley, A. (1981). The genetic contribution to neuroses. *British Journal of Hospital Medicine*, **25**, 185–90.

Murray, R. M., Lewis, S. W., and Reveley, A. M. (1985). Towards an aetiological classification of schizophrenia. *Lancet*, **i**, 1023–6.

Najlerahim, A. and Bowen, D. M. (1988*a*). Biochemical measurements in Alzheimer's disease reveal a necessity for improved neuroimaging techniques to study metabolism. *Biochemical Journal*, **251**, 305–8.

Najlerahim, A. and Bowen, D. M. (1988*b*). Regional weight loss of the cerebral cortex and some subcortical nuclei in senile dementia of the Alzheimer type. *Acta Neuropathologica*, **75**, 509–12.

Neary, D., Snowden, J. S., Mann, D. M. A., Bowen, D. M., Sims, N. R., Northen, B., Yates, P. O., and Davison, A. N. (1986). Alzheimer's disease: a correlative study. *Journal of Neurology, Neurosurgery and Psychiatry*, **49**, 229–37.

Nicoll, R. A. (1988). The coupling of neurotransmitter receptors to ion channels in the brain. *Science*, **241**, 545–51.

North, R. A., Williams, J. T., Surprenant, A., and Christie, M. J. (1987). μ and δ receptors belong to a family of receptors that are coupled to potassium channels. *Proceedings of National Academy of Sciences of the USA*, **84**, 5487–91.

Nutt, D. J. (1989). Altered central α₂-adrenoceptor sensitivity in panic disorder. *Archives of General Psychiatry*, **46**, 165–9.

Nutt, D. J. and Glue, P. (1989*a*). Clinical pharmacology of anxiolytics and antidepressants: a psychopharmacological perspective. *Pharmacology and Therapeutics*, **44**, 309–34.

Nutt, D. and Glue, P. (1989*b*). Monoamine oxidase inhibitors: rehabilitation from recent research? *British Journal of Psychiatry*, **154**, 287–91.

Nutt, J. G., Woodward, W. R., Hammerslad, J. P., Carter, J. H., and Anderson, J. L. (1984). The 'on–off' phenomenon in Parkinson's disease. Relation to levodopa absorption and transport. *New England Journal of Medicine*, **310**, 483–8.

O'Callaghan, E., Larkin, C., Kinsella, A., and Waddington, J. L. (1990). Obstetric complications, the putative familial–sporadic distinction and tardive dyskinesia in schizophrenia. *British Journal of Psychiatry*, **157**, 578–84.

O'Callaghan, E., Sham, P., Takei, N., Glover, G., and Murray, R. M. (1991). Schizophrenia after prenatal exposure to 1957 A2 influenza epidemic. *Lancet*, **337**, 1248–50.

O'Neill, R. D. and Fillenz, M. (1985). Simultaneous monitoring of dopamine release in rat frontal cortex, nucleus accumbens and striatum: effects of drugs, circadian changes and correlations with motor activity. *Neuroscience*, **16**, 49–55.

Oliver, C. and Holland, A. J. (1986). Down's syndrome and Alzheimer's disease, a review. *Psychological Medicine*, **16**, 307–22.

Olney, J. W. and Gubareff, T. (1978). Glutamate neurotoxicity and Huntington's chorea. *Nature*, **271**, 557–9.

Olsen, R. W. and Tobin, A. J. (1990). Molecular biology of GABA$_A$ receptors. *FASEB Journal*, **4**, 1469–80.

Oswald, I. (1990). Comparison of diazepam and buspirone. *British Journal of Psychiatry*, **155**, 866.

Owen, M. J. and Mullan, M. J. (1990). Molecular genetic studies of manic-depression and schizophrenia. *Trends in Neurosciences*, **13**, 29–31.

Ozawa, T., Tanaka, M., Sugiyama, S., Ino, H., Ohno, K., Hattori, K., Ohbayashi, T., Ito, T., Deguchi, H., Kawamura, K., Nakane, Y., and Hashiba, K. (1991). Patients with idiopathic cardiomyopathy belong to the same mitochondrial gene family as Parkinson's disease and mitochondrial encephalomyopathy. *Biochemical and Biophysical Research Communications*, **177**, 518–25.

Pain, S. (1988). Mad cows and ministers lose their heads. *New Scientist*, **119**, 27–8.

Palacios, J. M., Rigo, M., Chinagala, G., and Probst, A. (1990). Reduced density of striatal somatostatin receptors in Huntington's chorea. *Brain Research*, **522**, 342–6.

Palmert, M. R., Siedlak, S. L., Podlisney, M. B., Greenberg, B., Shelton, E. R., Chan, H. W., Usiak, M., Selkoe, D. J., Perry, G., and Younkin, S. G. (1989). Soluble derivatives of the β amyloid protein precursor of Alzheimer's disease are labelled by antisera to the β amyloid protein. *Biochemical and Biophysical Research Communications*, **165**, 182–8.

Pam, A. (1990). A critique of the scientific status of biological psychiatry. *Acta Psychiatrica Scandinavica*, **82** (suppl. 362), 1–35.

Parker, G. and Hadzi-Pavlovic, D. (1990). Expressed emotion as a predictor of schizophrenic relapse: an analysis of aggregated data. *Psychological Medicine*, **20**, 961–5.

Parker, W. D., Filley, C. M., and Parks, J. K. (1990). Cytochrome oxidase deficiency in Alzheimer's disease. *Neurology*, **40**, 1302–3.

Parnevalas, J. G. and Papadopoulos, G. C. (1989). The monoaminergic innervation of the cerebral cortex is not diffuse and non-specific. *Trends in Neurosciences*, **12**, 315–19.

Paykel, E. S. (1989). Treatment of depression: the relevance of research for clinical practice. *British Journal of Psychiatry*, **155**, 754–63.

Pearson, R. C. A., Esiri, M. M., Hiorns, R. W., Wilcock, G. K., and Powell, T. P. S. (1985). Anatomical correlates of the distribution of the pathological changes in the neocortex in Alzheimer disease. *Proceedings of the National Academy of Sciences of the USA*, **82**, 4531–4.

Penrose, R. (1989). *The emperor's new mind*. Vintage, London.

Perry, T. L. and Hansen, S. (1990). What excitotoxin kills striatal neurons in Huntington's disease? Clues from neurochemical studies. *Neurology*, **40**, 20–4.

Pinder, R. M. (1985). Adrenoceptor interactions of the enantiomers and metabolites of mianserin: are they responsible for the antidepressant effect? *Acta Psychiatrica Scandanavica*, **72** (suppl. 320), 1–9.

Popper, K. R. and Eccles, J. C. (1977). *The self and its brain*. Springer International, Berlin.

Price, L. H., Charney, D. S., Delgado, P. L., and Heninger, G. R. (1989). Lithium treatment and serotonergic function. *Archives of General Psychiatry*, **46**, 13–19.

Price, L. H., Charney, D. S., Delgado, P. L., and Heninger, G. R. (1990). Lithium and serotonin function: implications for the serotonin hypothesis of depression. *Psychopharmacology*, **100**, 3–12.

Procter, A. W., Lowe, S. L., Palmer, A. M., Francis, P. T., Esiri, M. M., Stratmann, G., Najlerahim, A., Patel, A. J., Hunt, A., and Bowen, D. M. (1988*a*). Topographical distribution of neurochemical changes in Alzheimer's disease. *Journal of Neurological Sciences*, **84**, 125–40.

Procter, A. W., Palmer, A. M., Francis, P. T., Lowe, S. L., Neary, D., Murphy, E., Doshi, R., and Bowen, D. M. (1988*b*). Evidence of glutamatergic denervation and possible abnormal metabolism in Alzheimer's disease. *Journal of Neurochemistry*, **50**, 790–802.

Procter, A. W., Wong, E. H. F., Stratmann, G. C., Lowe, S. L., and Bowen, D. M. (1990). Reduced glycine stimulation of [³H]MK801 binding in Alzheimer's disease. *Journal of Neurochemistry*, 53, 698–704.

Prusiner, S. B. (1982). Novel proteinaceous infectious particles cause scrapie. *Science*, 216, 136–44.

Pullen, R. G. L., Candy, J. M., Morris, C. M., Taylor, G., Keith, A. B., and Edwardson, J. A. (1990). Gallium-67 as a potential marker for aluminium transport in rat brain: implications for Alzheimer's disease. *Journal of Neurochemistry*, 55, 251–9.

Pycock, C. J. (1980). Turning behaviour in animals. *Neuroscience*, 5, 461–514.

Quinn, N. (1990). The modern management of Parkinson's disease. *Journal of Neurology, Neurosurgery, and Psychiatry*, 53, 93–5.

Quinn, N. P., Rossor, M. N., and Marsden, C. D. (1986). Dementia and Parkinson's disease—pathological and neurochemical considerations. *British Medical Bulletin*, 42, 86–90.

Quon, D., Wang, Y., Catalano, R., Scardina, J. M., Murakami, K., and Cordell, B. (1991). Formation of β-amyloid protein deposits in brains of transgenic mice. *Nature*, 352, 239–41.

Rakic, (1979). Genetic and epigenetic determinants of local neuronal circuits in the mammalian central nervous system. In *The neurosciences, Fourth Study Program* (ed. F. O. Schmitt and F. G. Worden), pp. 109–27. M.I.T. Press, Cambridge, Massachusetts.

Randrup, A. and Braestrup, C. (1977). Uptake inhibition of biogenic amines by newer antidepressant drugs: relevance to the dopamine hypothesis of depression. *Psychopharmacology*, 53, 309–14.

Rapoport, J. L. (1989). The biology of obsessions and compulsions. *Scientific American*, 260 (3), 62–9.

Rapoport, J. L. (1990). Obsessive compulsive disorder and basal ganglia dysfunction. *Psychological Medicine*, 20, 465–9.

Regier, D. A., Hirschfeld, R. M. A., Goodwin, F. K., Burke, J. D., Lazar, J. B., and Judd, L. C. (1988). The NIMH depression awareness, recognition, and treatment programme: structure, aims and scientific basis. *American Journal of Psychiatry*, 145, 1351–7.

Reid, I. C., Besson, J. A. O., Best, P. V., Sharp, P. F., Gemmell, H. G., and Smith, F. W. (1988). Imaging of cerebral blood flow markers in Huntington's disease using single photon emission computed tomography. *Journal of Neurology, Neurosurgery and Psychiatry*, 51, 1264–8.

Reiman, E. M., Raichle, M. E., Robins, E., Butler, F. K., Herscoritch, P., Fox, P., and Perlmutter, J. (1986). The application of positron emission tomography to the study of panic disorder. *American Journal of Psychiatry*, 143, 469–77.

Reiman, E. M., Fusselman, M. J., Fox, P. T., and Raichle, M. E. (1989a). Neuroanatomical correlates of anticipatory anxiety. *Science*, 243, 1071–4.

Reiman, E. M., Raichle, M. E., Robins, E., Mintun, M. A., Fusselman, M. J., Fox, P. T., Price, J. L., and Hackman, K. A. (1989b). Neuroanatomical correlates of a lactate induced anxiety attack. *Archives of General Psychiatry*, 46, 493–500.

Reynolds, G. P. (1983). Increased concentrations and lateral asymmetry of amygdala dopamine in schizophrenia. *Nature*, 305, 527–9.

Reynolds, G. P. (1989). Beyond the dopamine hypothesis. The neurochemical pathology of schizophrenia. *British Journal of Psychiatry*, 155, 305–16.

Reynolds, G. P., Pearson, S. J., Halket, J., and Sandler, M. (1988). Brain quinolinic acid in Huntington's disease. *Journal of Neurochemistry*, 50, 1959–60.

Rhee, S. G., Suh, P. G., Ryu, S. H., and Lee, S. Y. (1989). Studies of inositol phospholipid specific phospholipase C. *Science*, 254, 546–50.

Richardson, R. T. and Delong, M. R. (1988). A reappraisal of the functions of the nucleus basalis of Meynert. *Trends in Neurosciences*, 11, 264–7.

Rinne, U. I. (1985). Combined bromocriptine and levodopa therapy early in Parkinson's disease. *Neurology*, 35, 1196–8.

Riveros, N., Fiedler, J., Lagos, N., Munoz, C., and Orrego, F. (1986). Glutamate in rat brain cortex synaptic vesicles: influence of the vesicle isolation procedure. *Brain Research*, 386, 405–8.

Robbins, T. W. (1990). The case for frontostriatal dysfunction in schizophrenia. *Schizophrenia Bulletin*, 16, 391–402.

Robbins, T. W. and Everitt, B. J. (1987). Psychopharmacological studies of arousal and attention. In *Cognitive neurochemistry* (ed. S. M. Stahl, S. D. Iversen, and E. C. Goodman), pp. 135–70. Oxford University Press.

Roberts, G. W., Allsop, D., and Bruton, C. (1990). The occult aftermath of boxing. *Journal of Neurology, Neurosurgery and Psychiatry*, **53**, 373–8.

Rodbell, M. (1980). The role of hormone receptors and GTP-regulatory proteins in membrane transduction. *Nature*, **284**, 17–22.

Rodbell, M. (1985). Programmable messengers: a new theory of hormone action. *Trends in Biochemical Sciences*, **10**, 461–4.

Roland, P. E., Eriksson, L., Stone-Elander, S., and Widen, L. (1987). Does mental activity change the oxidative metabolism of the brain? *Journal of Neuroscience*, **7**, 2373–89.

Rolls, E. T., Thorpe, S. J., Boytim, M., Szabo, I., and Perrett, D. I. (1984). Responses of striatal neurons in the behaving monkey. 3-Effects of iontophoretically applied dopamine on normal responsiveness. *Neuroscience*, **12**, 1201–12.

Rose, S., Lewontin, R. C., and Kamin, L. J. (1984). *Not in our genes*. Penguin Books, Harmondsworth, UK.

Rosenthal, W., Hescheler, J., Trautwein, W., and Schultz, G. (1988). Control of voltage dependent Ca^{2+} channels by G protein coupled receptors. *FASEB Journal*, **2**, 2784–90.

Rossor, M. N., Iversen, L. L., Reynolds, G. P., Mountjoy, C. Q., and Roth, M. (1984). Neurochemical characteristics of early and late types of Alzheimer's disease. *British Medical Journal*, **288**, 961–4.

Roth, M. (1986). The association of clinical and neurological findings and its bearing on the classification and aetiology of Alzheimer's disease. *British Medical Bulletin*, **42**, 42–50.

Rowland, L. P. (1988). Clinical concepts of Duchenne muscular dystrophy. The impact of molecular genetics. *Brain*, **111**, 479–95.

Sahakian, B., Jones, G., Levy, R., Gray, J., and Warburton, D. (1989). The effect of nicotine on attention, information processing and short term memory in patients with dementia of the Alzheimer's type. *British Journal of Psychiatry*, **154**, 797–800.

Sandler, M. (1981). Monoamine oxidase inhibitor efficiency in depression and the cheese effect. *Psychological Medicine*, **11**, 455–8.

Saper, C. B., Wainer, B. H., and German, D. C. (1987). Axonal and transneuronal transport in the transmission of neurological disease: potential role in system degenerations including Alzheimer's disease. *Neuroscience*, **23**, 389–98.

Schapira, A. H. V., Cooper, J. M., Dexter, D., Clark, J. B., Jenner, P., and Marsden, C. D. (1990*a*). Mitochondrial complex I deficiency in Parkinson's disease. *Journal of Neurochemistry*, **54**, 823–7.

Schapira, A. H. V., Mann, V. M., Cooper, J. M., Dexter, D., Daniel, S. E., Jenner, P., Clark, J. B., and Marsden, C. D. (1990*b*). Anatomic and disease specificity of NADH Co Q, reductase (complex I) deficiency in Parkinson's disease. *Journal of Neurochemistry*, **55**, 2142–5.

Schimke, R. T. (1973). Control of enzyme levels in mammalian tissues. *Advances in Enzymology*, **37**, 135–87.

Schou, M. (1989). Lithium prophylaxis: myths and realities. *American Journal of Psychiatry*, **146**, 573–6.

Schultz, W., Ruffieux, A., and Aebischer, P. (1983). The activity of pars compacta neurones of the monkey substantia nigra in relation to motor activation. *Experimental Brain Resarch*, **51**, 377–87.

Schwarz, R., Okuno, E., White, R. J., Bird, E. D., and Whetsell, W. O. (1988). 3-hydroxyanthranilate oxygenase activity is increased in the brains of Huntington's disease victims. *Proceedings of the National Academy of Sciences of the USA*, **85**, 4079–81.

Sedvall, G., Farde, L., Persson, A., and Wiesel, F. A. (1986). Imaging of neurotransmitter receptors in the living human brain. *Archives of General Psychiatry*, **43**, 995–1006.

Seeman, P. (1987). Dopamine receptors in human brain diseases. In *Dopamine receptors* (ed. I. Creese and C. M. Fraser), pp. 233–46. A. R. Liss, New York.

Seeman, P. (1980). Brain dopamine receptors. *Pharmacological Reviews*, **32**, 229–313.

Seeman, P. and Niznik, H. B. (1990). Dopamine receptors and transporters in Parkinson's disease and schizophrenia. *FASEB Journal*, **4**, 2737–44.

Seeman, P., Niznik, H. B., and Guan, H. (1990). Elevation of dopamine D_2 receptors in schizophrenia is underestimated by radioactive raclopride. *Archives of General Psychiatry*, **47**, 1170–2.

Seguela, P., Watkins, K. C., and Descarries, L. (1989). Ultrastructural relationships of serotonin axon terminals in the cerebral cortex of the adult rat. *Journal of Comparative Neurology*, **289**, 129–42.

Selden, N. R. W., Everitt, B. J., Jarrard, L. E., and Robbins, T. (1991). Complementary roles of the amygdala and hippocampus in aversive conditioning to explicit and contextual cues. *Neuroscience*, **42**, 335–50.

Serby, M., Larson, P., and Kalkstein, D. (1991). The nature and course of olfactory deficits in Alzheimer's disease. *American Journal of Psychiatry*, **148**, 357–60.

Shepherd, G. M. (1988). *Neurobiology* (2nd edn), Oxford University Press.

Sherrington, C. S. (1906). *The integrative action of the nervous system*. Yale University Press, New Haven, Connecticut.

Sherrington, R., Brynjolfsson, J., Petursson, H., Pottor, M., Dudleston, K., Barraclough, B., Wasmuth, J., Dobbs, M., and Gurling, H. (1988). Localisation of a susceptibility locus for schizophrenia on chromosome 5. *Nature*, **336**, 164–7.

Sholl D. A. (1956). *Organisation of the cerebral cortex*. Methuen, London.

Shoulson, I. *et al.* (1989). Effect of deprenyl on the progression of disability in early Parkinson's disease. *New England Journal of Medicine*, **321**, 1364–71.

Simonds, W. F., Goldsmith, P. K., Woodward, C. J., Unson, C. G., and Spiegel, A. M. (1989). Receptor and effector interactions of G_s. *FEBS Letters*, **249**, 189–94.

Sims, N. R., Bowen, D. M., and Davison, A. N. (1981). [^{14}C]Acetylcholine synthesis and [^{14}C]carbon dioxide production from [U-^{14}C]glucose by tissue prisms from human neocortex. *Biochemical Journal*, **196**, 867–76.

Sims, N. R., Bowen, D. M., Neary, D., and Davison, A. N. (1983). Metabolic processes in Alzheimer's disease: adenine nucleotide content and production of $^{14}CO_2$ from [U-^{14}C]glucose *in vitro* in human neocortex. *Journal of Neurochemistry*, **41**, 1329–34.

Singer, T. P. and Ramsay, R. R. (1990). Mechanism of the neurotoxicity of MPTP. *FEBS Letters*, **274**, 1–8.

Singer, T. P., Trevor, A. J., and Castagnoli, N. (1987). Biochemistry of the neurotoxic action of MPTP. *Trends in Biochemical Sciences*, **12**, 266–70.

Smith, C. U. M. (1989). *Elements of molecular neurobiology*. Wiley, Chichester.

Smith, S. J. and Augustine, G. J. (1988). Calcium ions, active zones and synaptic transmitter release. *Trends in Neurosciences*, **11**, 458–64.

Smith, R. J. and Mindham, R. H. S. (1987). Dementia in disorders of movement. In *Dementia* (ed. B. Pitt). Churchill Livingstone, Edinburgh.

Soghomonian, J. J., Beaudet, A., and Descarries, L. (1988). Ultrastructural relationships of central serotonin neurons. In *Neural serotonin* (ed. N. N. Osborn and M. Hamon). Wiley, Chichester.

Somerville, R. A. (1985). Ultrastructural links between scrapie and Alzheimer's disease. *Lancet*, **i**, 504–6.

Speight, T. M. (ed.) (1987). *Avery's drug treatment* (3rd edn). Adis Press, Auckland, New Zealand.

Spencer, P. S., Nunn, P. B., Hugon, J., Ludolph, A. C., Ross, S. M., Roy, D. N., and Robertson, R. C. (1987). Guam amyotrophic lateral sclerosis–parkinsonism–dementia linked to a plant excitant neurotoxin. *Science*, **237**, 517–22.

Spencer, P. S., Allen, R. G., Kisby, G. E., and Ludolph, A. C. (1990). Excitotoxic disorders. *Science*, **248**, 144.

Srinivasan, Y., Elmer, L., Davis, J., Bennett, V., and Angelides, K. (1988). Ankyrin and spectrin associate with voltage dependent sodium channels in brain. *Nature*, **333**, 177–80.

Stamford, J. A. (1989). *In vivo* voltammetry—prospects for the next decade. *Trends in Neurosciences*, **12**, 407–12.

Starke, K. (1991). Selectivity of ethanol on ligand-gated ion channels. *Trends in Pharmacological Sciences*, **12**, 182.

Starkstein, S. E., Brandt, J., Folstein, S., Strauss, M., Berthier, M. L., Pearlson, G. D., Wong, D., McDonnell, A., and Folstein, M. (1988). Neuropsychological and neuroradiological correlates in Huntington's disease. *Journal of Neurology, Neurosurgery and Psychiatry*, **51**, 1259–63.

Storm, J. F. (1987). Action potential repolarisation and a fast after hyperpolarisation in rat hippocampal pyramidal cells. *Journal of Physiology* (London), **385**, 733–59.

Strange, P. G. (1987*a*). Dopamine receptors in the brain and periphery: 'state of the art'. *Neurochemistry International*, **10**, 27–33.

Strange, P. G. (1987*b*). Isolation and molecular characterisation of dopamine receptors. In *Dopamine receptors* (ed. I. Creese and C. M. Fraser), pp. 29–44. A. R. Liss, New York.

Strange, P. G. (1988). The structure and mechanism of neurotransmitter receptors. Implications for the structure and function of the central nervous system. *Biochemical Journal*, **249**, 309–18.

Strange, P. G. (1990). Aspects of the structure of the D_2 dopamine receptor. *Trends in Neurosciences*, **13**, 373–8.

Strange, P. G. (1991*a*). Neuroleptic drugs and dopamine receptors. *American Journal of Psychiatry*, **148**, 1101.

Strange, P. G. (1991*b*). Receptors for neurotransmitters and related substances. *Current Opinion in Biotechnology*, **2**, 269–77.

Strange, P. G. (1991*c*). Interesting times for dopamine receptors. *Trends in Neurosciences*, **14**, 43–5.

Strathmann, M. and Simon, M. I. (1990). G protein diversity: a distinct class of α subunits is present in vertebrates and invertebrates. *Proceedings of the National Academy of Sciences of the USA*, **87**, 9113–17.

Strittmatter, S. M., Valenzuela, D., Kennedy, T. E., Neer, E. J., and Fishman, M. C. (1990). G_o is a major growth cone protein subject to regulation by GAP-43. *Nature*, **334**, 836–41.

Suddath, R. L., Casanova, M. F., Goldberg, T. E., Daniel, D. G., Kelso, J. R., and Weinberger, D. R. (1989). Temporal lobe pathology in schizophrenia: a quantitative magnetic resonance imaging study. *American Journal of Psychiatry*, **146**, 464–72.

Sulser, F., Vetulani, J., and Mobley, P. L. (1978). Mode of action of antidepressant drugs. *Biochemical Pharmacology*, **27**, 257–61.

Sulzer, D. and Rayport, S. (1990). Amphetamine and other psychostimulants reduce pH gradients in midbrain dopaminergic neurons and chromaffin granules: a mechanism of action. *Neuron*, **5**, 797–808.

Swindale, N. V. (1990). Is the cerebral cortex modular? *Trends in Neurosciences*, **13**, 487–92.

Tamminga, C. A., Foster, N. L., Fedio, P., Bird, E. D., and Chase, T. N. (1987). Alzheimer's disease: low cerebral somatostatin levels correlate with impaired cognitive function and cortical metabolism. *Neurology*, **37**, 161–5.

Tanner, C. M. (1989). The role of environmental toxins in the aetiology of Parkinson's disease. *Trends in Neurosciences*, **12**, 49–54.

Tanzi, R. E., St George-Hyslop, P. H., and Gusella, J. F. (1989). Molecular genetic approaches to Alzheimer's disease. *Trends in Neurosciences*, **12**, 152–8.

Taylor, D. P. (1988). Buspirone, a new approach to the treatment of anxiety. *FASEB Journal*, **2**, 2445–52.

Taylor, F. K. (1989). The damnation of benzodiazepines. *British Journal of Psychiatry*, **154**, 697–704.

Taylor, A. E., Saint-Cyr, J. A., Lang, A. E., and Kenny, F. T. (1986*a*). Parkinson's disease and depression. *Brain*, **109**, 279–92.

Taylor, A. E., Saint-Cyr, J. A., and Lang, A. E. (1986*b*). Frontal lobe dysfunction in Parkinson's disease. *Brain*, **109**, 845–83.

Tetrud, J. W. and Langston, J. W. (1989). The effect of deprenyl (selegiline) on the natural history of Parkinson's disease. *Science*, **245**, 519–22.

Thase, M. E., Simons, A. D., Cahalane, J., McGeary, J., and Harden, T. (1991). Severity of depression and response to cognitive behaviour therapy. *American Journal of Psychiatry*, **148**, 784–9.

Thomas, N. and Isaac, M. (1987). Alois Alzheimer: a memoir. *Trends in Neurosciences*, **10**, 306–7.

Thompson, P. D., Berardelli, A., Rothwell, J. C., Day, B. L., Dick, J. P. R., Benecke, R., and Marsden, C. D. (1988). The coexistence of bradykinesia and chorea in Huntington's disease and its implications for theories of basal ganglia control of movement. *Brain*, **111**, 223–44.

Thompson, T. L., Filley, C. M., Mitchell, W. D., Culig, K. M., LoVerde, M., and Byynyl, R. L. (1990). Lack of efficacy of hydergine in patients with Alzheimer's disease. *New England Journal of Medicine*, **323**, 445–8.

Trimble, M. R. (1990). First rank symptoms of Schneider. A new perspective. *British Journal of Psychiatry*, **156**, 195–200.

Tsukita, S. and Ishikawa, H. (1980). The movement of membranous organelles in axons. *Journal of Cell Biology*, **84**, 513–30.

Turski, L., Bressler, K., Rettig, K. J., Loschmann, P. A., and Wachtel, H. (1991). Protection of substantia nigra from MPP neurotoxicity by N-methyl-D-aspartate antagonists. *Nature*, **349**, 414–16.

Tye, N. C., Everitt, B. J., and Iversen, S. D. (1977). 5-hydroxytryptamine and punishment. *Nature*, **268**, 741–3.

Tyrer, P. (1985). Neurosis divisible? *Lancet*, i, 685–8.

Tyrer, P. and Marsden, C. A. (1985). New antidepressant drugs: is there anything new they tell us about depression? *Trends in Neurosciences*, **8**, 427–31.

Tyrer, P. and Murphy, S. (1987). The place of benzodiazepines in psychiatric practice. *British Journal of Psychiatry*, **151**, 719–23.

Tyrer, P., Murphy, S., Kingdon, D., Brothwell, J., Gregory, S., Seivewright, N., Ferguson, B., Barczak, P., Darling, C., and Johnson, A. L. (1988). The Nottingham study of neurotic disorder: comparison of drug and psychological treatments. *Lancet*, ii, 235–40.

Volkow, N. D. and Tancredi, L. R. (1991). Biological correlates of mental activity studied with PET. *American Journal of Psychiatry*, **148**, 439–43.

Waddington, J. L. (1986). Behavioural correlates of the action of selective D-1 dopamine receptor antagonists: impact of SCH 23390 and SKF 83566 and functionally interactive D-1 : D-2 receptor systems. *Biochemical Pharmacology*, **35**, 3661–7.

Waddington, J. L. (1989). Sight and insight: brain dopamine receptor occupancy by neuroleptics visualised in living schizophrenic patients by positron emission tomography. *British Journal of Psychiatry*, **154**, 433–6.

Waddington, J. L. (1990). Sight and insight: regional cerebral metabolic activity in schizophrenia visualised by positron emission tomography, and competing neurodevelopmental perspectives. *British Journal of Psychiatry*, **156**, 615–19.

Watson, S. and Abbott, A. (1992). Receptor nomenclature supplement. *Trends in Pharmacological Sciences*, **12**, 1–36.

Watt, D. C. and Edwards, J. H. (1984). DNA and Huntington's chorea. *Psychological Medicine*, **14**, 729–32.

Watt, D. C. and Edwards, J. H. (1991). Doubt about evidence for a schizophrenia gene. *Psychological Medicine*, **21**, 279–85.

Weinberger, D. R. (1987). Implications of normal brain development for the pathogenesis of schizophrenia. *Archives of General Psychiatry*, **44**, 660–9.

Weinberger, D. R. (1988). Schizophrenia and the frontal lobe. *Trends in Neurosciences*, **11**, 367–70.

Weissman, C. (1991). The prion's progress. *Nature*, **349**, 569–71.

Weissman, M. M., Leaf, P. J., Tischler, G. L., Blazer, D. G., Karno, M., Bruce, M. L., and Florio, L. P. (1988). Affective disorders in five United States Communities. *Psychological Medicine*, **18**, 141–53.

Westaway, D., Carlson, G. A., and Prusiner, S. B. (1989). Unravelling prion diseases through molecular genetics. *Trends in Neurosciences*, **12**, 221–7.

Westlund, K. N., Denney, R. M., Rose, R. M., and Abell, C. W. (1988). Localisation of distinct mono-amine oxidase A and monoamine oxidase B cell populations in human brainstem. *Neuroscience*, **25**, 439–56.

Wexler, N. S., Young, A. B., Tanzi, R. E., Travers, H., Starosta-Rubinstein, S., Penney, J. B., Snodgrass, S. R., Shoulson, I., Gomez, F., Arroyo, M. A. R., Penchaszadeh, G. K., Moreno, H., Gibbons, K., Faryincarz, A., Hobbs, W., Anderson, M. A., Bonilla, E., Conneally, P. M., and Gusella, J. F. (1987). Homozygotes for Huntington's disease. *Nature*, **326**, 194–7.

White, N. M. (1989). A functional hypothesis concerning the striatal matrix and patches: mediation of S–R memory and reward. *Life Sciences*, **45**, 1943–57.

Wilcock, G. K., Esiri, M. M., Bowen, D. M., and Hughes, A. O. (1988). The differential involvement of subcortical nuclei in senile dementia of the Alzheimer's type. *Journal of Neurology, Neurosurgery and Psychiatry*, **51**, 842–9.

Wilson, C.J. (1986). Postsynaptic potentials evoked in spiny neostriatal projection neurones by stimulation of ipsilateral and contralateral neocortex. *Brain Research*, **367**, 201–13.

Wischik, C. M., Novak, M., Edwards, P. C., Klug, A., Tichelaar, W., and Crowther, R. A. (1988). Structural characterisation of the core of the paired helical filament of Alzheimer Disease. *Proceedings of the National Academy of Sciences of the USA*, **85**, 4884–8.

Wolf, M. E. and Roth, R. H. (1987). Dopamine autoreceptors. In *Dopamine receptors* (ed. I. Creese and C. M. Fraser), pp. 45–96. A. R. Liss, New York.

Wong, S. K. F., Parker, E. M., and Ross, E. M. (1990). Chimeric muscarinic cholinergic: β-adrenergic receptors that activate G_s in response to muscarinic agonists. *Journal of Biological Chemistry*, **265**, 6219–24.

Wong, Y. H., Federman, A., Pace, A. M., Zachary, I., Evans, T., Pouyssegur, J., and Bourne, H. R. (1991). Mutant α subunits of G_{i2} inhibit cyclic AMP accumulation. *Nature*, **351**, 63–5.

Wonnacott, S. (1990). The paradox of nicotinic acetylcholine receptor upregulation by nicotine. *Trends in Pharmacological Sciences*, **11**, 216–19.

Wood, A. J. and Goodwin, G. M. (1987). A review of the biochemical and neuropharmacological actions of lithium. *Psychological Medicine*, **17**, 579–600.

Wright, A. F. and Whalley, L. J. (1984). Genetics, ageing and dementia. *British Journal of Psychiatry*, **145**, 20–38.

Wu, K. and Siekewitz, P. (1988). Neurochemical characteristics of a postsynaptic density fraction isolated from adult canine hippocampus. *Brain Research*, **457**, 98–112.

Wurtman, R. J. and Wurtman, J. J. (1989). Carbohydrates and depression. *Scientific American*, **260** (1), 50–7.

Yamane, H. K., Farnsworth, C. C., Xie, H., Howald, W., Fung, B. K. K., Clarke, S., Gelb, M. H., and Gloniset, J. A. (1990). Brain G protein γ subunits contain an all *trans* geranylgeranyl cysteine methyl ester at their carboxyl terminal *Proceedings of the National Academy of Sciences of the USA*, **87**, 5868–72.

Yankner, B. A., Duffy, L. K., and Kirschner, D. A. (1990*a*). Neurotrophic and neurotoxic effects of amyloid β protein: reversal by tachykinin neuropeptides. *Science*, **250**, 279–82.

Yankner, B. A., Caceres, A., and Duffy, L. K. (1990*b*). Nerve growth factor potentiates the neurotoxicity of β-amyloid. *Proceedings of the National Academy of Sciences of the USA*, **87**, 9020–3.

Yatani, A. and Brown, A. M. (1989). Rapid β-adrenergic modulation of cardiac calcium channel currents by a fast G protein pathway. *Science*, **245**, 71–4.

Yatani, A., Codina, J., Imoto, Y., Reeves, J. P., Birnbaumer, L., and Brown, A. M. (1987). A G protein directly regulates mammalian cardiac calcium channels. *Science*, **238**, 1288–92.

Young, A. B., Greenamyre, J. T., Hollingworth, Z., Albin, R., D'Amato, C., Shoulson, I., and Penney, J. B. (1988). NMDA receptor losses in putamen from patients with Huntington's disease. *Science*, **241**, 981–3.

Zigmond, R. E., Schwarzschild, M. A., and Rittenhouse, A. R. (1989). Acute regulation of tyrosine hydroxylase by nerve activity and by neurotransmitters via phosphorylation. *Annual Review of Neuroscience*, **12**, 415–61.

Zipser, D. and Andersen, R. A. (1988). A back propagation programmed network that simulates response properties of a subset of posterior parietal neurons. *Nature*, **331**, 679–84.

Zorumski, C. F. and Isenberg, K. E. (1991). Insights into the structure and function of GABA–benzodiazepine receptors: ion channels and psychiatry. *American Journal of Psychiatry*, **148**, 162–73.

Zubrzycka-Gaarn, E. E., Bulman, D. E., Karpati, G., Burghes, A. H. M., Belfall, B., Klamut, H. J., Talbot, J., Hodges, R. S., Ray, P. N., and Worton, R. G. (1988). The Duchenne muscular dystrophy gene product is localised in sarcolemma of human skeletal muscle. *Nature*, **333**, 466–9.

Index